CW01483560

PRACTICAL ECHOCARDIOGRAPHY

GMM

© 1999

Greenwich Medical Media Limited
219 The Linen Hall
162-168 Regent Street
London
W1R 5TB

ISBN 1 900 151 863

First Published 1999

Apart from any fair dealing for the purposes of research or private study, or criticism or review, as permitted under the UK Copyright Designs and Patents Act 1988, this publication may not be reproduced, stored, or transmitted, in any form or by any means, without the prior permission in writing of the publishers, or in the case of reprographic reproduction only in accordance with the terms of the licences issued by the appropriate Reproduction Rights Organisations outside the UK. Enquiries concerning reproduction outside the terms stated here should be sent to the publishers at the London address printed above.

The right of Catherine Walsh and Peter Wilde to be identified as authors of this work has been asserted by them in accordance with the Copyright Designs and Patents Act 1988.

The publisher makes no representation, express or implied, with regard to the accuracy of the information contained in this book and cannot accept any legal responsibility or liability for any errors or omissions that may be made.

A catalogue record for this book is available from the British Library.

Distributed worldwide by Oxford University Press

Typeset by Saxon Graphics Ltd, Derby

Printed in China

PRACTICAL ECHOCARDIOGRAPHY

By

Catherine A Walsh

DipRad (Australia) DMU

Senior Radiographer
Department of Clinical Radiology
Bristol Royal Infirmary, Bristol, UK

Peter Wilde

BSc Hons, MRCP, FRCR

Consultant Cardiac Radiologist
Bristol Royal Infirmary, Bristol, UK

with contributions by

Alison Heads

ONC, HNC
REGIONAL TUTOR IN
PERINATAL
ECHOCARDIOGRAPHY

*Freeman Hospital
Newcastle upon Tyne*

Jayshree Joshi

BSc Hons
SENIOR CHIEF
TECHNICIAN

*Department of Echocardiography
Hammersmith Hospital
London*

Stephen Evans

BSc MRCP PhD
FELLOW IN INTERVEN-
TIONAL CARDIOLOGY

*Green Lane Hospital
Auckland
New Zealand*

CONTENTS

CHAPTER 5

CHAPTER 6

CHAPTER 7

PREFACE

Many textbooks on cardiac ultrasound have been written, so why have we produced another one? The rapid clinical application of echocardiography in more and more departments means that a greater number of people need to learn the skills required to be a competent echocardiographer. Many books are much too comprehensive and daunting for the beginner, containing much new research material or details of rare and complex cases. Other well illustrated atlases show excellent images of common pathologies but do not go into the practical detail required by the student.

We have aimed to produce a working text (a "bench book") for those who have started to scan but need to consolidate their knowledge and skills. It is not intended to be a comprehensive atlas, nor is it intended to be an authoritative opinion on all aspects of the subject. We feel that the content should be appropriate for both medical and technically trained sonographers.

If it is found to be a useful aid to developing echocardiographers who then want to go on and learn more, then we shall have been successful.

C.W.

P.W.

Bristol, September 1998

1

INTRODUCTION TO ECHOCARDIOGRAPHY

Brief history
Present clinical applications
Preparing to scan

Brief history

Ultrasound had its first non-medical uses during World War II. In 1952, the first paper on ultrasound imaging in the medical field was published. The first echocardiogram was a purely M-mode recording of myocardial movement recorded by Edler in 1954. Despite improvements in the recording of the images, it was not until over 10 years later that the next major advancement was reported – 1967 saw the beginnings of real-time scanning. However, due to the transducer size, it was not suitable for cardiac work. By 1974, two-dimensional real-time scanning of the heart became a reality. Equipment was still bulky, but the rapid expansion in the field of microcomputers led to the equipment becoming both more compact and much faster. By 1985 machines producing real-time, high resolution images had become widely available. This imaging was initially achieved by the use of rotating or oscillating crystals, but the introduction of phased array transducers with no moving parts allowed many technical innovations to be introduced. Both types of transducer are still in use, but the improved solid-state technology with its ever faster microprocessor control has led to the phased array type instrument being the most widely available on present systems.

The Doppler effect was first described, and named after, Christian Johann Doppler, an Austrian physicist who noted, in 1843, that stars moving relative to the Earth emitted a certain colour depending on the direction in which they were travelling, due to a change in frequency of the wavelength. The principle is true for all sources of radiation (including sound waves) when there is relative movement between the source and the observer. In 1956, this principle was applied to the measurement of aortic blood flow. However, it was not until 1978, when the first duplex scanners (combining real-time imaging with pulsed wave Doppler interrogation) were made available, that interest arose in the detailed study of blood flow within the heart. It is by chance, rather than by design, that the frequency shift recorded by Doppler ultrasound is within the audible range.

The beginnings of colour flow Doppler were reported in 1981. In 1985, real-time imaging, incorporating colour flow, became available. Recently, colour Doppler imaging of the myocardial movement has been marketed commercially. The first transoesophageal echocardiogram was performed in Japan in 1977. The original system was bulky, but rapid development of this modality has occurred, leading to today's small multiplane transducers. More recent advances include higher frame rates, and smaller faced and multifrequency transducers. Endocardial mapping and colour kinesis have made interpretation of images easier. Real-time three-dimensional imaging may be the next step to look forward to.

Modern echocardiography systems are a 'multi-modality' package with access to real-time and M-mode imaging and all forms of Doppler interrogation. They have the capacity to run a variety of transducers, including transoesophageal transducers. They are integrated with sophisticated computer software for analysis of results, and nowadays have a variety of outputs including hardcopy, video and computer disc. These systems are immensely powerful if used correctly, but operators need to be knowledgeable in a wide range of areas if they are to make useful and accurate diagnoses.

Present clinical applications

With today's technology, examination of the structure and function of the heart and great vessel structure by ultrasound is becoming of increasingly better quality. Due to the non-invasive nature of ultrasound and the expansion of the roles of cardiac technicians and radiographers, ultrasound scanning is becoming a fast and readily available modality, which is able to give immediate results at a relatively low cost. It is a technique that is used by medical and non-medical personnel alike and, whilst the basic skills are common to all, each discipline can bring its own benefits to the technique.

Common indications include:

- cause of heart murmur
- cause of cardiac failure
- assessment of left ventricular function
- diagnosis of infective endocarditis
- diagnosis of pericardial effusion/tamponade
- cardiac source of emboli (TIA)
- monitoring known cardiac lesions
- assessment of prosthetic valves and repairs
- monitoring and/or assessment of congenital heart disease.

Alternatives to echocardiography include:

- angiography
- magnetic resonance imaging (MRI)

- computed tomography (CT)
- MUGA scan (radio isotope assessment of ejection fraction)
- electrocardiography (not an imaging technique)

Preparing to scan

Ultrasound of the heart is a difficult but fulfilling talent to have. It is a challenge to master, and even those who are proficient in other areas of ultrasound scanning will find it a difficult technique to learn. There should be no such thing as 'a quick echo'. It is important that a complete and methodical scan is completed each time an examination is done. Even the most experienced of cardiologists requesting an echo may be mistaken in their clinical diagnosis. Many of the examinations performed will have been requested by clinicians other than cardiologists and some even by general practitioners. Multiple abnormalities are common and even experienced echocardiographers can be surprised by some findings.

Patient preparation

No patient preparation, apart from a proper explanation of the procedure, is needed for a transthoracic echo. It is important for the patient to know who they are being scanned by. It is good practice to introduce yourself and to give your job title. Many patients are quite anxious prior to the echo, partly due to the examination itself, but mostly due to the results; heart disease may be a routine part of the day's work for the echocardiographer, but it is often new and frightening for the patient. A brief description of what will actually take place during the scan, and perhaps an indication of how the scan will help in their management, will help to put the patient at ease. It is important, however, that the operator does not go too far in explaining results if they themselves do not have clinical responsibility for the patient. Often reassurance about who will review the results and how the patient will hear about them is all that is needed.

There is no absolute contraindication for an echo, but over inflated lungs (e.g. patients with chronic obstructive airways disease), very obese patients or those who are very ill, unconscious or on a ventilator, will often make the examination more difficult.

All patients will need to change for their echo as clothes may hinder the scan and will inevitably end in jelly-stained clothing. A screened changing area is helpful. While most men do not mind baring their chests, women are more reluctant to do so and should be provided with a gown with a front opening for the scan. Although it is almost impossible to keep a female patient completely covered at all times throughout the scan, an effort should be made to allow reasonable modesty whenever possible. In the apical four chamber view the operator's hand will inevitably come in contact with the female patient's left breast, and indeed at times this will have to be lifted for the transducer to be placed in position. The patient should always be warned that this is going to happen. If the operator, either male or female, envisages that this may be a problem, a chaperone may be necessary.

Ultrasound jelly is available in different viscosities. Thick jelly tends to be more practical for echocardiography. Because the patient is turned on one side, runny jelly tends to end up on the bed rather than on the patient!

The echo room

The couch on which the patient lies is an important piece of equipment in the echo room, and thought should be given to it. It should be of adjustable height so that patients can get on and off easily, and so that the height can be altered to suit the operator. The head end of the bed should be adjustable so that it can range from almost flat for subcostal views to semi-upright for parasternal views. It should be possible to lay the head end completely flat in an emergency, which can occasionally happen due to the nature of the patients that will be scanned. It is also important that the couch is reasonably comfortable, as the patient will be on it for up to 30 minutes and an uncomfortable patient will fidget, hindering the scan. To add to the patient's comfort and to reduce muscle tension, a pillow is necessary both to support the patient's head and to provide extra support behind their back.

In a similar way, thought should be given to the operator's chair. The chair should be of adjustable height to match the height of the couch. During most of the scanning, the patient will be on his or her left side, causing the operator to reach well around the patient to place the transducer into the desired position. Make sure that you always think of your back in such situations. A chair positioned at the same height as the couch will allow the user to slide closer towards the patient and onto the couch without twisting his or her spine.

The majority of echo scanning in the UK is right-handed. This means sitting on the right side of the

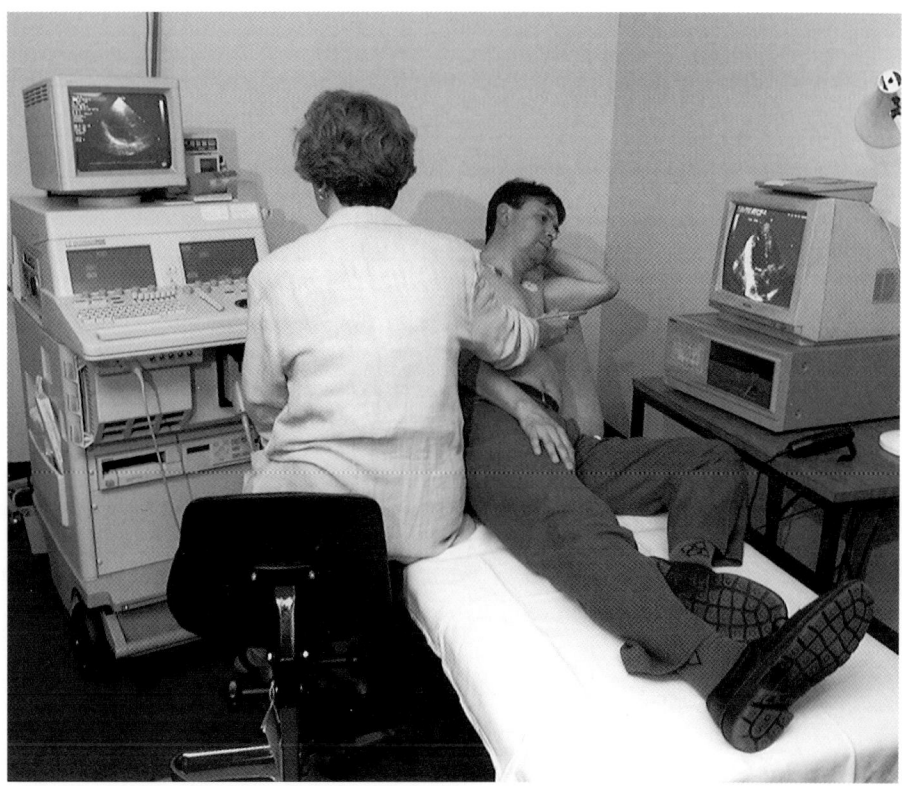

Figure 1.1 – A typical echo room, showing the right-handed operator with the ultrasound machine to her left. The patient rests comfortably with a secondary monitor to view.

patient, facing them, and reaching across with the transducer to the left side of the patient's chest (Figure 1.1). The machine controls are manipulated with the left hand. The advantages of this technique are that the dominant (and stronger) hand in most people is used for the more precise work of manipulating the transducer. In addition the right wrist rests on the patient's chest, giving stability to the transducer position, which may have to be maintained for extended periods. The main disadvantages of this technique are that the patient sometimes feels 'excluded' as they turn away from the screen (see below), and the operator has to stretch over a little more in larger patients. Some operators express a preference for scanning with their left hand, sitting on the opposite side of the couch. The technique of left-handed scanning will not be discussed in this book but it is perfectly feasible and is commonly used in some countries. However, it is practical for a convention to be established by all operators in one department, in order to avoid frequent rearrangement of equipment in the room.

Many patients are interested in watching their own scan. To keep the patient on their left side and not looking back over their right shoulder (causing muscle tension), a separate monitor placed to the left side of the couch is suggested. A much cheaper version of this is to have an adjustable mirror aimed towards the monitor for the patient to watch. A brief explanation, even just some basic anatomy, is all that is needed to satisfy most patients' curiosity.

Subdued lighting is essential for the best possible viewing of the echo. This reduces the amount of reflected light off the monitor and increases the contrast viewed from the screen. A couple of carefully placed lamps are all that is needed if specialised lighting is not fitted in the room.

Record keeping

Diligent record keeping is vital in an efficient echocardiography department. As the heart is a moving structure, a real-time recording on video is necessary. This will allow for a comparison with subsequent scans on patients and for clinicians to view abnormalities/contractility before they treat the patient. For this reason it is very important to ensure that the correct patient name and identification number is on each scan and that the quality of the recording is as good as possible. It is surprising how difficult it is to obtain a short but meaningful recording for a patient. Reviewing the video after the patient has left is good practice for the first few examinations recorded, as you may find that you are not recording a certain point of interest for long enough or, conversely, for too long. A record of which patients' scans are on a particular tape will need to be kept. If you are working in a large hospital, it may be useful to record brief findings in a database for both audit and research purposes. Videos should be kept for 7 years.

Recent advances have meant that digital images can be stored on the hard disk of the ultrasound machine and backed up on optical or compact disc. Images saved may be static, but complete heart cycles can be stored, giving the impression of real-time. This can be extremely useful when comparing previous studies or for stress echoes. Digital storage of images means that there is no loss of image quality as there is with video recording, and random access to files saves time. The digital format also allows for a large range of post-processing, an area where advances are proceeding at a rapid rate. At present, however, technical limitations mean that archiving of routine work on disc is not usually possible.

Reports on findings should be made immediately after the scan has been completed. At the end of a long list of patients it is difficult to remember each individual case. Even reviewing the video may not give rise to the same ideas that were originally formed. The examination is not complete until the report has been written. It is preferable to document the findings on a system that allows production and retrieval of the report without access to the patient's clinical notes (e.g. a computer database system). This allows quick access to the findings of the report when the notes are not easily to hand. Of course important findings will also be written in the clinical notes. A guide to report writing is included in the Appendices.

Transducers

The frequency of the transducer used for an examination will depend on the individual patient. A higher frequency transducer will give better resolution and detail but less penetration depth. Conversely, a lower frequency transducer will give greater penetration but less resolution. Many companies now have multifrequency transducers where the frequency of a transducer may be raised or lowered at the press of a button. As a general rule, the thinner the patient, the higher the frequency

can be used. It should also be remembered that, when scanning a large patient using a low frequency transducer, it is sensible to change to higher frequency when looking at structures in the near field (e.g. the apex in the case of apical thrombus). In general, there will be a transducer that is suitable for most patients, particularly in an adult practice, and changing of transducers is not usually necessary during most examinations.

Although the size and shape of different transducers still varies markedly, all transducers used for cardiac scanning have a small face, termed 'the footprint'. This is so the transducer can be fitted between the ribs to reduce shadowing artefacts. Consequently, this means that the image in the near field is very small. The beam is steered through an arc in order to produce a wide sector, typically 90°. The beam steering is achieved either electronically or mechanically. There are advantages and disadvantages of both types of transducer, and these are discussed in the Appendices. A more detailed description of transducers is given in the Physics Appendix.

Printers

Commonly, stationary images from echoes are recorded on thermal paper. Most of these images are simply used to record measurements and so can be recorded on (cheap) black and white thermal paper. Printers may be set to print white on black or black on white. Most machines are now fitted with colour thermal printers so that images of colour flow Doppler examinations can be recorded. These images are much more expensive, and thought should be given to when such images are taken. Some older machines are fitted with a Polaroid camera, but the image quality of these is usually less good than that provided by the best colour thermal printers. More modern equipment allows for the digitised image to be displayed on a computer, which means that post-processing can be performed on the image before it is finally printed. Digitised images can be stored, and printed using laser or thermal colour printers.

Electrocardiogram

An electrocardiogram (ECG) records the electrical activity of the heart. A trace is recorded at either the top or bottom of the monitor in synchronisation with the real-time, two-dimensional, M-mode and Doppler recordings (Figure 1.2). This allows the operator to determine precisely when in the cardiac cycle a certain movement or blood flow occurs (i.e. in systole or dias-

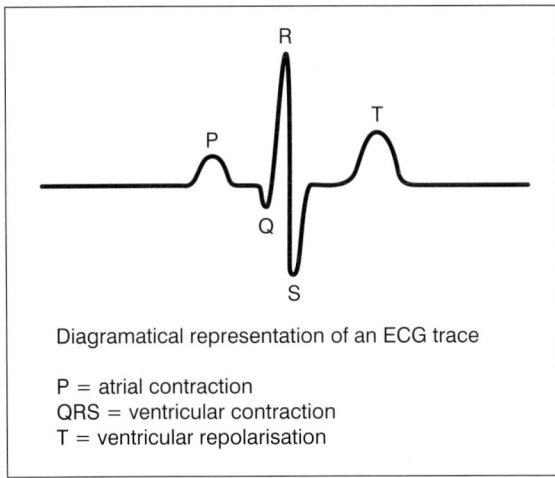

Diagramatical representation of an ECG trace

P = atrial contraction
QRS = ventricular contraction
T = ventricular repolarisation

Figure 1.2 – Diagrammatical representation of an ECG trace.

tole). It can also be used to compare the timing of events recorded separately. All modern systems use the electrocardiogramatic signal to give a continuous display of the current heart rate, which may be useful diagnostically and in some calculations. The connection of electrodes is described in Chapter 4.

Insurance

If you are working within a hospital situation, the hospital should indemnify you, as long as they are aware that you are performing echocardiograms unsupervised and/or issuing your own reports. In the majority of departments this is the normal situation. The British Society of Echocardiography suggests that if you are working outside the cover of a hospital it is prudent to check that your employer has insurance to cover the work you do and, if not, invest in your own medical indemnity insurance.

2

ANATOMY AND
PHYSIOLOGY OF
THE HEART

Pericardium and external relationships
Internal cardiac anatomical relationships
Anatomical features of individual structures
Intracardiac flow and pressure
Electrocardiogram
Nomenclature for cardiac description

Pericardium and external relationships

The heart lies immediately posterior to the sternum in the anterior mediastinum. It is surrounded by two layers of pericardium, one being the thick lining of the fibrous pericardial sac (the parietal pericardium) and the second being the thin layer covering the heart itself (the visceral pericardium). The heart is freely mobile within these layers except at the entry point of the systemic and pulmonary veins and the exit point of the two great arteries, the aorta and the pulmonary artery. The heart is relatively fixed in these areas. There is normally a small amount of fluid between these layers to allow free movement during the cardiac cycle. There is a small recess between the pulmonary veins, the *oblique sinus*, and a larger space, the *transverse sinus*, lies between the great veins and the great arteries. The latter is sometimes seen on good-quality scans. There is often a quite substantial layer of fat on the surface of the heart and there may also be fatty pads lying outside the pericardium (Figure 2.1).

Inferiorly the pericardium is continuous with the central tendinous portion of the diaphragm. The fundus of the stomach lies immediately below the diaphragm to the left of the midline. The two lungs lie close to the heart on each side, partially extending round the anterior surface of the heart itself and the great arteries, leaving only a small part of the heart in direct relationship with the sternum (mostly the right ventricular wall). Posteriorly the middle mediastinal structures lie close to the heart, in particular the oesophagus lies close to the left atrium and the trachea, and the bronchi lie close to the pulmonary artery bifurcation.

Access to the heart is relatively limited from the front of the chest due to the ribs, the sternum and the intervening air. It is, however, possible to create some changes in the anatomy by certain manoeuvres. Inspiration will fill the lungs more and will decrease the amount of cardiac tissues that lie close to the sternum. In contrast, expiration will increase this area. This applies to the anterior chest wall, but in the subxiphoid area inspiration will bring the diaphragm down and may give better access to the heart. The air in the lungs of a supine patient will tend to rise and will thus act against the echocardiographer who must avoid air between the transducer and the organ of interest. Rotation of the patient to the left will tend to deflate the left lung and will often give better access to the heart as the ventricular apex will come close to the chest wall. The heart itself, being slightly mobile within the chest, may drop a little to the left and aid the examiner (Figure 2.2).

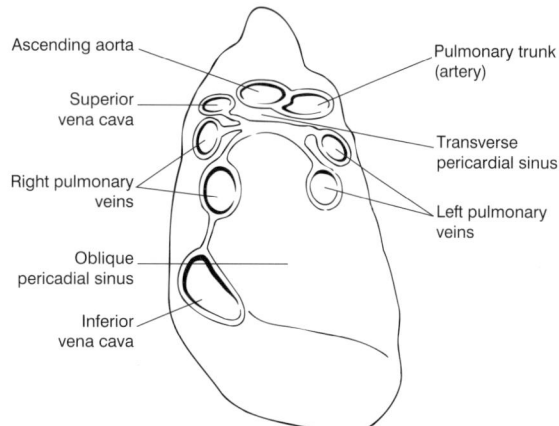

Figure 2.1 – The anatomy of the pericardium. Frontal view of the pericardial cavity with the heart removed, showing the major vessels and pericardial reflections.

The aortic arch rises up in the anterior mediastinum, slightly to the right of the midline, and then curves posteriorly and to the left in the superior mediastinum just below the level of the suprasternal notch. The descending aorta lies in the posterior mediastinum on the anterior and left aspect of the thoracic vertebral bodies (Figure 2.3).

The arch encloses the pulmonary artery bifurcation and the tracheal bifurcation, the latter lying more posteriorly. The left and right pulmonary arteries thus pass into the lungs from the middle mediastinum. The anatomy of the two pulmonary arteries is slightly asymmetrical, the right pulmonary artery lying immediately posterior to the ascending aorta and anterior to the right main bronchus. The left pulmonary artery arches superiorly over the top of the left main bronchus. The aorta above the aortic root and the distal pulmonary trunk and its bifurcation lie outside the pericardial cavity (Figures 2.4 and 2.5).

Internal cardiac anatomical relationships

The internal cardiac anatomy (Figure 2.6) is best appreciated by starting with the left ventricle. This chamber has substantially more muscle in its wall than any other chamber, as it needs to generate sufficient pressure to pump blood into the high-resistance systemic circulation. The apex of the ventricle is directed inferiorly,

11

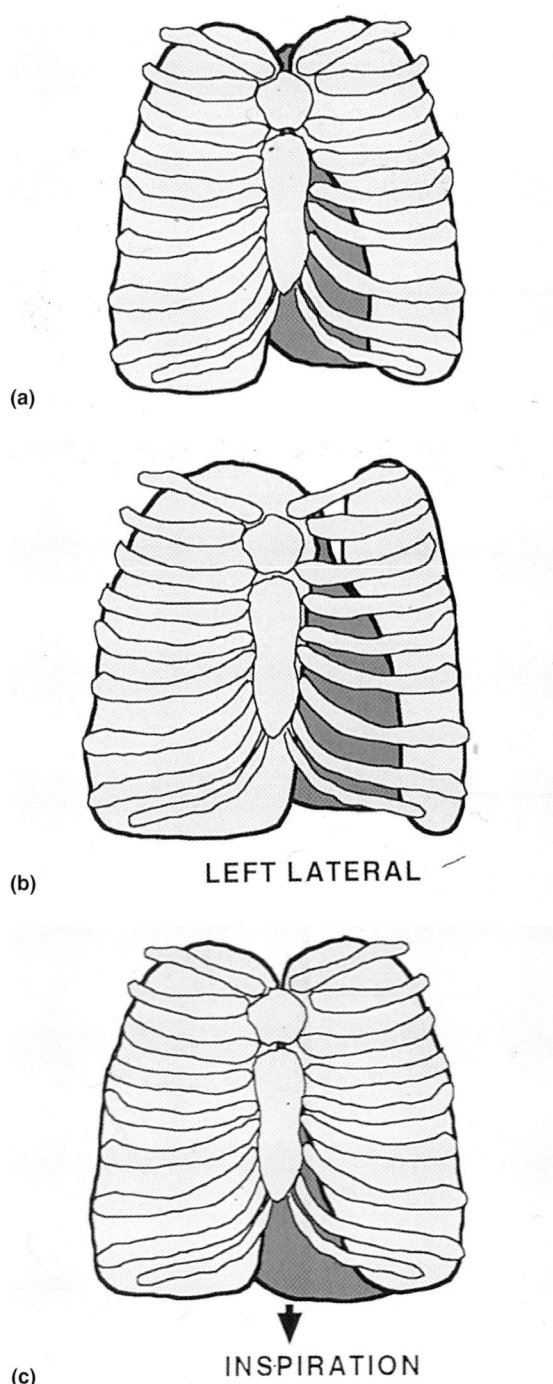

(a)

(b) LEFT LATERAL

(c) INSPIRATION

Figure 2.2 – (a) The position of the heart behind the ribs and sternum and partially obscured by the lungs. (b) A left lateral position allows better contact of the heart with the left chest wall. (c) With inspiration there is loss of access to the heart in the parasternal area, but the subcostal access is improved.

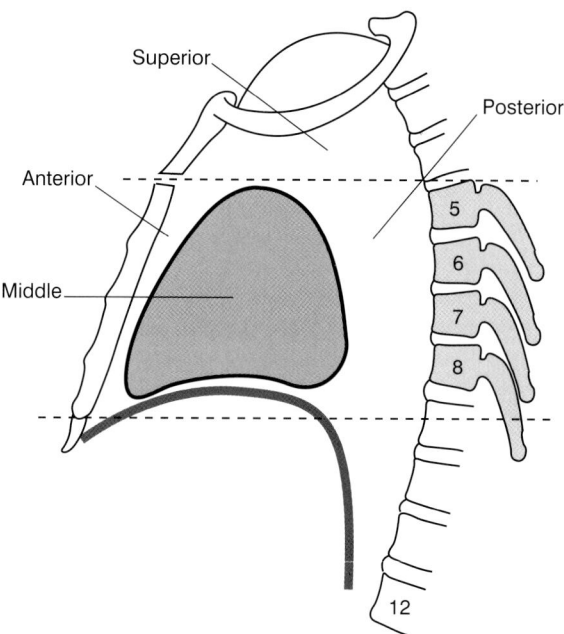

Figure 2.3 – Lateral projection showing the regions of the mediastinum.

anteriorly and leftward, and lies close to the sixth interspace in the midclavicular line. The base of the left ventricle (the base implies the opposite end of the heart from the apex, not the inferior surface) lies at a slightly higher level, just to the left of the midline. The cross-section of the left ventricle is circular and has walls that are typically 10 mm thick in diastole in an average adult.

The structure of the heart is dominated by this muscle mass. The right ventricle has an entirely different structure, lying anteriorly and 'wrapping around' the posteriorly positioned left ventricle. Only a small proportion of the left ventricular apex forms part of the anterior surface of the heart. The common muscle lying between the two ventricular chambers is the interventricular septum and, although forming a wall of both ventricles, its shape and thickness are structured as if they are part of the left ventricle. The walls of the two ventricles beyond the septum are termed the *free walls*. In the case of the left ventricle this free wall continues the thick circular shape of the chamber. The free wall of the right ventricle is much thinner and forms the majority of the front of the heart. The consequence of the right ventricle 'wrapping around' the left is that its cross-section is crescent shaped.

Each inlet valve lies between the collecting chamber (atrium) and the pumping chamber (ventricle). On the

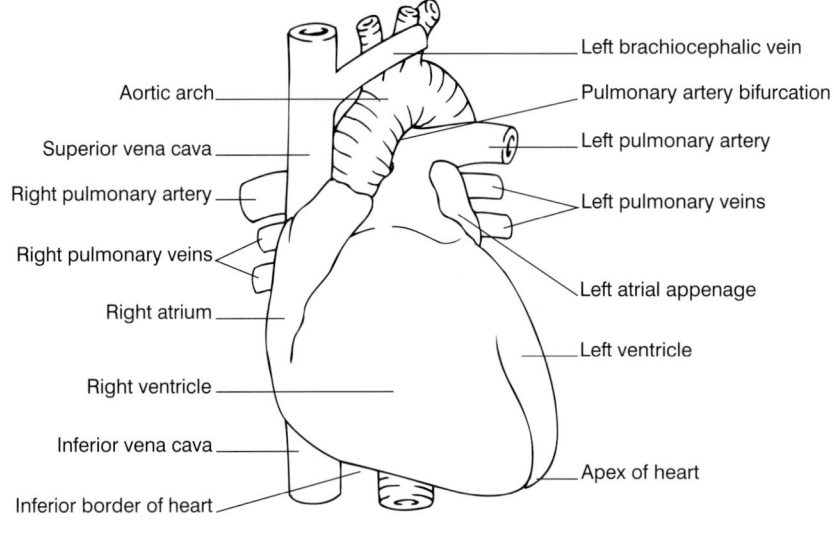

(a)

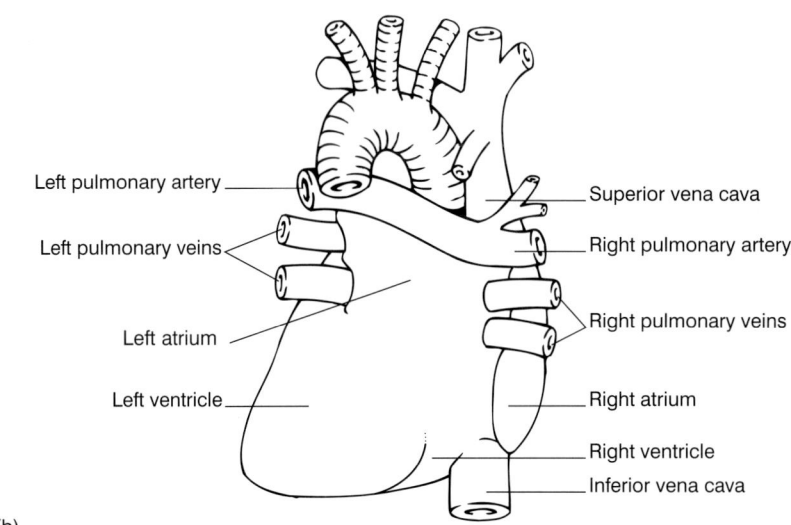

(b)

Figure 2.4 – (a) Frontal view of the external surface of the heart and great vessels. The right ventricle forms much of the anterior surface of the heart. The aortic arch passes from right to left as it arches over the pulmonary bifurcation. (b) Corresponding posterior view of the external surface of the heart.

left side, the left atrium empties through the mitral valve to the left ventricle, and on the right side the right atrium empties through the tricuspid valve to the right ventricle. The two atria have thin muscular walls and lie side by side, separated by the interatrial septum. The right atrium is to the right and more anterior than the left atrium, which occupies a slightly more superior position and forms a major part of the posterior surface of the heart. The right atrium receives inlet veins, which drain systemic blood from below the diaphragm, the inferior vena cava, the superior mediastinum and

the superior vena cava. The pulmonary veins, usually an upper and lower one on each side, drain into the left and right posterior aspects of the left atrium.

The great arteries arise from the ventricles, the aorta from the left ventricle and the pulmonary artery from the right ventricle. The two arteries twist around each other in a characteristic way. The pulmonary artery, arising from the anterior ventricle, must pass posteriorly to bifurcate into left and right pulmonary arteries in the middle mediastinum. It achieves this by passing

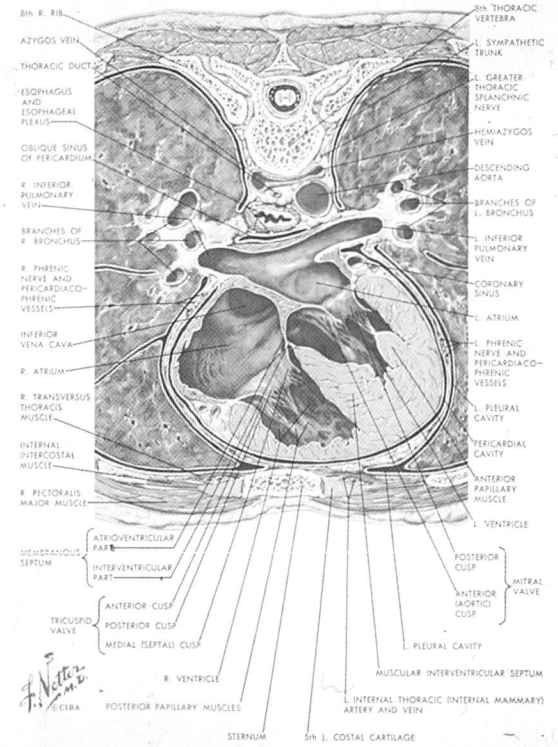

Figure 2.5 – Transverse section of the thorax at the level of the mitral valve, showing the relationship of the heart to the sternum anteriorly, the hilar regions of the lungs laterally, and the vertebral column and oesophagus posteriorly.

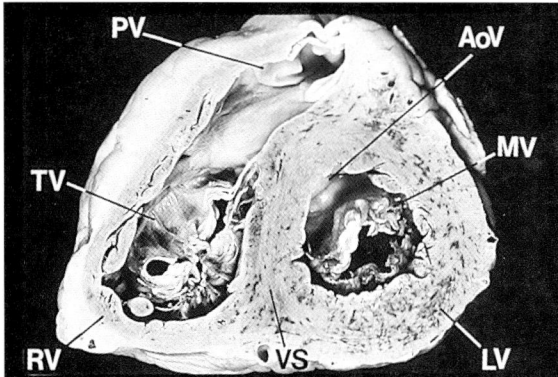

Figure 2.6 – Short axis section of a heart specimen showing the thick walled circular left ventricle (LV) with the right ventricle (RV) 'wrapping' around it anteriorly. The tricuspid valve (TV) and mitral valves (MV) can both be seen in the bases of the ventricles. The aortic valve (AoV) is just visible superior to the mitral valve. The pulmonary valve (PV) can be seen at the distal end of the right ventricular outflow tract, lying superior to the left ventricle and aortic valve.

round to the left side of the ascending aorta. The aorta itself, arises from the posterior (left) ventricle and passes forwards and to the right as it ascends to the upper mediastinum. The two outlet valves, pulmonary and aortic, lie close together but are orientated differently, the pulmonary valve allowing flow posteriorly and the aortic valve allowing flow superiorly.

It is necessary to define two important anatomical planes when describing the cardiac anatomy:

- the atrioventricular groove, the indentation running around the heart, which separates the atrial chambers from the ventricular chambers;

- the interventricular groove, separating the left ventricle from the right ventricle.

Anatomical features of individual structures

Right and left atrium

The right atrium has inflow from three sources: the inferior vena cava from below, the superior vena cava from above, and the coronary sinus from a low position close to the interatrial septum and the tricuspid valve. The coronary sinus is the main draining vein of the coronary circulation and runs round in the inferior leftward part of the atrioventricular groove. The postero-leftward wall of the right atrium is the interatrial septum. This, when viewed from the right side, has a fossa ovalis (an impression related to the embryonic patent foramen ovale), where the septum is particularly thin. The right atrial appendage is a broad-based recess which wraps around the anterior aspect of the heart from the upper part of the right atrium. The left atrium has a left atrial appendage which wraps around the left heart border from the upper aspect of the left atrium. The pulmonary veins are the only normal inflow to the left atrium.

Inlet valves and ventricles

The right ventricle is rhomboid in shape and has an inner surface which has coarse trabeculations (muscle bundles). One of these muscle bundles, the moderator band, is particularly prominent and runs across the chamber. The anterior wall is relatively thin compared with the left ventricular walls. The inlet valve from the right atrium is the tricuspid valve, which has an anterior, a septal and an inferior leaflet. A number of chordae (strings) attach the edge of the valve leaflets to a number of small papillary muscles which arise from the inner aspect of the chamber walls. The right ventricle has a muscular outflow tube (infundibulum) leading up from the main body of the chamber towards the pulmonary valve; this tube wraps around the superior aspect of the left ventricle. The outflow pulmonary valve is thus some distance from the inlet valve.

In contrast, the much thicker walled left ventricle has finer trabeculations and two large papillary muscles which are attached to the chordae on the free edges of the mitral valve, the inlet from the left atrium. The mitral valve has two leaflets: a deep anterior leaflet and a shallower posterior leaflet. The points at which the two leaflets come together are the commissures, one anterolateral and one posteromedial. The outflow valve of the left ventricle, the aortic valve, lies close to the inlet mitral valve and is described as being in fibrous continuity with it. In other words, the two valves are not separated by a muscular tube. The aortic valve lies superior and anterior to the mitral valve.

Although the tricuspid and mitral valves lie side by side with parallel orientated flow through them both, it is important to recognise that they are not at exactly the same level. The septal leaflet of the tricuspid valve is positioned slightly more apically than the anterior leaflet of the mitral valve, which means that a small portion of the septum of the heart lies between the left ventricle and the right atrium. This is known as the ventriculoatrial septum (Figure 2.7).

The interventricular septum itself is essentially part of the left ventricle, which is circular in the majority of its cross-section. A small part of the interventricular septum near the upper part of the tricuspid valve annulus (supporting structure) is very thin and is called the membranous septum. The muscle at the left ventricular apex is relatively thin compared with the remainder.

The interventricular septum is conveniently described in several parts:

- the inlet septum, which lies close to the inlet or atrioventricular valves (tricuspid and mitral);
- the membranous septum;
- the midmuscular septum, which occupies the main area between the bodies of the two ventricles;
- the apical septum near the apex;
- the outflow septum, which lies in the 'roof' of the left ventricle as the right ventricular outflow tract wraps round over the left ventricle – this portion of septum lies close to the aortic and pulmonary valves.

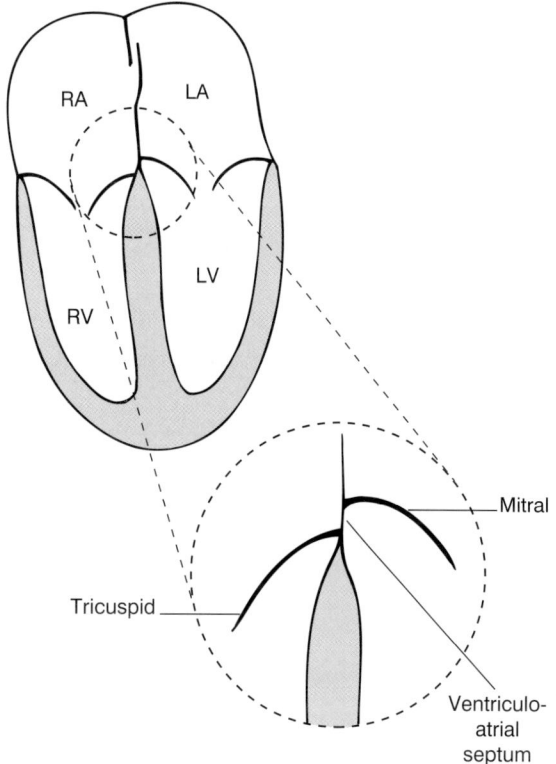

Figure 2.7 – The ventriculoatrial septum

Outlet valves and great arteries

Both outlet valves are described as semilunar valves. They do not rely on muscular action to close properly (as do the tricuspid and mitral valves), as the pressure of blood is sufficient to close the three hammock-shaped pockets, which are similar in shape for the pulmonary and aortic valves. The three leaflets of each valve arise from slightly bulbous parts of the proximal great arteries. These areas are known as the sinuses. In the case of the aortic valve, two of the three sinuses of Valsalva give rise to the origins of the coronary arteries. The two outlet valves lie close together, with flow in the pulmonary valve being directed posteriorly and flow in the aorta being directed superiorly, anteriorly and slightly rightward. The left coronary artery arises from the left posterior sinus (traditionally termed the left coronary sinus) and the right coronary artery arises from the anterior sinus (traditionally called the right coronary sinus). The coronary arteries are not usually visualised beyond their origins by ultrasound, and their detailed anatomy will not be described further

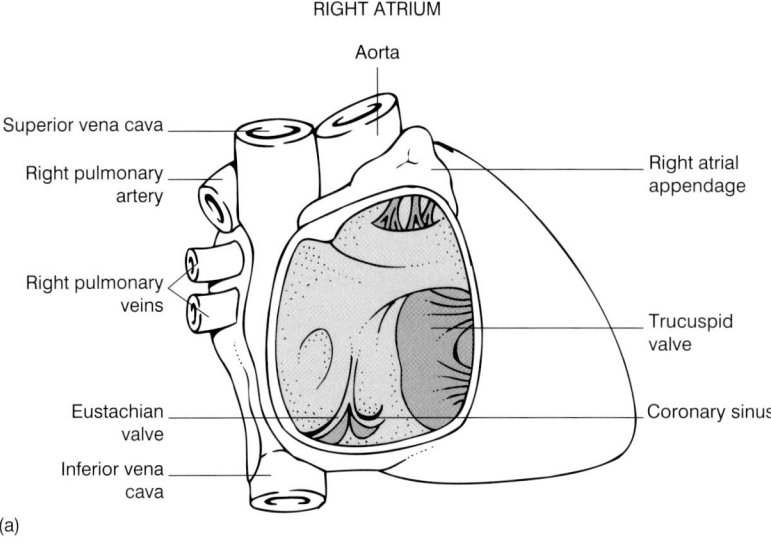

RIGHT ATRIUM

Aorta

Superior vena cava

Right pulmonary artery

Right pulmonary veins

Eustachian valve

Inferior vena cava

Right atrial appendage

Trucuspid valve

Coronary sinus

(a)

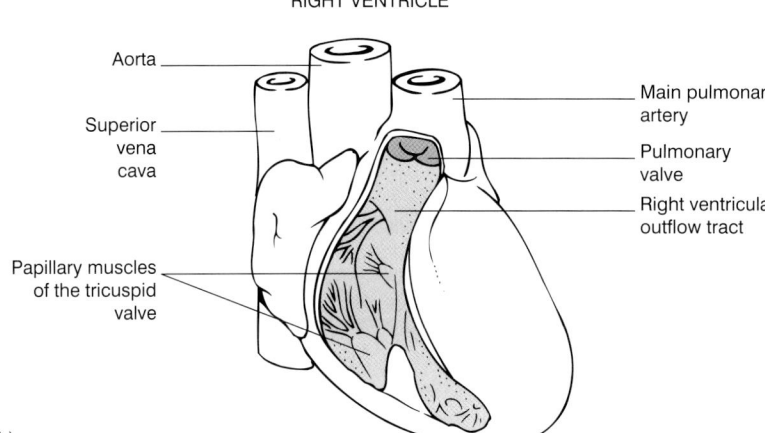

RIGHT VENTRICLE

Aorta

Superior vena cava

Papillary muscles of the tricuspid valve

Main pulmonary artery

Pulmonary valve

Right ventricular outflow tract

(b)

Figure 2.8 – (a) Anterior view with the right atrium opened. (b) Anterior view with the right ventricle opened.

The pulmonary artery is a simple tube running posteriorly to the left of the ascending aorta and dividing (bifurcating) into right and left main divisions. The left pulmonary artery passes over the left main bronchus into the hilum of the left lung and the right pulmonary artery passes posterior to the ascending aorta and then anterior to the right main bronchus as is passes into the hilum of the right lung. The fetal arterial duct enters the superior aspect of the proximal left pulmonary artery.

The aorta passes superiorly after giving off the coronary arteries and ascends slightly to the right of the midline before curving posteriorly to form the aortic arch in the upper mediastinum. The arch passes down to the left of the thoracic spine as the descending aorta. The arch itself gives off the brachiocephalic arteries, which supply the head and neck. The first branch is the right brachio-cephalic artery, which divides to form the right common carotid artery and the right subclavian artery. The second branch is the left common carotid artery and the third branch is the left subclavian artery. There can be a number of minor variations from this pattern including the right sided aortic arch. (Figures 2.8 and 2.9).

Intracardiac flow and pressure

In a normal resting adult the heart pumps 4 to 5 l of blood per minute around the body at a rate of about 70 bpm. This means that with every beat the heart ejects about 60 ml of blood; this is called the *stroke volume*. Of course this volume is ejected simultaneously to the aorta from the left ventricle and to the pulmonary artery from the right ventricle. The ventricular pump-

LEFT VENTRICLE AND LEFT ATRIUM
(MITRAL VALVE EXCISED)

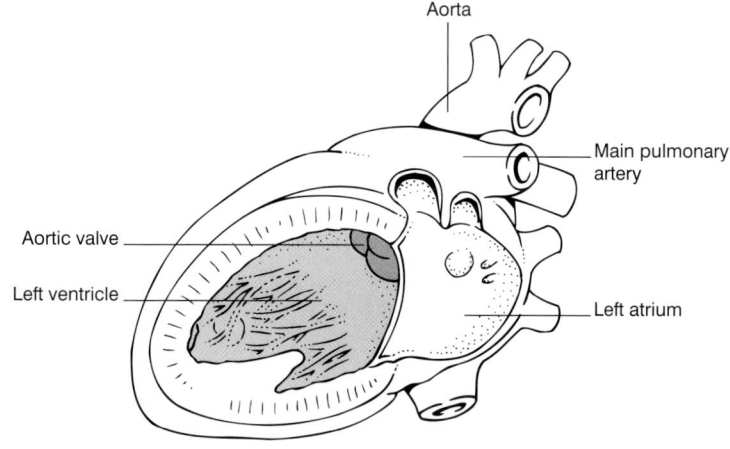

(a)

LEFT VENTRICLE

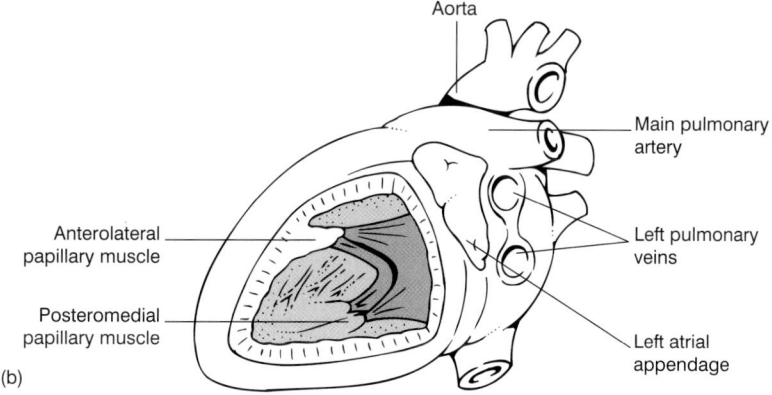

(b)

Figure 2.9 – (a) Posterior view with the mitral valve removed, and both the left atrium and the left ventricle opened. (b) Posterior view with only the left ventricle opened. The mitral valve is intact and the papillary muscles and chordae can be seen.

ing action is called *systole*. The pressure needed to perform this pumping action is determined by the 'resistance' of the vascular system into which the blood is being pumped. In the case of the aorta, supplying the 'systemic' circulation, the resistance is high due to the nature of the vessels in all the end-organs, and so the pressure needed to drive the blood must be high. In the case of normal adults a *systolic* pressure of approximately 120 mmHg is required to pump blood round the body. The blood vessels in the lungs have a much lower resistance and so the same volume of blood can be pumped at a much lower pressure. The right ventricle needs to generate only about 25 mmHg to pump blood round the lungs. The difference in these pressures explains the obvious difference in the amount of muscle in the left ventricular wall compared with the right. In both cases, however, the circulation is a high-pressure arterial circuit. At the end of systole the ven-

tricles stop contracting, their pressure falls below the level in the great arteries and so the aortic and pulmonary valves shut. This period of ventricular relaxation is termed *diastole*. During diastole, the closed semilunar valves allow pressure to be maintained in the arterial circuits and this pressurised blood steadily 'runs off' into the systemic or pulmonary vessels. As this run-off occurs the pressure steadily falls until it is boosted by the next systolic cycle. Typically the pressure falls to 80 mmHg in the aorta and 15 mmHg in the pulmonary artery. These changes account for the normal arterial pressures of around 120/80 mmHg in the aorta and 25/15 mmHg in the pulmonary artery.

Venous return is a relatively passive phenomenon, the venous blood 'draining' back to the left atrium from the pulmonary veins and to the right atrium from the systemic veins. The atria act as collecting chambers and remain at low pressure, normally less than 10 mmHg and often less than 5 mmHg. These low pressure chambers act as collection chambers, preparing to fill the ventricles during each cycle. Atrial filling occurs throughout the period of ventricular systole. The ventricular muscle has a capacity to relax completely after each contraction. Not only does this allow recovery, it also is essential in maintaining the circulation. Only if the ventricular diastolic pressure falls lower than the atrial pressure can the inlet valves open and allow filling of the ventricles from the atria. The inlet valves have a complex function. They must open freely and widely to allow a large volume of flow to pass across in a short time under a low driving pressure, after which they must close completely and withstand the much higher systolic pumping pressures. The filling of the ventricles is aided by contraction of the atria when the ventricles are relaxed.

There is a strict sequence of changes relating these pressure changes to the opening and closing of valves. These are listed for the left side of the heart but are essentially similar on the right side.

1. Left ventricular contraction starts.
2. Left ventricular pressure rises higher than left atrium.
3. *Mitral valve shuts*.
4. Left ventricular pressure continues to rise.
5. Left ventricular pressure exceeds aortic pressure.
6. *Aortic valve opens*.
7. Flow across aortic valve.
8. Left ventricle stops contracting.
9. Left ventricular pressure falls below aortic pressure.
10. *Aortic valve shuts*.
11. Left ventricular pressure continues to fall.
12. Left ventricular pressure falls below left atrial pressure.
13. *Mitral valve opens*.
14. Flow across mitral valve
15. Back to (1) to continue the cycle.

Note that between stages 3 and 6 both valves are shut while the pressure builds up. This is known as the phase of *isovolumic contraction*, i.e. no blood is moving out of the ventricle. Between stages 10 and 13 there is again no flow; this is the period of *isovolumic relaxation*.

Electrocardiogram

The electrocardiogram (ECG) is an electrical recording of the wave of electrical discharge that passes across the heart with each cycle. It can be used in many ways, but the echocardiographer only needs to know the normal

pattern and common variations in order to allow timing of the cardiac cycle.

The contraction of the heart is co-ordinated by electrical activity, generated by the natural 'pacemakers' in the heart. In the wall of the atria lies the sinoatrial node, which generates the desired cardiac rate and rhythm. This causes a wave of contraction to pass through the atrial walls, accompanied by a wave of electrical discharge in the heart muscle cells. When the electrical

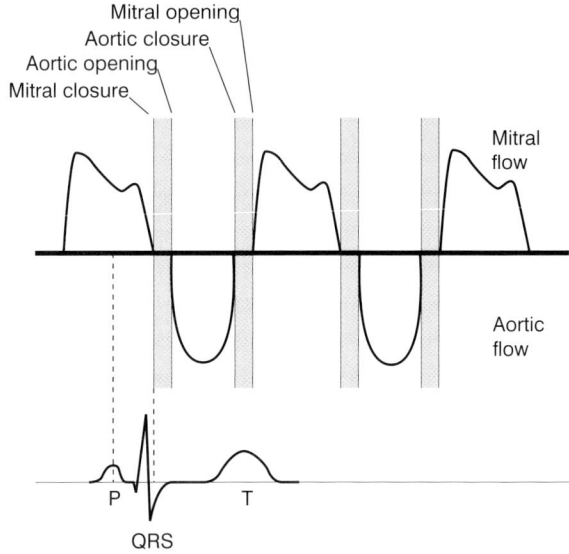

Figure 2.10 – Timing of valve opening and closure and a corresponding ECG trace. The dotted lines show how the 'P' wave of the ECG precedes the atrial component of mitral flow and the 'QRS' complex precedes the main systolic contraction of the ventricle.

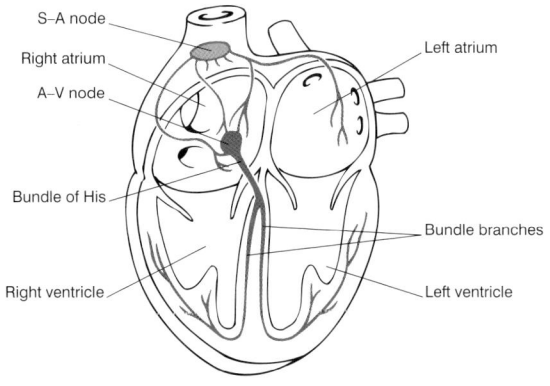

Figure 2.11 – The pattern of depolarisation passing through the heart.

wave reaches the atrioventricular node in the base of the interventricular septum, a strong new impulse is generated. This new impulse is spread through a complex conducting system (starting at the bundle of His) through a network of fibres that ensures that there is synchronous contraction of all the ventricular muscle, which in turn produces effective pumping action. There are a number of abnormalities of this electrical conduction system, but the normal rhythm is called *sinus rhythm*.

The normal electrical activity is represented by a diagram. The *P wave* represents the atrial depolarisation or discharge. The higher amplitude *QRS complex* shows the main ventricular depolarisation, and the *T wave* represents the recovery or repolarisation phase for the ventricles. The QRS complex precedes the onset of ventricular contraction by a few milliseconds and can be used as a marker of the end of diastole or the beginning of systole. The end of systole is not exactly identifiable from the ECG trace. (Figures 2.10 and 2.11).

Nomenclature for cardiac description

Unfortunately, history has led to rather confusing terminology in the description of cardiac anatomy, perhaps due to the obvious oblique orientation of the heart in the thorax. Cardiologists and anatomists in the past have developed a system of nomenclature that is not entirely consistent with that used elsewhere in the body. In addition to this, the nomenclature is not always used consistently in texts and publications.

Standard orientation uses the term *superior* to mean towards the head and *inferior* to mean towards the feet.

Anterior is taken to mean towards the sternum and *posterior* to mean towards the spine. *Left lateral* and *right lateral* relate simply to the left and right sides of the body. (For example, superior mediastinum or anterior mediastinum, left lobe of the liver, and posterior segment of the lung.)

In cardiac nomenclature the following terms are often used a little differently. For example: -

- *Left and right ventricles*: In the case of the left ventricle this means left but also posterior. The right ventricle is correspondingly right and anterior.

- *Left ventricular regions*:

  - *Anterior*. Often the anterior surface of the left ventricle is used to mean the superoanterior surface of the chamber, as in 'anterior myocardial infarct'.

  - *Lateral*. The lateral wall of the left ventricle is actually orientated posterolaterally.

  - *Posterior*. The posterior wall of the left ventricle lies close to the diaphragm, almost inferiorly.

  - *Inferior*. This part of the left ventricle is close to the posterior area but is even further round.

These terms are shown diagramatically in Figure 9.3 in Chapter 9, where they are used in the context of stress echo techniques.

Do not be too confused by these descriptions. The cardiological terms are in such common use that you will soon become familiar with them. The main thing is not to expect the words to mean exactly the same as they do elsewhere.

3

INTRODUCTION TO ECHOCARDIOGRAPHY MODALITIES

Nature of ultrasound
Two-dimensional imaging
M-mode (time–motion) imaging
Doppler ultrasound studies
Other basic equipment details

Nature of ultrasound

All sound waves are pressure waves. The frequency of a sound wave is the number of cycles per second (hertz ; Hz). Audible sound is in the range 2–20 kHz (1000 Hz = 1 kilohertz (1 kHz)). Frequencies above this are referred to as ultrasound. Imaging ultrasound frequencies range from 2 MHz (1 megahertz (1 MHz) = 1 000 000 Hz) for imaging of deep tissues to 40 MHz (e.g. for specialist intravascular imaging).

The wavelength is the distance travelled by a wave during one cycle. The shorter the wavelength, the better the resolution of the ultrasound image. The speed of sound, C, is related to both the frequency, F, and the wavelength, λ (Figure 3.1):

$$C = \lambda F.$$

It should be remembered that, although C is assumed to be fairly constant for any one type of tissue, there are in fact small variations.

When a short electrical pulse is applied to a transducer crystal, the crystal expands and compresses the molecules in the adjacent tissues. After expansion, the crystal then contracts, thus decreasing the pressure in the molecules. This produces a pressure wave that travels through the tissues. The number of times that the crystal is excited every second is termed the *pulse repetition frequency* (PRF). Pressure waves returning to the crystal undergo an opposite effect, being converted into a voltage which is then amplified and used to create an image or a Doppler signal. The phenomenon of a using a crystal to convert an applied pressure to a voltage, and vice versa, is called the *piezoelectric effect.*

The radiation of pressure waves from any one source is in a longitudinal direction. Close to the source the intensity of the ultrasound beam is maintained. As the distance from the source increases the intensity of the beam decreases rapidly as it diverges and curves (Figure 3.2). Sound waves travel though tissues by the transfer of pressure waves from one vibrating particle to the next, in the direction of the wavefront. A pulse of ultrasound passes through homogenous tissue with no change in velocity (Table 3.1). The average velocity of ultrasound through soft tissue is 1540 m/s. All ultrasound machinery assumes this speed to compose a two-dimensional image, for measurements and for Doppler traces.

As the beam passes through tissue it is attenuated by reflection, refraction and absorption, and thus echoes returning from greater distances are weaker. To overcome this problem, echoes returning from deeper structures (i.e. those that take longer to return) are amplified more. This is achieved by means of the swept time compensation (STC) facility also often called time gain compensation (TGC), which can be found on all imaging ultrasound machines.

Reflection

When the incident beam hits a large flat target, the reflection is termed specular (Figure 3.3). In specular reflection the intensity of reflection equals the angle of incidence. The bigger and flatter the interface, the greater the intensity of reflection. Therefore, when visualising a structure, the best images are gained when the incident beam is at right angles to that structure. In this situation a relatively high proportion of the ultrasound energy is returned to the transducer. Specular reflection is generally used in imaging techniques.

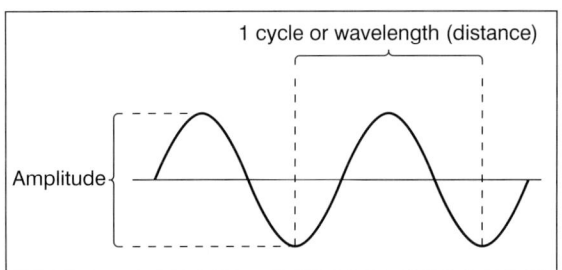

Figure 3.1 – Diagrammatic representation of a sinusoidal wave demonstrating the amplitude, cycle and wavelength

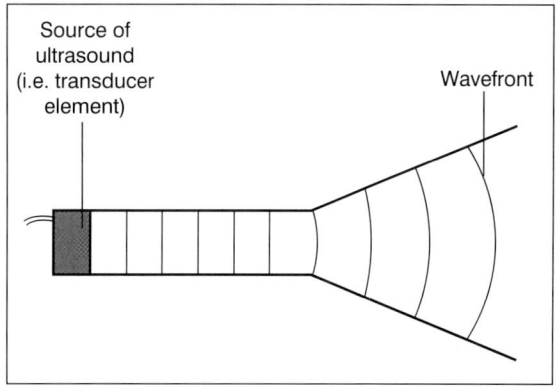

Figure 3.2 – The change in the shape of an ultrasound beam over a distance.

Table 3.1 – The velocity of sound in different tissues

Medium	Velocity (m/s)
Air	330
Water (20°C)	1480
Blood	1570
Fat	1460
Bone	3500
Soft tissue	1540

Scattering

When the incident beam hits a small target non-specular reflection (or scattering) occurs, with radiation in all directions (Figure 3.4). In this situation a very small proportion of the ultrasound energy is returned to the transducer. Scattered reflection is generally used in Doppler techniques.

Refraction

If the ultrasound beam travels at different velocities in two tissues, the beam is bent (refracted) at the boundary (Figure 3.5). This causes misregistration of data, as the collection equipment assumes that the returning signals have travelled along straight lines.

Attenuation

Attenuation is the weakening of the ultrasound beam that limits its penetration. Attenuation is due to:

● beam divergence

● reduction of power due to scattering, reflection and refraction

● absorption (which gives rise to heat).

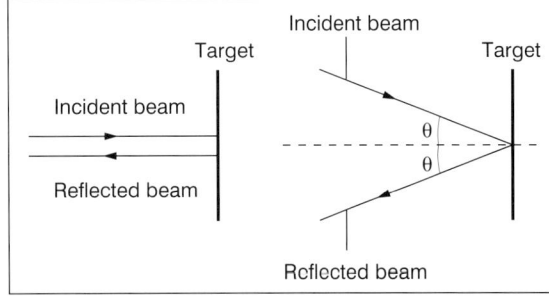

Figure 3.3 – Specular reflection: diagrammatic representation of an ultrasound beam hitting a large interface.

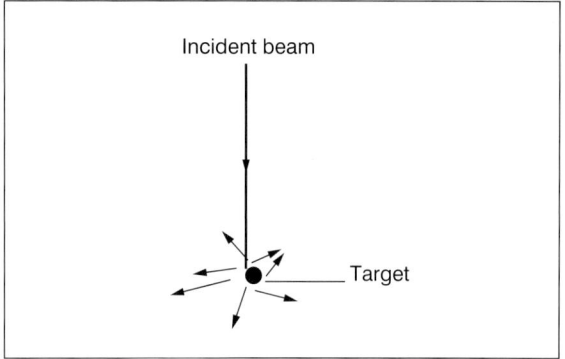

Figure 3.4 – Scattering: diagrammatic representation of an ultrasound beam hitting a small target.

Each tissue has a different attenuation coefficient. The attenuation coefficient, μ, for most soft tissues is approximately 1 decibel per centimetre per megahertz (dB/cm/MHz). Therefore the higher the frequency of the transducer the greater the attenuation.

Two-dimensional imaging

Two-dimensional imaging is sometimes referred to as B-mode, real-time or sector scanning.

Reflections from interfaces, (both large and small reflections) make up the two-dimensional ultrasound image. The time taken for an echo to return is used to calculate how far from the transducer the interface is: the further away from the transducer an interface is, the longer it will take for the reflection (echo) to return. The transducer sends out a pulse of ultrasound and then waits for echoes to return. When all echoes have returned, the transducer emits another pulse of ultrasound. The time between the pulses being emitted is, to a degree, controlled by the user, in the sense that the further from the transducer the sonographer wants to interrogate, the longer the time between pulses.

Several different kinds of transducer are used for echocardiography (for a description see the Appendices). All have a small 'footprint' in order to fit between the ribs. This means that the field of view at the transducer face is small. The beam is steered through a wide sector to give a large field of view distal

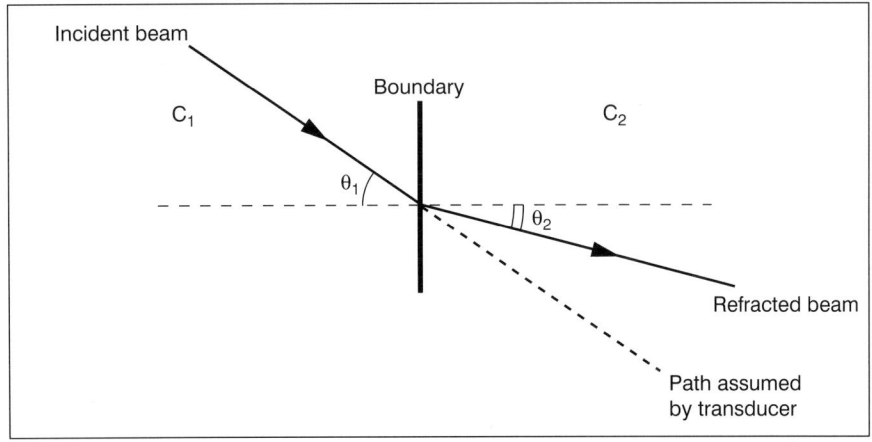

Figure 3.5 – Diagrammatic representation of an ultrasound beam passing through two adjacent tissues with different velocities, resulting in refraction of the beam. C_1, C_2, Velocity of the beam in tissues 1 and 2; θ_1, angle of incidence; θ_2, angle of refraction.

to the transducer. The near field contains the same number of scan lines as the far field. The image of an area at some distance from the transducer is of poorer quality due to attenuation of the ultrasound beam and divergence of the beam distal to the focal zone. Transducers used in general applications are not suitable for cardiac examinations, as their larger 'footprint' configurations (e.g. curvilinear or linear) mean that many of the useful lines making up the image will lie opposite ribs and will be of no practical use.

A scan converter is used to change the incoming analogue data, which is in the form of radial scan lines, to a digital matrix. The digital matrix is made up of picture elements, or 'pixels', and this is a form of image that can be handled by a microcomputer. Once in the digital matrix form, various functions are performed on the data (e.g. smoothing, to eliminate the actual scan lines) to produce the image we see on the monitor. An ultrasound machine must contain a scan converter in order to have a freeze-frame facility and to allow for post-processing.

Resolution

The *temporal resolution* is the time an ultrasound machine takes to gain enough information to display an imaging sector and hence to obtain the necessary number of frames per second (frame rate) to make a real-time image. The temporal resolution is inversely proportional to the number of scan lines in each sector and the depth to which penetration is required.

Spatial resolution is the ability of the machine to display structures that are situated close together as separate entities. It is divided into lateral and axial resolution. *Lateral resolution* refers to structures that are side by side horizontally and depends on the number of scan lines in a sector, the width of the beam (improves with focusing) and the amount of averaging or smoothing that the machine applies. Typical lateral resolution is 1–3 mm.[1] *Axial resolution* is the ability to resolve structures along the length of the beam, and depends on the length (in distance) of the ultrasound pulse. It tends to be more accurate than lateral resolution, (0.5–2 mm), which is why distance measurements are more accurate vertically than horizontally. The best application of this principle, therefore, is in measurements made on M-mode traces.

The higher the frequency of the transducer, the better the axial and lateral resolution. Higher frequencies give shorter pulse lengths, and smaller crystals give rise to narrower beams.

Imaging moving structures

Imaging fast-moving structures, such as the heart, requires a high frame rate so that continuous movement is seen by the eye and there is no obvious jump or jerkiness from one frame to the next. An acceptable rate is 20–40 frames/s. The fast frame rate is also necessary for frame-by-frame cineloop review so that no important information is missed. A fast heart rate will require a higher frame rate for equivalent diagnostic information to be obtained (e.g. if the frame rate is 30 Hz, an adult heart rate of 60 bpm will mean 30 images of every cardiac cycle, but in a neonate with a heart rate of 150 bpm there will only be 12 images of every cardiac cycle). Some machines offer the option of altering the angle of the scan sector; reducing the size will increase the frame rate.

M-mode (Time-motion) imaging

Although M-mode imaging is not considered the important tool it once was at the beginning of echocardiogram history, it is still a very useful facility and a complete examination cannot be performed without it. M-mode traces are used to measure the movement of fast moving structures. The M-mode graph is made up of information collected along one scan line only. In other words, the same single line is sampled over and over again. The advantage of this is that a much higher sampling rate can be used (than for two-dimensional imaging) for a particular structure and this results in a very accurate representation of movement. Often an M-mode trace will display movement that is too fast for the eye to detect (e.g. aortic valve opening). The position of the M-mode sampling line is usually guided by the two-dimensional image, and both the image and the M-mode trace can be visualised simultaneously with phased array systems. Typical M-mode traces are taken of the aortic valve, mitral valve and the left ventricle (for systolic and diastolic measurements).

How it works

The M-mode cursor, or line, is positioned through the area of interest (e.g. atrioventricular leaflet tips). This cursor represents the position of a corresponding beam that will collect the information. In a phased array system with simultaneous 'live' two-dimensional imaging and M-mode tracing, alternate pulses are used to build up the two-dimensional sector image and the M-mode trace. The resultant M-mode trace is a one-dimensional line recording but, because the M-mode image is recorded on the monitor by an electron beam swept across the screen, the actual movement is recorded as a continually updated graph and becomes two-dimensional (the distance moved in the direction of the incident beam versus time). The distance a structure moves in the direction of the sample line is displayed on the vertical axis, and the time taken to perform the movement is displayed on the horizontal axis (Figure 3.6). The sweep speed of the screen can be changed on all cardiac ultrasound machines. A faster sweep speed is useful in patients with a fast heart rate (tachycardia), as it stretches out the otherwise closely spaced movement. If the two-dimensional image is 'frozen' all the lines can be used for the M-mode trace and an even higher temporal resolution can be achieved.

The speed of a moving interface (e.g. mitral valve) is given by the slope of the trace. The size and motion of a structure is accurately recorded only if it is in line with the sample line. Stationary structures will be displayed as horizontal lines.

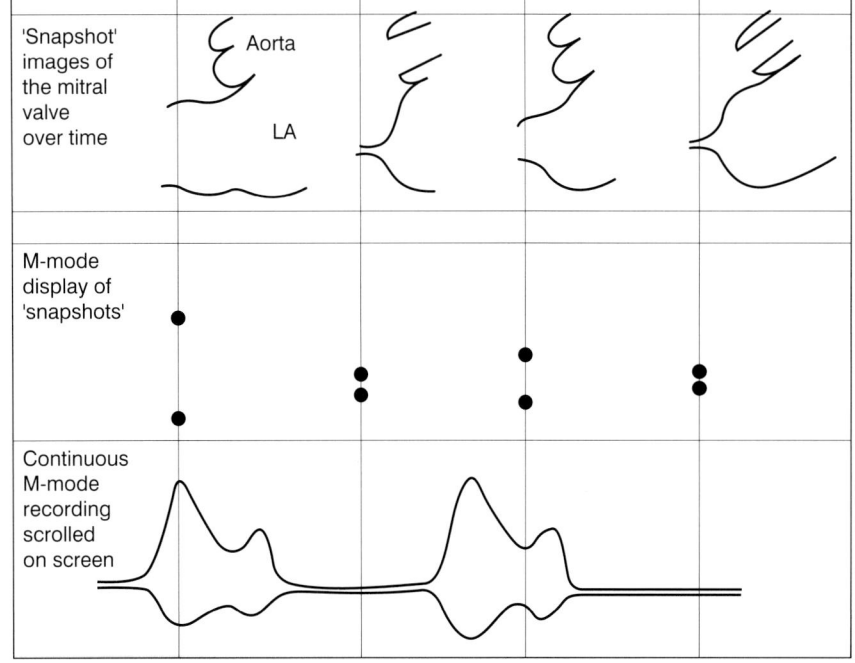

Figure 3.6 – Simplified diagram showing how an M-mode trace is made. A single line through the anatomical structure is repeated rapidly to show movement.

Colour M-mode combines both an M-mode trace and colour flow Doppler (see later) information from the same cursor line (Figure 3.7). It is useful for determining the timing, site, direction and velocity of flow at any point on the M-mode line.

Doppler ultrasound studies

Doppler studies are most commonly used to measure blood flow. The Doppler effect is defined as a shift in the observed frequency of radiated wave motion when there is relative movement between the source of radiation and the observer. In the case of medical ultrasound, the transducer is the 'observer' and the 'source of radiation' is moving blood cells (or myocardium in the case of Doppler tissue imaging).

The transducer emits sound at a known frequency (e.g. 3 MHz). The transducer expects the returning waves (echoes) to be at the same frequency, which they will be if they are reflected from stationary interfaces. When the transmitted wave interacts with moving blood the returning frequency will be lower than 3 MHz if the blood is moving away from the transducer, and higher if it is moving towards the transducer (Figure 3.8).

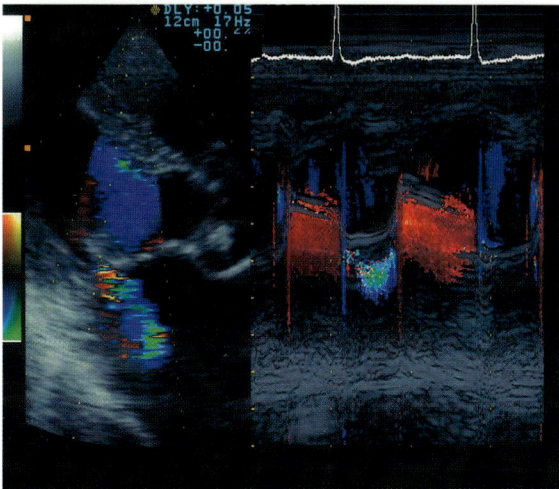

Figure 3.7 – Example of colour M-mode. In this case M-mode sampling is through the mitral valve and demonstrates mitral regurgitation (blue and aqua) when the valve is closed. When the valve is open in diastole, the forward flow is shown in red. The angulation of this recording allows both flows to be demonstrated optimally.

Doppler Equation

The difference in frequency (frequency shift) is termed Δf

$$\Delta f = \frac{2vf \cos \theta}{C}$$

where v is the velocity of the blood, f is the transmitted frequency (in our case 3 Mhz), θ is the angle between the direction of blood flow and the beam (machine assumes 0° unless told otherwise by the operator), C is the velocity of ultrasound in tissue (1540 m/s).

Δf is measured by the machine's software from the returning echoes, so the velocity of the blood can be calculated as:

$$v = \frac{\Delta f \, C}{2f \cos \theta}$$

As cos 0° = 1 (maximum value), the maximum velocity will be recorded when the blood is flowing directly towards or directly away from the transducer. As cos 90° = 0, flow perpendicular to the transducer has a calculated velocity of 0 m/s. In other words, flow perpendicular to the beam will not be detected (Figure 3.9).

In most cardiac studies, when calculating the velocity v the software is set to assume that there is an angle of 0°, unless told otherwise by the operator. It is the component of velocity along the ultrasound beam that produces the Doppler shift (Figure 3.10). Therefore, if the beam is at any angle other than 0°, the velocity will be underestimated. So, when performing Doppler traces one should always try to get the Doppler beam parallel with the flow. Colour flow Doppler (see later) can give an indication of the direction of flow through the heart valves. Angle correction is not normally used when performing cardiac Doppler studies, as large inaccuracies have been shown to occur with angle correction calculations in turbulent flow.

By chance, the range of 'shift' frequencies produced by moving blood and other biological structures (assigned to Δf) are usually within the range of sound that can be detected by the human ear (2–20 kHz). It is Δf that is heard on medical ultrasound machines, not the *actual* pulse sound. With a little practice, a sonographer can pick up flow signals just by listening to these sounds. All returning signals will demonstrate multiple frequency shifts, but the more organised the flow, the fewer the shifts that will be detected (Figure 3.11). Turbulent flow results in a broad range of detected frequency shifts.

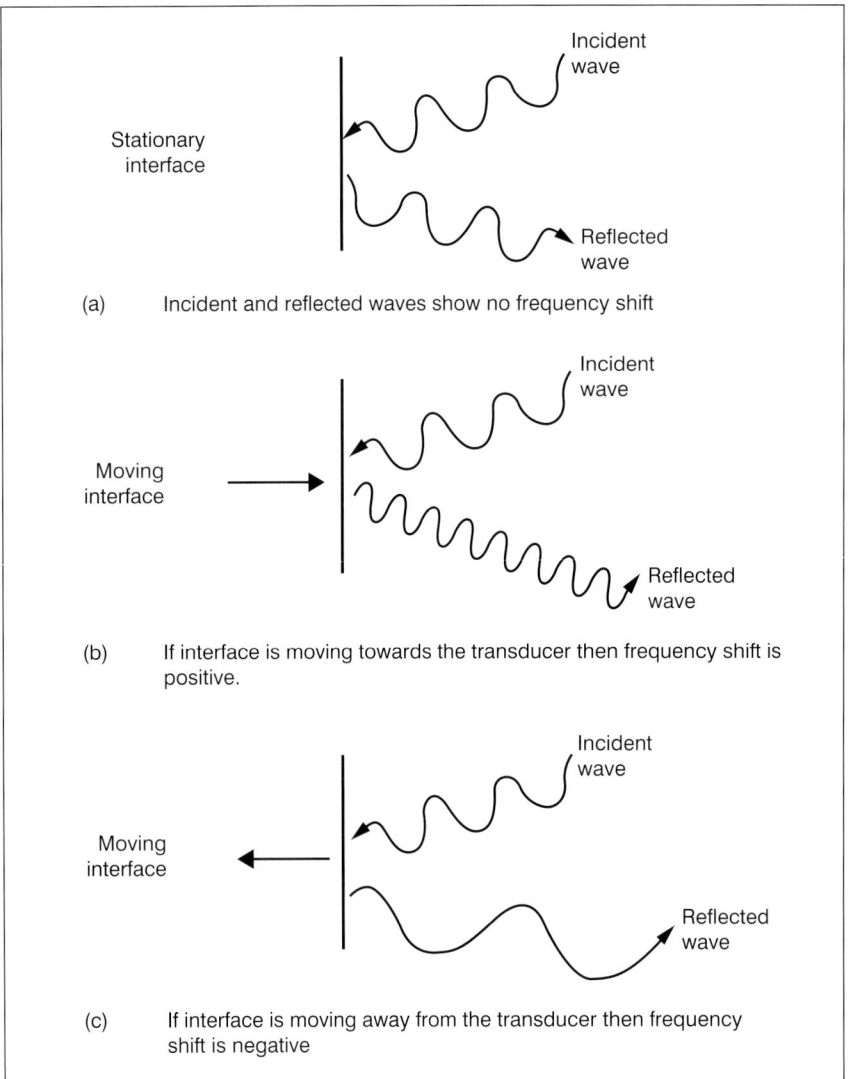

Stationary interface

Incident wave

Reflected wave

(a)   Incident and reflected waves show no frequency shift

Moving interface

Incident wave

Reflected wave

(b)   If interface is moving towards the transducer then frequency shift is positive.

Moving interface

Incident wave

Reflected wave

(c)   If interface is moving away from the transducer then frequency shift is negative

Figure 3.8 – The Doppler effect.
(a) Stationary interface
(b) and (c) Moving interfaces

The Doppler spectrum can be considered to show three components of blood flow. Velocity and timing are the two most obvious components. The third component is the intensity of the signal, which reflects the volume of flow. Unfortunately, the intensity can normally be used only as a qualitative rather than a quantitative measure.

Spectral Analysis

The returning Doppler signal has to be digitised and plotted in such a way that useful information can be obtained from it. The function that is first applied to the returning signal is to separate flow towards (positive frequency shifts) and flow away from (negative shifts) the transducer. This is performed by a phase quadrature detector. Further analysis is then performed by a mathematical algorithm called fast fourier transform which splits the waveform into its individual frequency components. A zero crossing detector is an older and less accurate method used to analyse the returning waveform. The standard format of a spectral Doppler display represents zero flow as a central horizontal baseline with flow towards the transducer being shown above the line and flow away being shown below the line. The frequency shift (related to velocity) is the distance from

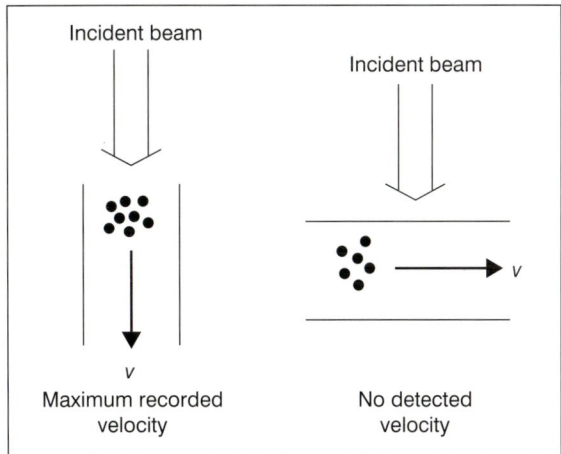

Figure 3.9 – Doppler interpretation of flow at right angles and parallel to the beam. If the beam is incident at angles between 0° and 90°, different velocities will be recorded even though the actual velocity of the blood is the same.

the baseline. Time runs horizontally across the trace. The intensity of signal is usually represented by the density of recording at any point on the spectral trace (Figure 3.12).

Equipment Controls for Spectral Doppler Studies

POWER OUTPUT

The power output on the machine may need to be increased when performing Doppler studies in order to

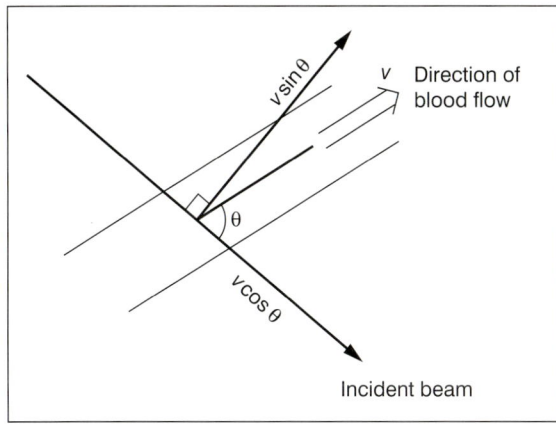

Figure 3.10 – The velocity component measured by the ultrasound system is $v \cos \theta$.

obtain the best results possible but the operator should try to keep this as low as possible, especially for paediatric patients. Power output is higher when using Doppler than for two-dimensional imaging due to the concentration of power in a smaller area and the use of scattered reflected energy. Pulsed and colour flow Doppler have a higher output power than continuous wave Doppler and should be used for as short a time as possible due to potential biological hazards (discussed in the Appendix). Increasing the Doppler gain (see below) to just below the noise limit before altering the power gives an optimal spectral trace.

DOPPLER GAIN

If the Doppler gain is set too high a lot of noise occurs in the Doppler signal and 'cross talk' (mirroring) of the

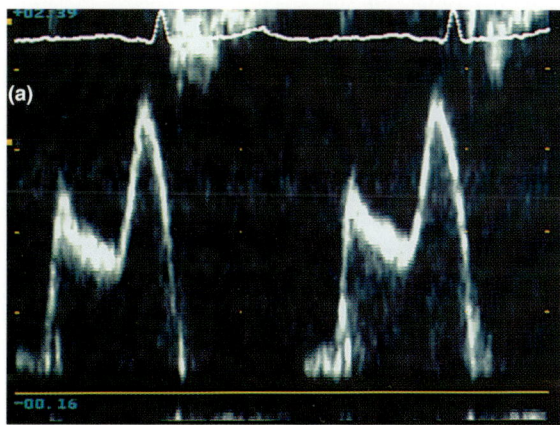

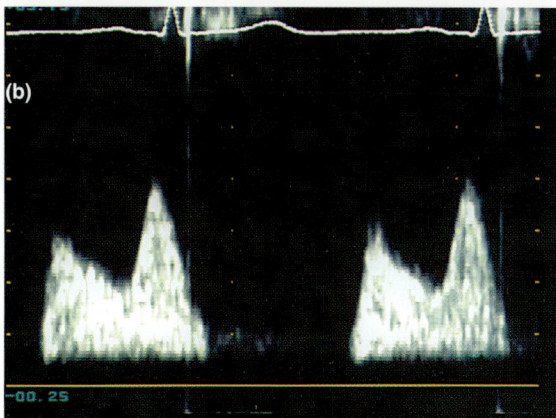

Figure 3.11 – (a) A narrow spectrum of 'shift' frequencies has a crisp outline and a corresponding crisp audible sound. (b) A broad spectrum shows fill-in of the spectral trace, relating to the wide range of velocities detected at any one point in time.

Doppler signal may occur. Cross talk occurs when there is a reflection of high intensity signals on the opposite side of the zero line. Turning down the gain should help to sort this out if the mirroring is an artefact or real flow. If the Doppler gain is set too low it is possible to miss important low intensity flow signals.

LOW FREQUENCY FILTER

Movements of the valves and myocardium produces low velocity, high intensity signals that will flood the useful audio and spectral signal of the blood flow. Increasing the filter threshold will eliminate the low-velocity portion of the Doppler spectrum. This will be seen as a signal-free area on both sides of the zero line on the spectral trace (Figure 3.13). Most machines have a range of filters that can be chosen, typically from 100 Hz to 1000 Hz. As a general rule, the higher the velocity being sampled, the higher the frequency of the filter should be used in order to concentrate on the maximum velocity. Beware though, as a filter that is set too high can also filter out the legitimate low velocity flow. (*Note*: A low frequency filter is often referred to as just a 'filter'.)

COMPRESSION AND REJECTION

These two controls alter the dynamic range of the spectral trace. Increasing the compression and/or rejection will give rise to a very 'contrasty', black and white trace,

and decreasing it will give a softer trace encompassing a wider dynamic range.

BASELINE SHIFT

Because the direction of blood flow in the heart is both towards and away from the transducer it is necessary to move the zero velocity line (baseline) either up or down so that an entire envelope of the valve flow can be displayed. Although this can apparently help to reduce or eliminate 'aliasing', it does not truly eliminate the effect, but rather alters the display (see below). On some machines the zero line on colour flow Doppler can be shifted to alter the colour display in an analogous way.

SCALE

The velocity scale of the spectral trace can be altered to study both low and high velocity flow in detail within the limits of the technique being used. In the case of pulsed wave Doppler studies, there is a limit that is quickly reached.

Pulsed Wave Doppler Studies

Pulsed wave Doppler examination is used when it is necessary to measure the blood flow at a selected depth along the line of Doppler interrogation. It is commonly used to evaluate forward mitral flow (especially in mitral stenosis), flow in the left ventricular outflow

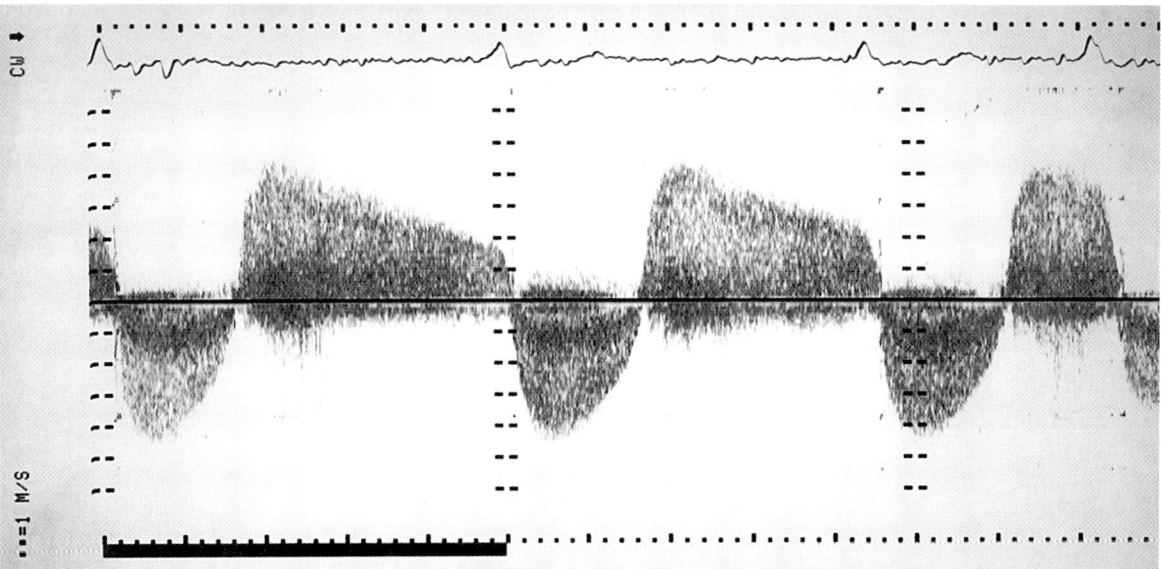

Figure 3.12 – Continuous wave apical recording of aortic flow. Flow above the zero line demonstrates flow towards the transducer, and in this case illustrates moderate aortic regurgitation. Flow below the zero line demonstrates flow away from the transducer, in this case forward aortic flow illustrating severe aortic stenosis.

tract, flow through the pulmonary valve to calculate pulmonary acceleration time, and flow in the descending aorta when assessing amount of aortic regurgitation. The cursor on the screen usually has a cross-marker to indicate the site selected (sometimes called the 'sample volume').

A very short pulse of ultrasound is emitted from the transducer, which is immediately turned off. A selected short period of time is allowed to elapse, after which the transducer is switched to receive mode. The length of time between the emitted pulse and the listening or receive period is determined by the operator, who chooses the position of the sample volume (or gate). The further from the transducer the sample volume position, the longer the time for which the transducer is switched off during the 'wait' period. A second variable, the length of the period of receive time, determines the length of the area being interrogated; this is called the 'sample volume'.

Aliasing

To measure the frequency shift (Δf) accurately, the signals must be sampled at least twice per cycle (of the sine wave). The minimum rate at which the signal must be sampled (sampling rate) for accurate measurement is twice the maximum Doppler shift:

$$\text{Sampling rate} = 2\Delta f \qquad \text{Nyquist limit}$$

If the sampling rate is less than this, then the frequency shift is inaccurately recorded (Figure 3.14). This occurs when the blood is moving quickly (i.e. Δf is larger) or when sampling at a great distance from the transducer

(it will take longer for echoes to return, thus decreasing the sampling rate).

To overcome this problem, which is known as aliasing, some machines use a technique known as 'high pulse repetition' Doppler interrogation. In this situation the system introduces additional sample volumes in response to adjusting the velocity range. The transducer will send out two or three pulses before there is time for the first pulse to have returned (Figure 3.15). Although this helps to solve the aliasing problem, misinterpretation can result due to the extra sample volumes recording flow at sites other than the site originally interrogated. Operators must be careful that the system has not 'sneaked in' another sample volume that has not been noticed.

Continuous Wave Doppler Studies

Continuous wave Doppler examination is used to measure fast-flowing blood, such as in aortic stenosis or mitral regurgitation, as it does not suffer from the aliasing that occurs when using pulsed wave Doppler. Two ultrasound transducers, usually mounted side by side in the one device, are used: one transducer continually emits ultrasound and the other continually receives the returning echoes. For this reason it is not possible to determine at what depth the returning signal is coming from, but the technique does have the advantage that very high velocity signals can be read.

In the normal heart, blood moves fastest through the valves, so it is not necessary to know at what depth the returning echoes are coming from as it can be assumed that they originate in the valves. Each valve has charac-

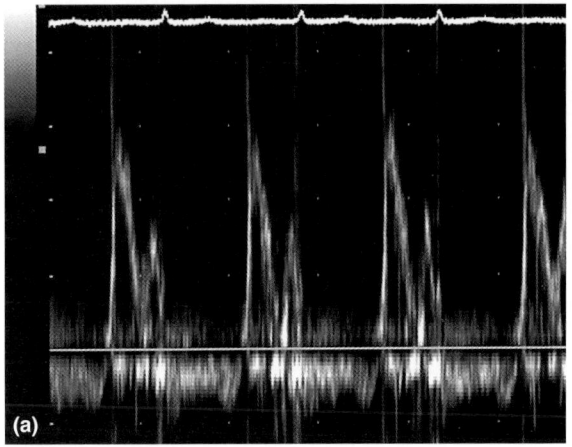
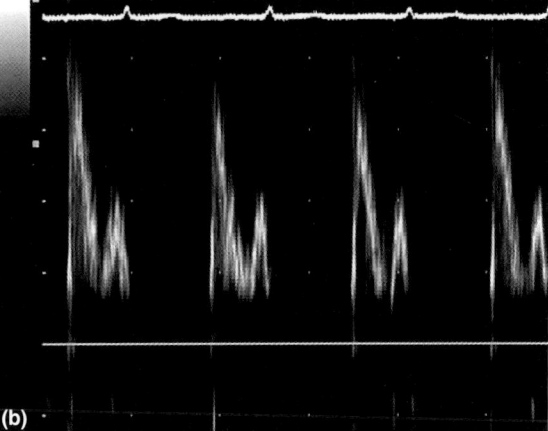

Figure 3.13 – Spectral trace of mitral flow with low (a) and high (b) filter settings.

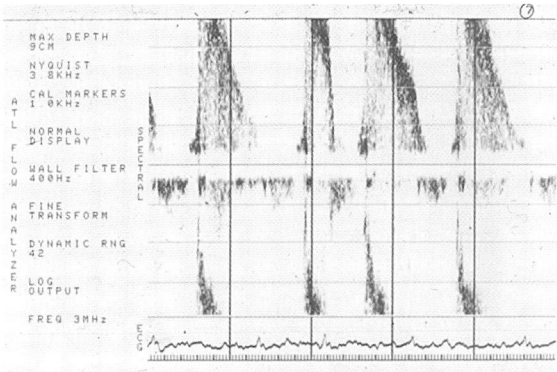

Figure 3.14 – The appearance of aliasing on a pulsed wave Doppler trace. The peaks of the cycles cannot be recorded accurately and appear at the bottom of the trace.

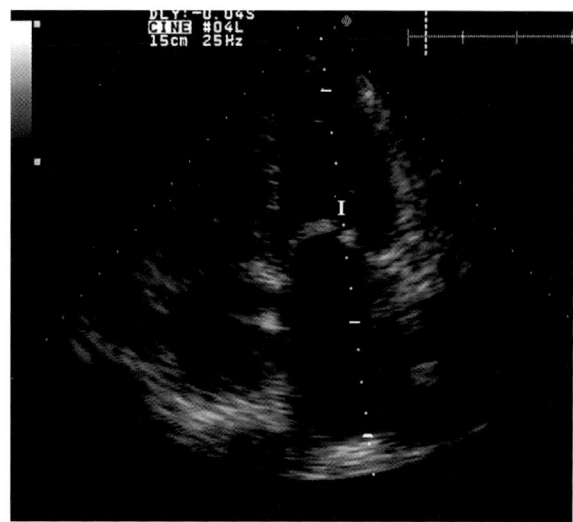

Figure 3.15 – Multiple pulsed wave Doppler gates introduced to overcome aliasing. The original site of interrogation is denoted by I; the extra gates are denoted by the horizontal lines.

teristic spectral Doppler traces. Some heart diseases (e.g. ventricular septal defect) will result in high-velocity flow arising from sites other than valves, but this results in characteristic traces (see Chapters 5 and 6). Pulsed wave Doppler studies can be used in conjunction with continuous wave Doppler measurements to determine an actual site of increased flow.

The intensity of the spectral trace depends on the number of blood cells moving in the same direction. For this reason, forward flow through all valves is always intense, while regurgitation (if mild) is often less intense. As the amount of regurgitation increases, so the trace becomes brighter, and this can be used to help grade the regurgitation (see Chapter 5).

Independent continuous wave Doppler scanning

Continuous wave Doppler can be used in two formats. (1) It can be used in *duplex scanning*, that is, in combination with the two-dimensional image for guided placement of the cursor. *Independent* continuous wave transducers display a spectral trace only, and practice is needed to use this technique. The advantages of using an independent continuous wave transducer include:

- it is more sensitive to weaker signals.

- the transducer face is very small and is set at an angle for better access between the ribs.

- the operator has to concentrate on the sound and spectral trace only, and thus is not tempted to place the cursor where he or she thinks the maximum flow *might* be.

Peak velocity

Peak velocity is measured simply by placing a cursor on the maximum point on the spectral trace. Cardiac measurement packages calculate the velocity automatically. The peak velocity (or the peak pressure drop (PPD)) is most commonly quoted in echocardiogram reports. It is a quick and simple measurement for the operator to perform. The peak velocity is a derived value, and depends on accurate alignment of the beam with the direction of flow. Most software combines the peak velocity with a derived pressure drop calculated using the modified Bernoulli equation.

Bernoulli equation

The physics of pressure and flow through narrow communications is very complicated and the original full Bernoulli equation attempts to describe this. Fortunately, it has proved possible in practice to use a simplified form of the equation under certain specific circumstances when:

- there is low velocity prior to the orifice, usually a large chamber,

- the orifice is short in length; and

- the ultrasound beam is well aligned with the jet.

The conditions are often met in the cardiac circulation, for example in stenotic valves, regurgitant valves and small ventricular septal defects.

A spectral Doppler trace through a valve displays the velocity of blood passing through the valve. This velocity is commonly converted to a pressure drop reading that is then compared with values obtained at cardiac catheterisation. Great care must be taken in the interpretation of these pressure values as catheter derived values are not usually exactly the same as Doppler derived values. In general, however, when the flow before the valve is less than 1m/s the pressure drop is calculated very simply (by the ultrasound machine) by a modified Bernoulli equation:

$$P \; (\mathrm{mmHg}) = 4 \, v^2$$

where P is the pressure drop and v is the velocity (m/s).

If a valve is obstructed the velocity will be increased and the pressure drop will increase. However, for an unobstructed valve, if the blood flow before the valve is increased to more than 1m/s (e.g. in severe regurgitation or increased cardiac output) then the forward velocity will also be increased significantly. This must be taken into consideration, otherwise the pressure drop will be overestimated. A slightly expanded equation must then be used (Figure 3.16):

$$P = 4(v_2^2 - v_1^2)$$

where v_2 is the peak flow through the valve and v_1 is the flow just prior to valve and must be measured by pulsed wave Doppler.

Mean velocity (average velocity calculation)

Mean velocity measurements are more time consuming to make than peak velocity measurements, but can give a more accurate indication of flow patterns. To obtain a mean velocity measurement the operator must trace around the margin of a spectral trace. The software then effectively measures the velocity at multiple points along the spectral trace and averages all these velocities (Figure 3.17). If two spectral traces with the same peak velocity are compared, the mean velocity will sometimes give more information about the actual flow or stenosis (Figure 3.18).

The mean velocity can be converted to a mean pressure drop (MPD) by using the Bernoulli equation (see above):

$$\mathrm{MPD} = 4 \, v_{\mathrm{mean}}^2$$

Colour flow Doppler studies

Colour flow Doppler imaging superimposes a colour representation of the blood velocity over the two-dimensional image. Separate software is used to display the two functions simultaneously. In order to be able to determine the velocity of the moving blood, several pulses (e.g. 3–7) must be sent down each line and compared. Points along the successive lines with slightly different signals are due to blood flow occurring at those points. Because of the longer dwell time needed for multiple lines to be interpreted, obtaining multiple samples over a large area means that the frame rate is decreased. The display of colour relates to the mean velocity within a particular sample region. As soon as blood reaches a set velocity it is given a designated colour hue. Only the velocity component in the direction of the incident beam can be used. Therefore, if no colour is displayed this does not necessarily mean that there is no flow (just as with other forms of Doppler examination). Indeed, there can be a large volume flow at a fast rate perpendicular to the incident beam and no colour will be assigned as there is no velocity component in the direction of the beam. A good example of this is in the arch of the aorta (Figure. 3.19). At cardiac settings, low-velocity blood flow will not be colour coded, regardless of volume (due to filter settings). Acoustic shadowing, such as occurs behind a prosthetic mitral valve, will prevent both colour display and the two-dimensional image (see Artefacts in the Appendices).

The widely accepted colour display codes flow towards the transducer as red and yellow hues, and flow away from the transducer as blue and aqua. The majority of ultrasound machines have different preset colour charts for the user to select. A typical choice is to display turbulent flow (or variance) in a different colour, typically green.

As with pulsed wave Doppler, aliasing occurs when flow reaches a velocity of more than half the sampling rate. With colour flow this is a definite advantage, as it draws the operator's eye to the bright mosaic pattern that is present in abnormal flow (e.g. ventricular septal defects and regurgitant jets). The aliasing is seen as a sudden change in colour in the fastest moving part of the flow area (Figure 3.20).

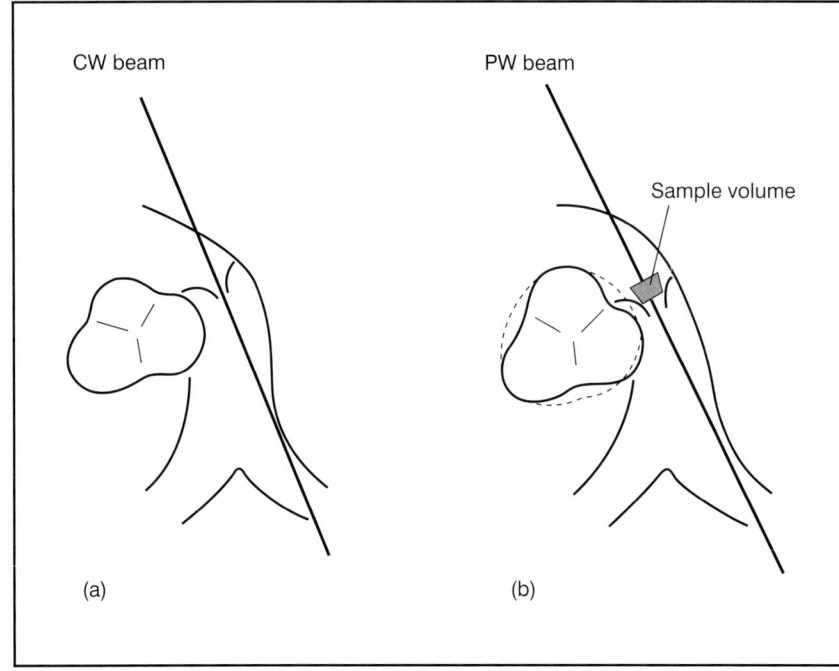

(a) (b)

Figure 3.16 – Application of the expanded Bernouilli equation for the calculation of the pressure drop across a vale when the blood flow is increased before it. (a) The velocity in the valve (v_2) is obtained using continuous wave (CW) Doppler. (b) The velocity in the RVOT just prior to the valve (v_1) is obtained using pulsed wave Doppler.

EQUIPMENT CONTROLS FOR COLOUR DOPPLER

Because the colour image is superimposed on the two-dimensional image it is important that variable settings for both modalities are set at their optimum levels. In order to achieve this:

- Select the colour flow map that displays the most information to you. Different operators will have different preferences.

- The gain of the two-dimensional image should be turned down to prevent 'white-out' obscuring the plotting of colour pixels.

- The gain of colour flow should be increased until the background noise is colour coded. The gain should then be decreased slightly until the noise just disappears.

- The area being sampled by colour Doppler should be decreased in width to the smallest reasonable size in order to increase the frame rate to its maximum.

- The frame rate can also be increased by decreasing the depth of the two-dimensional image, if possible.

- Increase the colour pixel size (i.e. reduce the resolution) to increase the frame rate.

- Some machines allow the user to change the filter

level of the colour display. If your machine allows for this, beware that the filter is not set too high, otherwise important low velocity flow may be missed.

- Some machines allow the sensitivity to be varied; however, usually, the more sensitive the recording the lower the aliasing limit. Changing the sensitivity may also affect the frame rate. This is usually achieved by altering the number of times each line is interrogated (sometimes referred to as 'packet size').

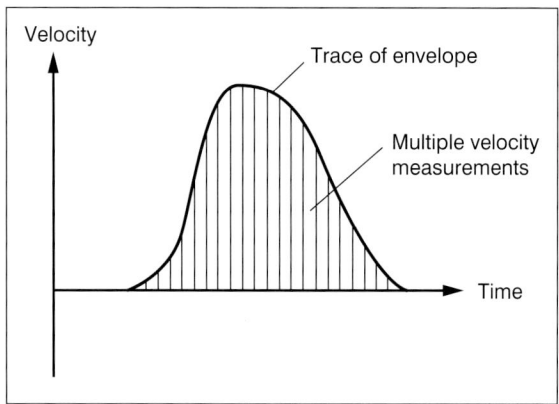

Figure 3.17 – Calculation of the mean velocity.

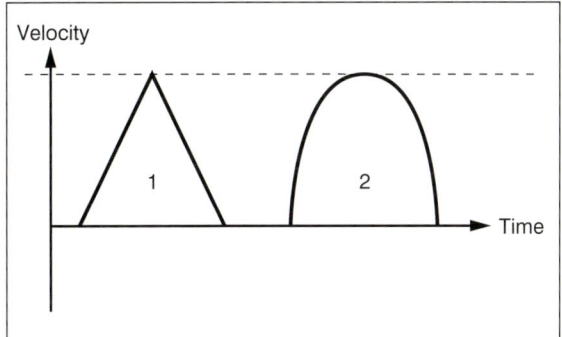

Figure 3.18 – Illustration of a case when the mean velocity is a more accurate measure than the peak velocity. Traces 1 and 2 both have the same peak height and last for the same length of time, but the mean velocity calculated from trace 2 is higher than that calculated from trace 1.

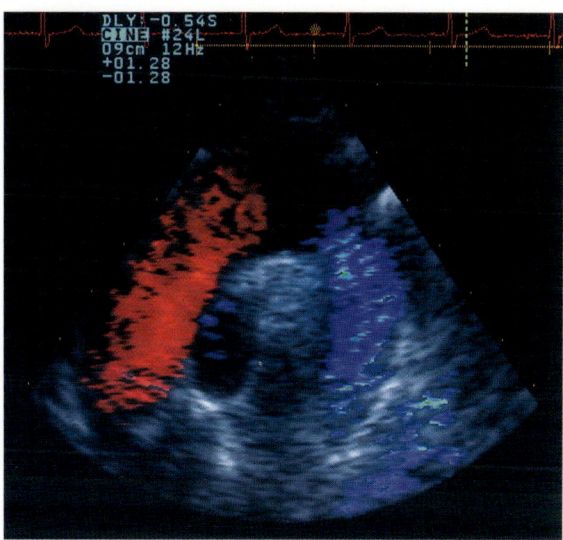

Figure 3.19 – Colour flow applied to the arch of the aorta. Blood flow towards the transducer in the ascending aorta is encoded red and flow away via the descending aorta is blue. In the transverse arch no colour is assigned, as flow is perpendicular to the beam.

The display size of regurgitant jets can be altered significantly by instrument factors, and care must be taken not to rely on this aspect alone when assessing abnormalities.

It must be remembered that colour flow Doppler is a qualitative rather than quantitative technique, and so actual velocities cannot easily be estimated from the colour assigned. This is because the flow displayed is just the velocity component in the direction of the beam, the velocity displayed is the mean value and not the peak, and the same colour hue is given to a range of different velocities.

Other basic equipment details

Depth

This increases or decreases the distance from which the returning echoes are collected. If the depth is increased, this means a longer time delay for the echoes to return. This is reflected in the frame rate, which decreases for longer interrogated depths. The same principle applies to colour flow and pulsed wave Doppler.

Gain

This controls the amplitude of the returning signals, either magnifying or compressing them. By increasing the overall gain, a brighter image will be obtained. Because echoes returning from a distance will be

reduced by attenuation, all ultrasound machines also have the facility of magnifying the signals from the far field more than those from the near field. This control is called *time gain compensation* or *swept gain control*. It is a set of about 10 sliding controls in a vertical row that can be altered independently of each other. On some new machines the lateral gain can be altered by increasing the amplitude of the returning echoes along the length of a scan line (in reality, several grouped scan lines). Again, sliding controls are used, but these are in a horizontal row.

Measurement packages

A cardiac ultrasound machine must have the ability to perform simple distance measurements as well as more complex ones such as calculations of the ejection fraction and cardiac output. The operator should be aware of how the results are calculated so that he or she can minimise errors (see Measurement Calculations in the Appendices).

Invert

This facility can be used to turn the image upside down on the display. This inversion is quite obvious. A more insidious inversion is left to right which is not always immediately apparent and can cause much confusion. It

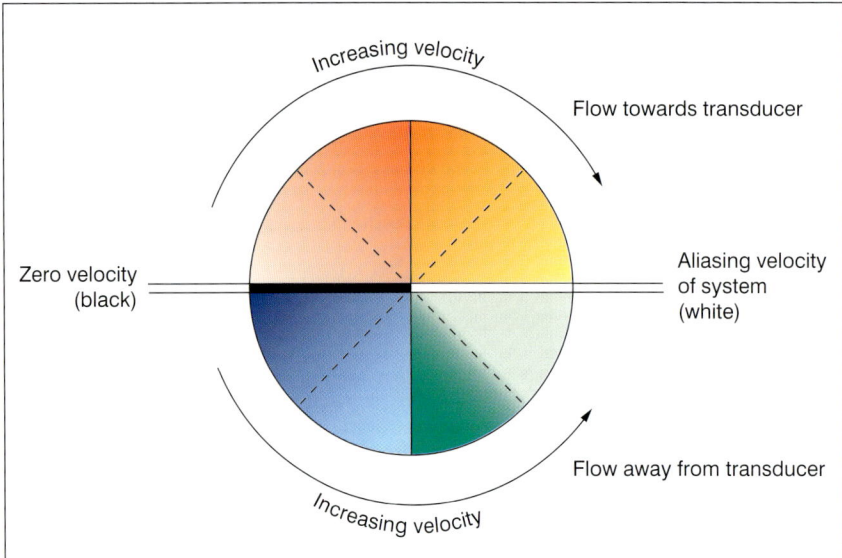

Figure 3.20 – An illustration of aliasing in colour flow Doppler.

is suggested that the machine is always operated at the standard setting and the transducer rotated through 180° if this kind of inversion is required.

Sweep speed

The operator can choose the speed at which the scrolling screen is swept for M-mode and Doppler traces. The speed is usually selected according to the patient's heart rate so that a meaningful trace can be obtained. The speed may be increased to study a trace in more detail. Some machines have the useful facility that the speed can be altered after the trace has been frozen.

Cine loop

After a few seconds of scanning the image may be frozen; the last few frames are stored in digital memory and can be reviewed. On most machines this process is immediate and can be accessed simply by rolling the track ball. Some machines are slightly more complex and a separate cine loop button is provided to activate this facility. Typically 30–60 images are stored. The cine loop is a very helpful facility, as it allows the operator to retrieve an image that has just passed.

Reference

1. Hendrick WR, Hykes DL, Starchman DE. *Ultrasound Phyics and Instrumentation*, 3rd edn. Mosby, St Louis, 1995.

4

PRACTICAL SCANNING
TECHNIQUE

Choice of transducer
Windows
Electrocardiogram
Distance measurements
Standard full examination

Choice of transducer

The transducer chosen for each examination very much depends on the build of the patient. Low frequencies, for example 2.5 MHz, are typically used for large patients, where more penetration is required. The frequency used for average patients is 3.0 – 3.75 MHz. Children can be scanned using 5 MHz, and neonates 7 MHz. The higher the frequency, the better the resolution (image quality), but penetration is reduced. Transducers are designed with an optimal focal depth (sometimes dynamically variable on phased array transducers) at which image quality is likely to be optimal. In general, higher frequency transducers have a shorter focal depth to allow more superficial structures to be imaged better. Even when scanning a large patient on a 2.5 MHz transducer, it is often useful to change to a higher frequency (and lower focal depth) to interrogate structures in the near field (e.g. changing to 5 MHz when looking in the left ventricular apex for thrombus).

Doppler interrogation is more sensitive when used at lower frequencies, and less aliasing of pulsed wave spectral traces and colour flow imaging will occur. Most transducers have a Doppler frequency slightly lower than the imaging frequency. In some cases the Doppler emitting frequency can be changed.

Newer machines have multifrequency transducers (where the same transducer is capable of emitting and receiving different frequencies) or broad-band transducers (where a range of returning frequencies is used to create the image, giving rise to good resolution in the near field and also penetration to the far field).

All cardiac transducers have a small face that can fit between the ribs. On each transducer there is an orientation mark, which may be in the form of a ridge, dot or light, so that the transducer can be aligned correctly on the chest. Most phased array transducers have a square or rectangular face, which can be slightly awkward to use when rotation 'on the spot' is required to view another plane from the same window. Mechanical transducers generally have a circular face (often slightly smaller), which is easier to rotate in rib interspaces.

Windows

When performing an echo scan, the operator should envisage the three-dimensional heart within the chest. If this can be achieved, it will make comprehension of the scan much easier, and it will be easier to improvise views to interrogate a structure of interest. Due to the location of the ribs and overlying lung, there are only a few sites on the chest wall where the transducer can be placed to produce an image of the heart. These are called 'windows'. There are three commonly used windows (left parasternal, apical and subcostal), each with two planes at right angles to each other, that are used to view the heart (Table 4.1). Once an operator is familiar with this slightly simplistic approach to cardiac anatomy from the three 'standard windows' there is no reason why non-standard windows and planes should not be used to interrogate a structure. A commonly used view is the suprasternal window. This is generally used to examine the aortic arch and other superior mediastinal structures. The right parasternal window is used for continuous wave Doppler assessment of the ascending aorta only, and is generally not used for imaging except where the ascending aorta is enlarged or the heart is displaced to the right.

The aim initially is to position the transducer such that the three standard projections, or planes, can be viewed (Figure 4.1a-f). Different transducer angles will be needed for each patient as the heart is positioned differently within each individual's chest. Each projection is orientated by convention. As you begin to scan, by moving the transducer, it will become apparent how the different cardiac structures are related and thus the transducer should be moved to obtain the required image. By convention, paediatric scans are viewed with the image inverted (upside down) compared with conventional adult scan viewing.

Electrocardiogram

An electrocardiogram (ECG) should be recorded for every patient in order to determine the timing of cardiac events. A very basic description of an ECG waveform is given in Chapter 1. The ECG electrodes should be placed such that the right terminal is on the right upper

Table 4.1 – The three commonly used windows and the associated planes of visualisation

Window	Planes
Left parasternal	Long-axis
	Short axis
Apical	Four chamber
	Long-axis
Subcostal	Four chamber
	Short axis

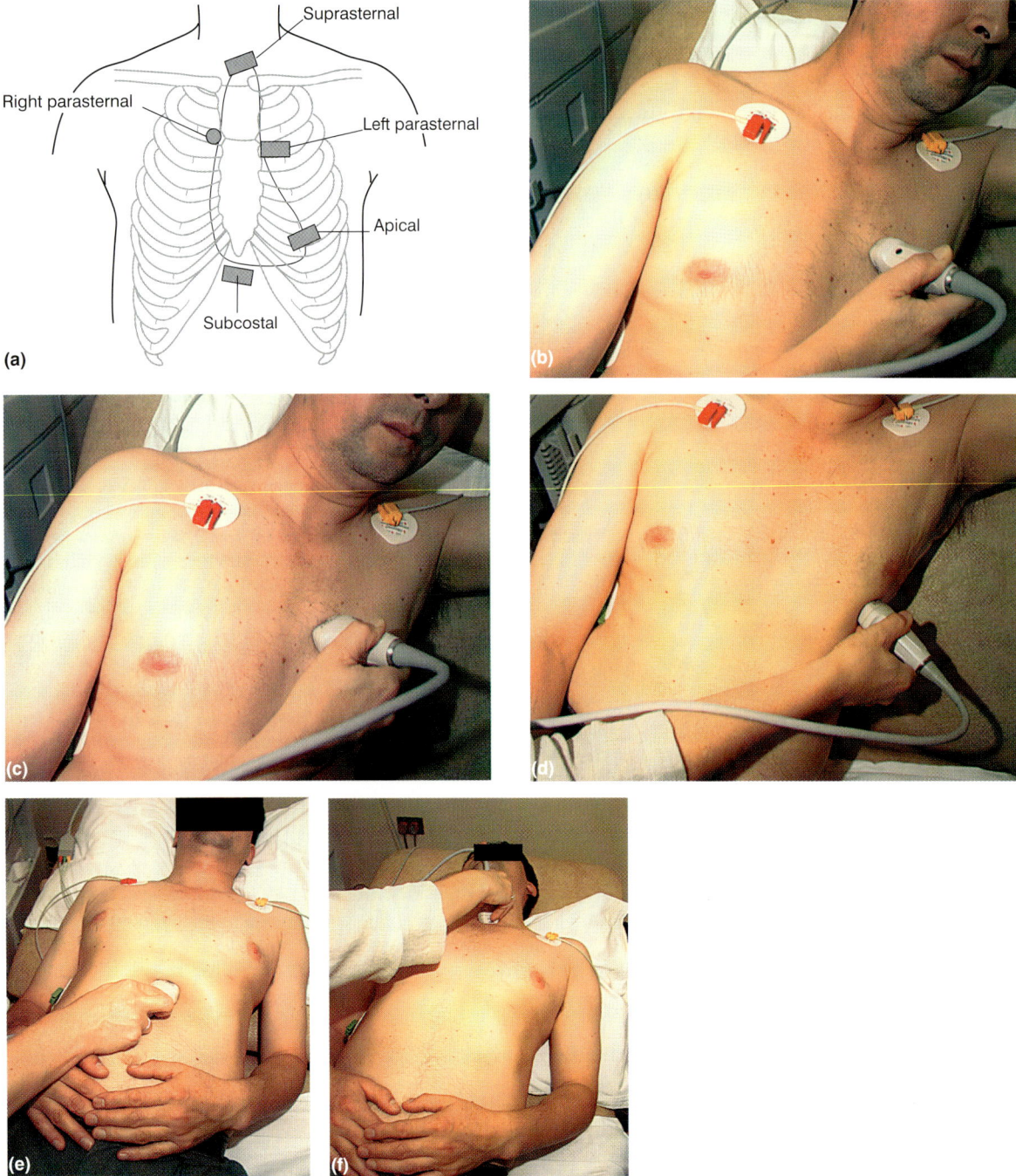

Figure 4.1 – (a) Diagram showing approximate positions of the transducer for visualising the standard windows. (b) Position of the left parasternal window. The transducer orientation marker is directed towards the patient's right shoulder to produce the long axis plane (c) Position of the left parasternal window with the transducer rotated clockwise through 90° to produce the short axis plane. The orientation marker (no longer visible) is now directed towards the patient's left shoulder. (d) The apical window. The transducer is orientated almost transversely with the marker directed posteriorly. This produces the apical four chamber view. (e) The patient now lies flat for the subcostal window. A little pressure may need to be applied to obtain a satisfactory window. The four chamber and short axis planes can both be obtained from this position. (f) The patient's head is now extended slightly over the pillow to allow access to the suprasternal window.

chest or shoulder and the left terminal is just below the apex. Sometimes it may be convenient to place one or both of the terminals on the patient's back. It should be appreciated that a line drawn between these two leads should follow the approximate axis of the heart. The earth lead can be placed anywhere, but is typically sited on the left upper chest or shoulder. Perhaps the most important thing to remember when positioning the electrodes is to site them well away from the echo windows. Try to attach the electrodes in hair-free areas, for both a better trace and easier removal. For more information on ECGs, see Chapter 2.

Jelly

Interfaces between materials of greatly different acoustic properties will lead to considerable reflection and, consequently, to poor penetration beyond the interface. There is a lot of reflection of the ultrasound beam at rib and lung interfaces; of course, some sound is propagated through these tissues, but at vastly different speeds than through soft tissue or blood. Ultrasound jelly is used to match the speed of sound through the face of the transducer to that through the skin, and to ensure that there is no air between the transducer/skin interface. The slippery nature of such jelly means that the transducer can be moved easily across the skin surface. Be generous with the amount of jelly used. Good images cannot be gained if too little is used. Ideally, the jelly should be fairly viscous, not only to prevent it running over the curve of the chest, but also to allow in-filling of any gaps if the face of the transducer has to be set at an angle to the skin surface. The jelly currently used for echo work fulfils these requirements, as well as being water soluble and non-staining.

Distance measurements

It is generally accepted that when making echocardiographic measurements that cavities (such as the cardiac chambers and aorta) are measured from inside edge to inside edge and solid structures (such as the myocardium and masses) are measured from outside edge to outside edge. The borders of a structure need to be clearly defined for accurate placement of the calipers.

Two-dimensional image

The image is frozen and the cine loop is used to move 'back in time' until the structure of interest is at its optimal position in the cardiac cycle (e.g. end diastole for septal thickness). The line between the two calipers

needs to be at right angles to the long axis of the structure. If making a second measurement to obtain a two-dimensional measurement of a structure (e.g. the left atrium) the second pair of callipers needs to be placed at right angles to the first.

M-mode trace

In theory, distance measurements made on the M-mode trace are more accurate due to the faster frame rate, which gives a recording of continual movement. It must be remembered, however, that the measurement will only be accurate if the M-mode beam is passing through the structure of interest at 90° and both distance callipers are placed on the trace at the same time in the heart cycle (i.e. the line between the two calipers is exactly vertical).

Standard full examination

The non-technical aspects of the examination are described in Chapter 1. The order in which the cardiac structures are examined is purely a personal choice. It is important to choose your own approach and then routinely adhere to it so that no part of the examination is forgotten. A suggested system is described below.

Parasternal long axis

The parasternal long axis view (Figure 4.2) is the typical starting point for recording an echocardiogram. The head end of the bed should be laid almost flat and the patient turned partly or completely on their left side.

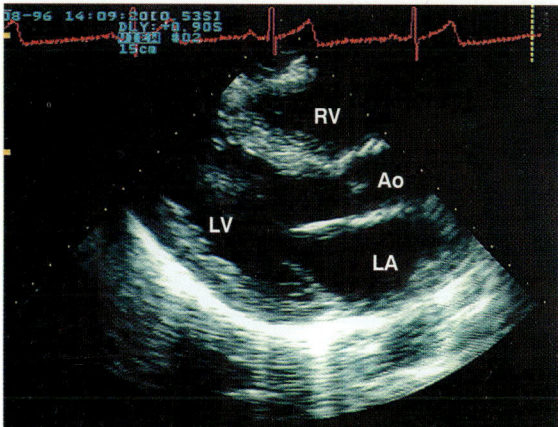

Figure 4.2 – Parasternal long axis image recorded during diastole, showing open mitral valve leaflets and closed aortic leaflets. Ao, aorta; LA, left atrium; LV, left ventricle; RV, right ventricle.

When on their side, encourage the patient to rest his or her right shoulder on a supporting pillow (without rolling back) so that the soft tissues of the chest are relaxed and in an open position. The transducer is then placed between the third and fourth ribs, directly to the left of the sternum. The orientation marker is towards the right shoulder (Figure 4.1b).

It may be necessary to angle (tilt) the transducer slightly upwards (cephalad) or downwards (caudad). To visualise both the mitral and the aortic valves on the same image it may be necessary to rotate the transducer gently, clockwise or anticlockwise in order to align the imaging plane with the long axis of the structures on the left side. This will also have the effect of elongating or shortening the left ventricular cavity. In some cases the interspace will have to be changed if the alignment is not appropriate for achieving the plane (i.e. if you cannot get the mitral valve and aortic valve well imaged at the same time, try a higher interspace).

If the left ventricle is seen to be pointing anteriorly (Figure 4.3), rather than lying horizontally, accurate M-mode measurements of the ventricle cannot be performed. There are several things that can be done to make the left ventricle appear more horizontal:

- position the patient so that their head is lying completely flat

- turn the patient further onto their side (sometimes, rolling the patient slightly forward will help)

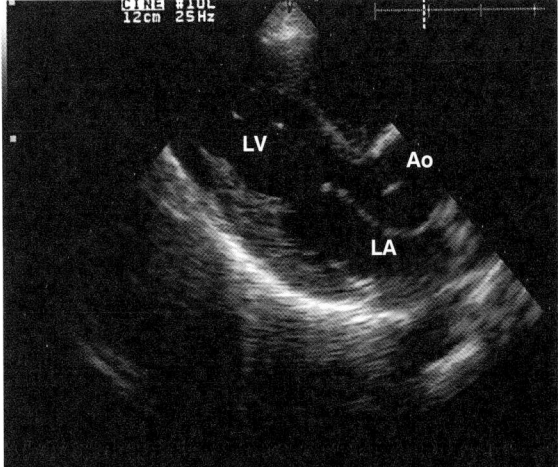

Figure 4.3 – Parasternal long axis image in which the left ventricle is oriented too anteriorly for accurate M-mode traces to be obtained.

- move the transducer up one rib space and gently angle the transducer back down towards the heart

- slide the transducer closer to the sternum.

If lung is a problem, turning the patient further onto their side, or even slightly forwards and partly onto their front, can help.

Better images can often be obtained on obese women if they sit more upright and roll slightly backwards; this helps reduce the amount of soft tissue beside the sternum.

DIFFICULTY IN FINDING AN IMAGE

If no image at all can be obtained, the patient's heart may particularly high or low sited. For example, in patients with chronic lung disease a good parasternal view can often be found using a subcostal position. Bold movements with the transducer and lots of jelly will need to be used. Start with the transducer just below the clavicle on the left. Slide the transducer slowly down along the length of the sternum to just below the ribs. If the heart is not found in this movement, start once more at the top of the chest, but this time more laterally towards the left shoulder, and again slide the transducer slowly down to the bottom of the ribs. If the heart still cannot be located, it is a good idea to look at a previous chest radiograph if one is available, which may explain the difficulty. A few patients do not have a parasternal window (especially those patients with a pectus excavatum), and the apical view can then be sought. As a last resort, the patient can be turned on their right side and a right parasternal view can be attempted. Patients with a pneumonectomy or dextrocardia can often be imaged this way.

The following structures should be visualised and measured on the parasternal long axis view, but not necessarily in the order listed. Always keep in mind that the structures you are looking at are three-dimensional and a full understanding of a patient's anatomy and pathology can only be obtained by sweeping the beam (by moving the transducer) across the entire structure under interrogation. Do not just find the classic view and then not move the transducer. This applies to all the modalities of echocardiography (imaging and Doppler).

AORTA

In the majority of patients, only the very proximal part of the ascending aorta can be visualised, unless it is dilated, in which case, it becomes more obvious. First observe the walls to check for any flaps or false aneurysm. The diameter should be measured either on the two-dimensional image or from an M-mode trace (Figure 4.4). The aortic root needs to be studied and checked for any overriding of the right ventricle.

AORTIC VALVE

Observe the leaflets for their thickness and amount of movement. On the long axis view only two of the three leaflets can be seen at any one time. The anterior leaflet is always the right coronary cusp. The two posterior leaflets cannot be differentiated in this view. An M-mode trace should then be performed (Figure 4.5). The cursor must be placed at the leaflet tips, not through the body of the leaflets, otherwise maximal opening will not be demonstrated. The shape of the resultant trace then needs to be studied for the amount of leaflet excursion and to check for any early closure. Most normal aortic leaflets flutter as the blood is passing through them in systole.

Colour flow Doppler should now be applied to the aortic valve, aortic root and left ventricular outflow tract (LVOT). If any aortic regurgitation is present it can usually be visualised at this stage. Colour flow on the aortic root will highlight a sinus of valsalva fistula if one is present. Colour applied to the LVOT is used to assess the perimembranous region of the interventricular septum in order to check for defects. The flow will be shown in red, towards the right ventricle, but take care not to confuse this with the forward tricuspid flow which is adjacent to this area. The colour box can then be moved along the length of the interventricular septum, this time concentrating on the right ventricle to check for any septal defects.

LEFT VENTRICULAR OUTFLOW TRACT

The diameter of the LVOT is measured on this projection (Figure 4.6) if needed for cardiac output or continuity equation measurements. The callipers should be placed immediately proximal to the aortic valve at right angles to the outflow tract.

LEFT ATRIUM

Although the left atrium can be clearly seen in the parasternal long axis view, the entire chamber cannot be fully assessed from this one view. Some sonographers advocate the measurement of the left atrium using this view from an M-mode trace. However, this is only a one-dimensional measurement, and with the patient turned on their side the left atrium is compressed against the spine. It has been suggested[1] that the left atrium should be measured in two planes on the apical four chamber view instead, in order to represent its true size more accurately. Certainly, the left atrium can be studied in this view, and this is particularly useful in patients who have had their mitral valve replaced as there tends to be less artefact in this projection than in others.

MITRAL VALVE

Observe the valve leaflets for their thickness and amount of movement. Also observe the annulus; the posterior mitral annulus is often thickened. To represent the mitral leaflet movement accurately an M-mode trace must be performed (Figure 4.7). The cursor should be placed through the leaflet tips, not the body of the leaflets. The anterior leaflet can usually be identified very clearly. The posterior leaflet is not necessar-

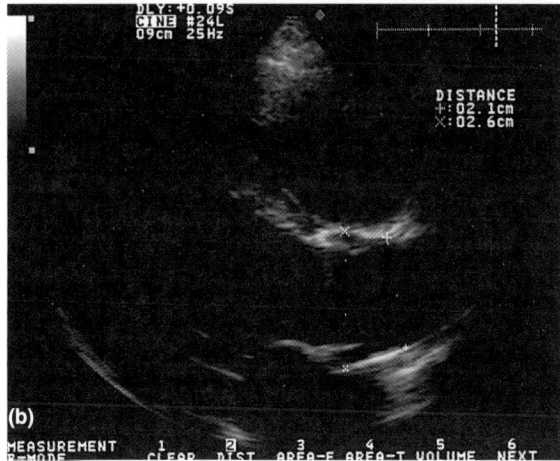

Figure 4.4 – (a) The measurements show the annulus size across the valve hinge points (left) and the sinus of Valsalva (right). (b) this shows the sino-tubular junction measurement to the right of the sinus of Valsalva.

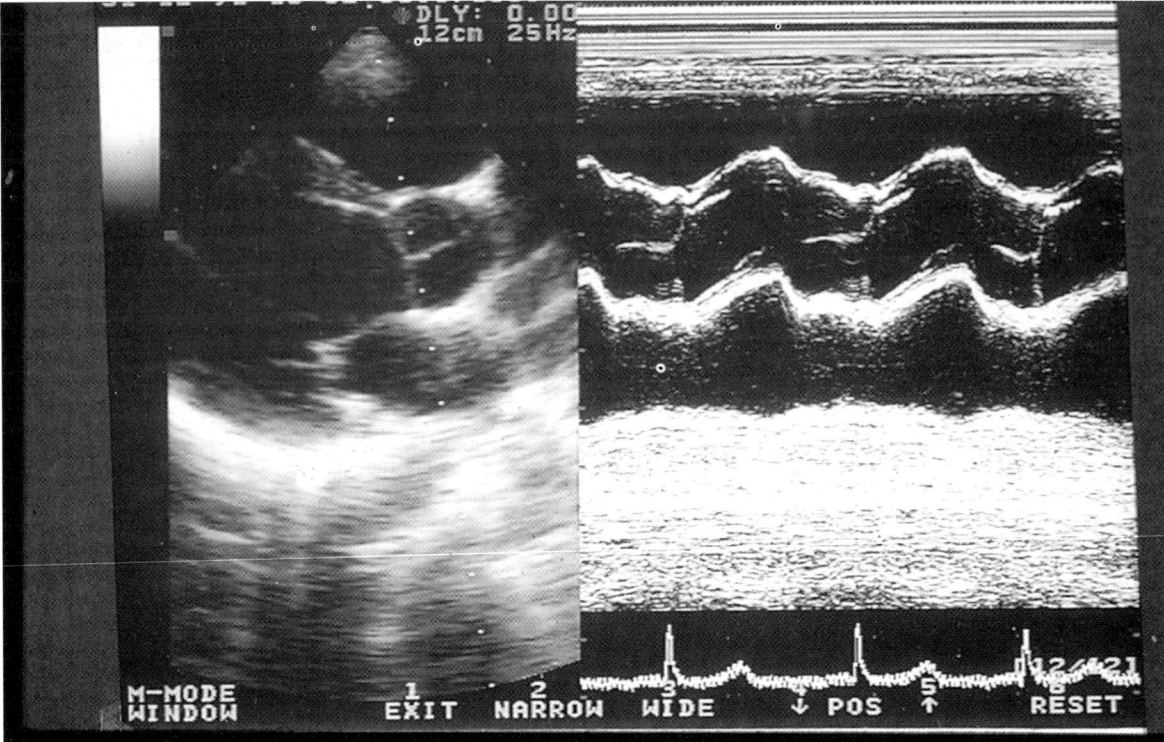

Figure 4.5 – M-mode trace of the aortic valve (commonly described as a 'box'). Note the flutter of the posterior leaflet.

ily identified on the M-mode trace as it is smaller than the anterior leaflet, so the excursion is not so great and

the anterior leaflet is highly reflective; the posterior leaflet is often acoustically shadowed.

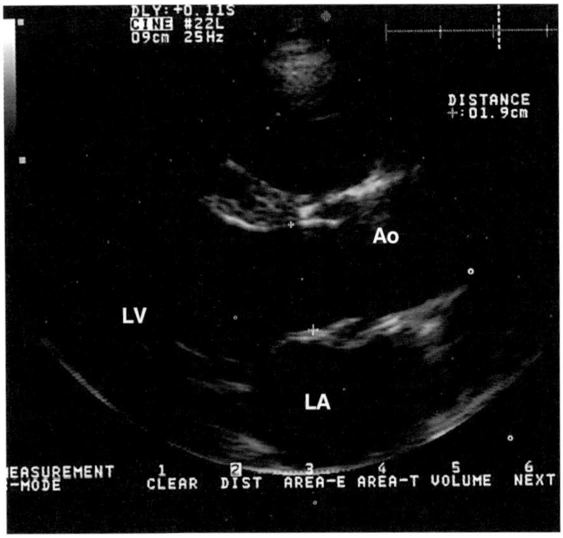

A normal M-mode trace displays an M shape due to the biphasic flow through the mitral valve in diastole. The systolic portion of the trace (when the leaflets are closed) should be a straight line, usually sloping gently upwards. Colour flow Doppler can be applied over the mitral valve, but this is usually disappointing as regurgitation is usually perpendicular to the beam, unless it is eccentric.

LEFT VENTRICLE

The left ventricle needs to be assessed for its size, contractility and myocardial thickness. The cavity size of the left ventricle can be measured on the two-dimensional image, but a good quality M-mode image, if it can be obtained is more accurate as there is no ambiguity as to when end systole and end diastole occur. The M-mode cursor is positioned just beyond the mitral leaflet tips (Figure 4.8). The corresponding trace may therefore include echoes from the chordae. The cursor must be at right angles to the long axis of the left ven-

Figure 4.6 – Measurement of the diameter of the left ventricular outflow tract.

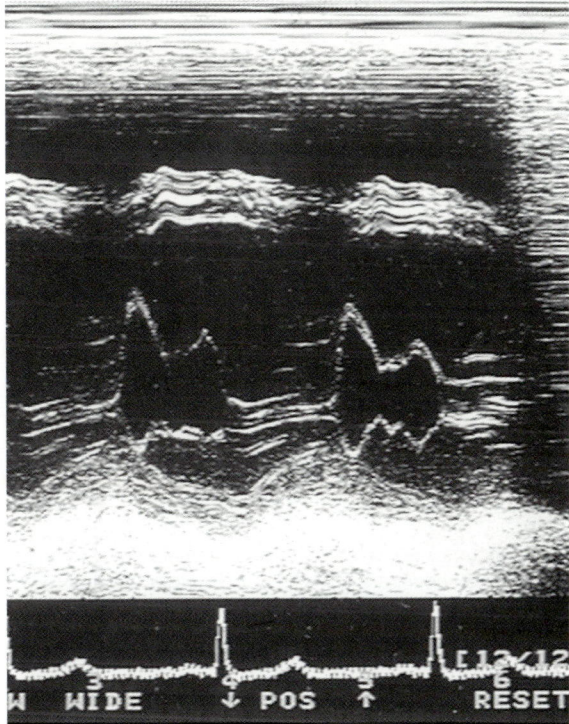

Figure 4.7 – M-mode trace of the mitral valve. Note the biphasic flow.

tricle (i.e. along the line from the point of the mitral-aortic continuity to the apex).

The end systolic (ESD) and end diastolic diameters (EDD) should be measured during the same cardiac cycle and as late during diastole as possible (Figure 4.9).

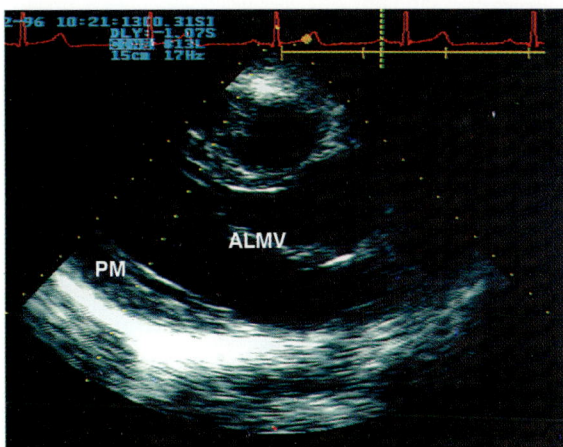

Figure 4.8 -The correct position of the M-mode beam for measuring the diameter of the left ventricle. ALMV, anterior leaflet mitral valve; PM, papillary muscle.

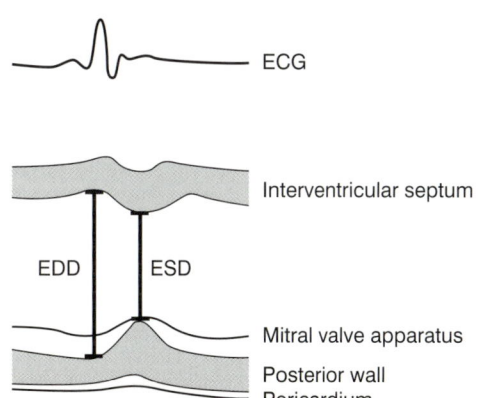

Figure 4.9 – Measurement of the end-systolic (ESD) and end diastolic (EDD) diameters.

Diastole is defined as the maximum diameter of the ventricle. This can be assessed directly from the M-mode trace, but some prefer to time diastole at the point of the R-wave on the ECG, which is electrically the latest point electrically before contraction begins. Systole is, more simply the smallest ventricular diameter; it cannot be defined electrically. The diameter should always be measured at the same point in time on the septum and posterior wall; that is, the line between caliper points must be exactly vertical.

Cardiac measurement software packages will convert these two measurements (ESD and EDD) into an ejection fraction and various other factors such as stroke volume and fractional shortening (these measurements are discussed in the Appendices). Various mathematical equations can be used to convert these two one-dimensional measurements into a three-dimensional ejection fraction. However, Many assumptions are made in the calculations and thus the results include errors. Certainly, the two diameters are accurate and can be quoted. There is currently much controversy about whether and/or when ejection fractions should be quoted. It is up to each department to decide upon which measurements and calculations are included in the report. If an accurate measurement cannot be made, for example if the left ventricle is oriented too anteriorly DO NOT make M-mode measurements. You can do the patient a disservice by quoting inaccurate measurements. Instead, if the endocardium can be clearly visualised, a measurement made directly from the image can be used as a guide of the size of the left ventricle. Measurements of both the ESD and EDD can be made in this way, but should be done so during the same cardiac cycle by using the cine loop.

The rules for left ventricular volume studies (especially of ejection fractions) are as follows:

- The M-mode line must be correctly placed: perpendicular to the long axis of the left ventricle, centrally across the maximum diameter of the left ventricle, and between the mitral leaflet tips and the tip of the papillary muscle.

- The endocardial boundaries must be clear and unambiguous on the trace (i.e. not 'Which line do you think is the septum?').

- There must be no regional wall motion abnormalities (to ensure this you must assess the ventricle fully in all views).

- The left ventricle must be normal in shape (i.e. not globular if very dilated or distorted by pathology).

If these rules are fulfilled then useful calculations can be made. If any rule is not fulfilled you will probably be calculating completely unreliable values.

The assessment of the left ventricular contractility is probably the most difficult technique to learn, as it is a highly subjective measure. It is only by performing many examinations that you can become confident in this area. When assessing contractility, remember that each view only shows the heart in two dimensions and that the overall contractility can only be estimated after observing the ventricle from every view in order to get a three-dimensional impression. First, mentally divide the left ventricle into segments. In our own practice we have divided the left ventricle into nine segments, as illustrated in Figure 4.10. Although the published literature suggests dividing the left ventricle into 16 segments, this requires both a lot of time and a lot of experience. The nine segment model covers the entirety of the left ventricle in a reasonable amount of detail, without being too complicated and time consuming, and is suitable for assessing the majority of routine departmental echocardiograms. More detailed studies of left ventricular function should be based on the 16 segment model, for example when performing stress echocardiographic studies (see Chapter 9).

The long axis parasternal view demonstrates the anterior septum, anterior free wall and the inferior wall. It is rare to be able to image the apex in this position. Observe

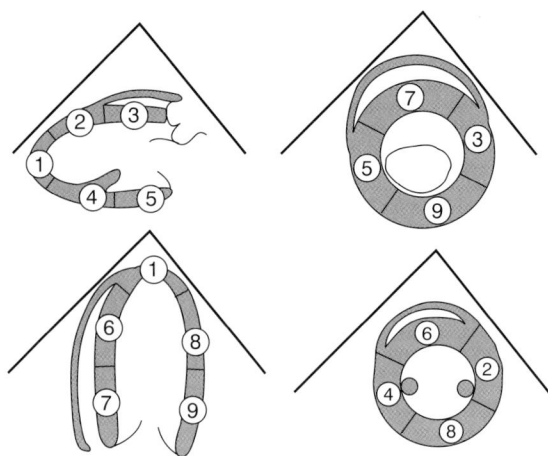

1 Apical region	–	generally LAD territory
2 Midanterior	–	generally LAD territory
3 Basal anterior	–	generally LAD territory
4 Midinferior region	–	generally RCA or Cx
5 Basal inferior region	–	generally RCA or CX
6 Midseptum	–	generally LAD
7 Basal septum	–	generally LAD +/– PDA
8 Midpostero-lateral free wall	–	generally Cx
9 Basal postero-lateral free wall	–	generally Cx

- LAD = Left anterior descending artery
- RCA = Right coronary artery
- Cx = Circumflex artery
- PDA = Posterior descending artery

Figure 4.10 – Nine segment model for assessing left ventricular function, as used at the Bristol Royal Infirmary. Each segment corresponds to the supply from a specific coronary artery, although individuals may differ in coronary anatomy. Cx, circumflex artery; LAD, left anterior descending artery; PDA, posterior descending artery; RCA, right coronary artery.

each section over several cardiac cycles to decide on the type of contractility – normal, hypokinetic (impaired but still contracting), akinetic (not contracting at all) or dyskinetic (moving abnormally, usually in the opposite direction). Hypokinetic contractility can be further divided into mild, moderate or severe hypokinesia. Do bear in mind that, when there are regional wall motion abnormalities, even if one segment is contracting better than the others, it may still have impaired contractility (but by contrast *appears* normal). When each of the regions has been assessed, consider the overall contractility. The M-mode trace can help demonstrating the amount of systolic excursion and also the amount of myocardial thickening in systole.

The thickness of the myocardium is measured at end-diastole to assess whether there is hypertrophy. It can be measured on the M-mode trace if the borders are clearly defined. However, it can be quite difficult to differentiate right ventricular trabeculations from the true edge of the myocardium. This is easier to determine on a frozen two-dimensional image where a measurement can be made perpendicular to the line of the septum. The inferior wall can be measured in the same way. Check that the papillary muscle is not included in the measurement.

PERICARDIUM

Increase the depth of penetration and check the pericardium behind the left ventricular inferior wall for fluid or any masses. A pleural effusion on the left side may also be detected on this projection (see Chapter 6). The descending aorta can sometimes be visualised behind the left atrium.

RIGHT VENTRICULAR OUTFLOW TRACT, PULMONARY VALVE AND MAIN PULMONARY ARTERY

By gently tilting the transducer cephalically, the right ventricular outflow tract and pulmonary valve come into view (Figure 4.11). If the window is good, the main pulmonary artery can also be seen. These structures are more typically evaluated in the short axis view, but there is no reason why colour flow and continuous wave Doppler should not be applied to the pulmonary valve on this projection.

RIGHT VENTRICLE, RIGHT ATRIUM AND TRICUSPID VALVE

Tilt the transducer back down through the left ventricle and continue slightly caudally. The tricuspid valve can now be visualised (Figure 4.12). The thickness of the right ventricular myocardium is often obscured by a reverberation artefact, but if it can be delineated clearly, it can be measured.

If the tricuspid valve can be visualised reasonably clearly, colour flow Doppler should be used to assess the amount of tricuspid regurgitation and a continuous wave Doppler beam placed through the valve to measure the peak pressure drop of any tricuspid regurgitation. The peak pressure drop of any tricuspid regurgitation should be measured in every possible view to ensure that the maximum velocity has been recorded.[2] The reason for this is that the maximum velocity will only be recorded when the flow is directly parallel with the continuous wave beam and, as the tricuspid valve is a large valve, regurgitant jets may occur in any direction through any of the three coaptation lines.

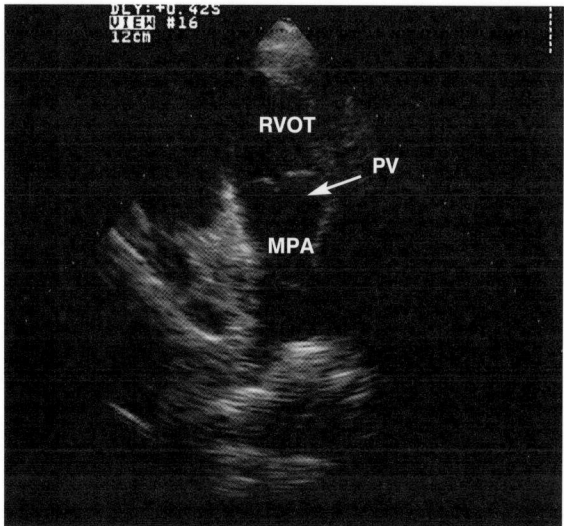

Figure 4.11 – Long axis projection of the right ventricular outflow tract, pulmonary valve and main pulmonary artery.

Parasternal short axis

When the best projection of a parasternal long axis has been achieved and studied, the transducer should be turned clockwise by 90° so that the orientation marker is pointing towards the left shoulder (Fig 4.1c). The patient's position remains the same. The transducer should be gently tilted cephalically. This brings the aor-

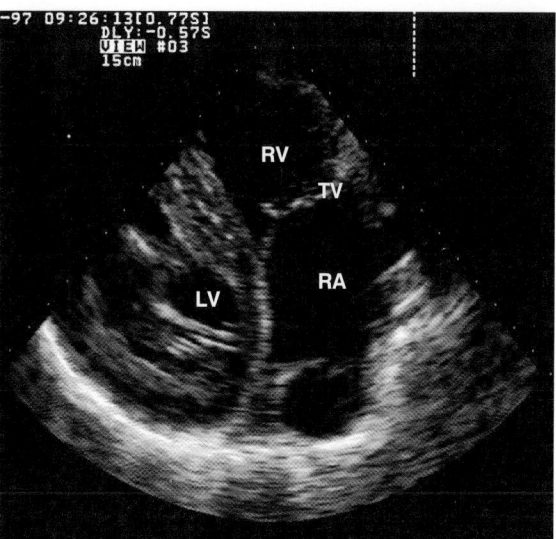

Figure 4.12 – Parasternal long axis view of the right ventricle, right atrium and tricuspid valve.

tic and pulmonary valves into view. It makes sense to start at the top and work systematically downwards (Figs. 4.13 and 4.14). The main pulmonary artery cannot always be visualised due to overlying lung. To reduce the amount of lung artefact the patient can be turned more onto their side. On this view the diameter of the pulmonary artery can be measured.

Continuous wave Doppler can be positioned through the pulmonary valve. The shape of the trace of both pulmonary valve forward flow and regurgitation is similar to that seen on traces of aortic valve flow. A forward velocity through the pulmonary valve greater than 2.5 m/s⁻¹ (peak pressure drop (PPD) 25 mmHg) may be due to either pulmonary stenosis or an increase in right-sided volume. To differentiate between the two, pulsed Doppler wave should be positioned just proxi-

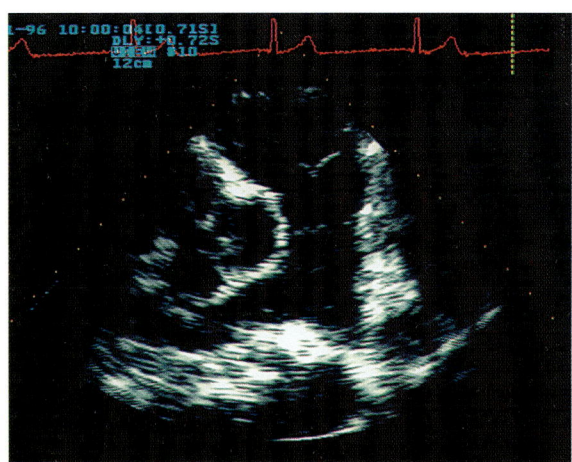

Figure 4.14 – Modified short axis view showing the pulmonary artery and a bifurcation. The right pulmonary artery lies behind the ascending aorta.

mal to the pulmonary valve and the peak forward velocity in this position measured. The following modified Bernoulli equation should be used to determine the cause of the increased velocity:

$$\text{PPD thru PV} = 4[\text{Peak forward velocity through PV (CW)}^2 - \text{Peak velocity proximal to PV (PW)}^2].$$

Note: Where PV denotes pulmonary valve, and CW and PW denote the continuous wave and pulsed wave Doppler measurements respectively. If the peak velocity recorded on the pulsed wave trace is 1.0 m/s⁻¹ or less, then it is negligible and the calculation does not need to be made.[3]

This projection is also the best position in which to measure the pulmonary acceleration time. A pulsed wave cursor should be positioned just beyond the pulmonary valve tips (Figures 4.15 and 4.16). The pulmonary acceleration time is the time it takes for pulmonary flow to reach its maximum velocity from the beginning of systole. This measurement does not quantify the degree of pulmonary hypertension as does the pressure drop of tricuspid regurgitation, but will indicate the presence or absence of clinically significant pulmonary hypertension in the absence of tricuspid regurgitation. The normal acceleration time in adults is above 100 m/s.[4]

The aortic valve is assessed on the short axis view for the number, thickness and mobility of leaflets. An M-mode through the aortic valve can also be performed in this projection. The colour flow box can be positioned

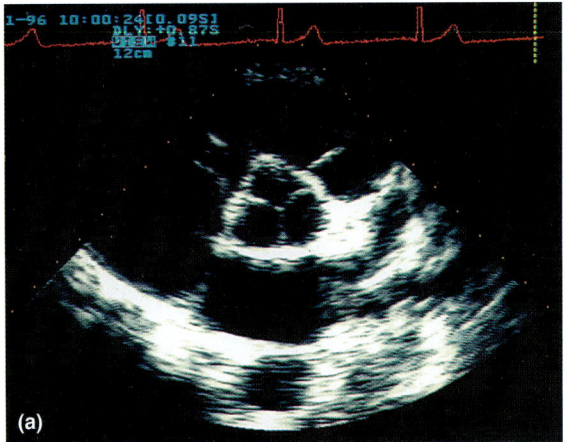

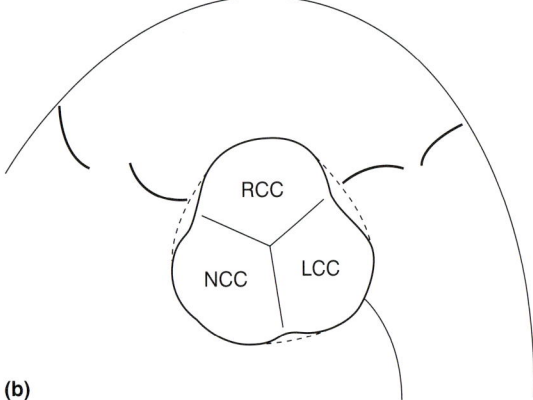

Figure 4.13 – (a) Short axis view of the aortic, pulmonary and tricuspid valves. (b) Sketch of the scan shown in (a), indicating the right coronary (RCC), left coronary (LCC) and non-coronary (NCC) cusps of the aortic valve.

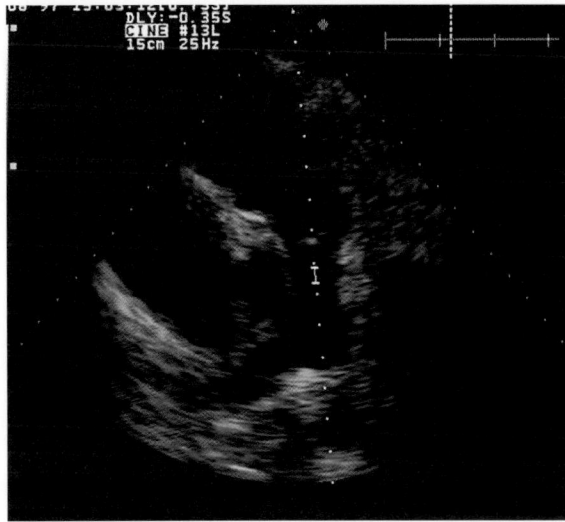

Figure 4.15 – Location of the pulsed wave sample volume for measuring the pulmonary acceleration time.

over the aortic valve to determine the site of origin of any regurgitation (e.g. centrally, between just two of the cusps, or through a perforation in a leaflet). At this same level the interatrial septum can be seen and assessed for any defect on both the 2D image and with colour flow.

Continue to angle the transducer down towards the apex, and the mitral and tricuspid valves come in to view. Colour flow Doppler should be applied to the tricuspid valve to look for the presence of any regurgitation. Continuous wave Doppler should then be

positioned through the regurgitant jet, if present, and the peak pressure drop recorded.

The mitral valve can now be studied. Planimetry of the orifice can be performed if stenosis is suspected. In this view, the commisures of the mitral valve can be visualised (Figure 4.17). It is important that the commisures are assessed for thickening and calcification if valvuloplasty of the mitral valve is being considered.

Colour flow can be applied to the mitral valve in this projection if the site of origin of mitral regurgitation is required (e.g. in cases of leaflet perforation).

Contractility of the myocardium at this level should also be assessed. By tilting the transducer very slightly towards the apex, the papillary muscles can be visualised (Figure 4.18). The contractility of the left ventricle should be assessed once more at this level. An M-mode measurement can also be made at this papillary muscle level. This can only be done accurately if the long axis view shows the left ventricle lying horizontally. As the beam is then angled further towards the apex, contractility can be assessed all the way down to the apex if possible. Tilting the transducer down towards the apex, there will come a position where rib will obscure the image. To overcome this, the transducer should be moved up the chest a couple of centimetres, which will allow for greater angulation towards the apex with less interference from the rib.

Apical four chamber view

Roll the patient slightly towards their back from the position used for the parasternal images. This allows

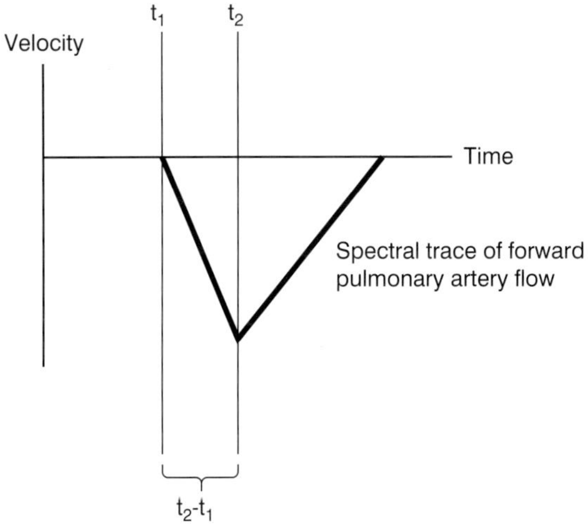

Figure 4.16 – Measurement of the pulmonary acceleration time.

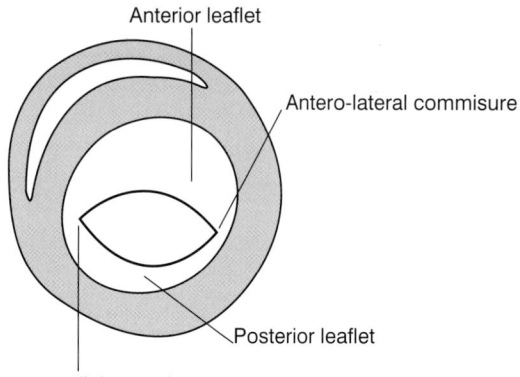

Figure 4.17 – Sketch of the short axis view of the mitral valve, showing the commisures.

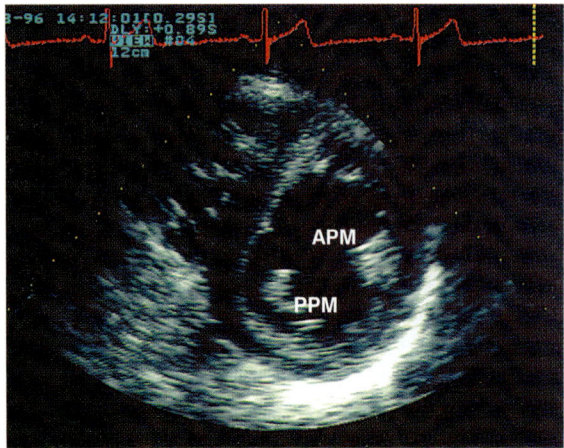

Figure 4.18 – Parasternal short axis view of the anterolateral (APM) and posteromedial (PPM) papillary muscles.

Obviously the position of the heart within the thorax varies from person to person. The transducer may need to be moved more centrally or more laterally. Occasionally the apex will be rib space or two higher or lower, and the transducer must be moved accordingly.

Probably the greatest difficulty in achieving a satisfactory four chamber view is to get a view of the heart at the correct angle within the sector. Although the two-dimensional appearance can be assessed equally well on the two images, Doppler studies will be suboptimal. To align the image of the heart more vertically, the transducer needs to be moved more around the patient's side. Imagine the heart as a central pivot point, and angle backwards towards it (Figures 4.19 and 4.20). Sitting the patient up (but still turned on their left) can sometimes give a better view of the heart. In addition, raising the patient's left arm behind their head can help to separate the ribs, giving more room to manoeuvre the transducer.

access to the lateral left ribs. The transducer is placed laterally between the sixth and seventh ribs over the apex of the heart. On a man, this is usually just to the left and below the left nipple (Fig 4.1d). On a woman, the transducer has to be positioned underneath the left breast, again towards the lateral side of the chest. Sometimes the breast tissue will have to be lifted by the examiner as the transducer is adjusted; image quality must not be compromised by embarrassment about moving the breast. The orientation of the transducer is towards the left shoulder, as for the parasternal short axis view.

LEFT VENTRICULAR CONTRACTILITY

The left ventricle is divided into the same segments described above for the parasternal views. Each segment should be studied individually and assessed for contractility (as described for the parasternal views). In broad terms the segments of the left ventricle displayed on the apical four chamber view are the septal, apical and lateral regions. The apex is not usually seen on the parasternal views so take a close look at it on the four chamber view. Take some time to consider the images in order to obtain an overall impression of the left ventricular function. Make sure you move the transducer

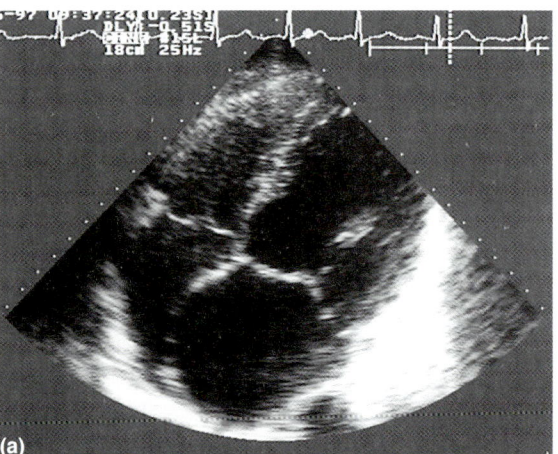

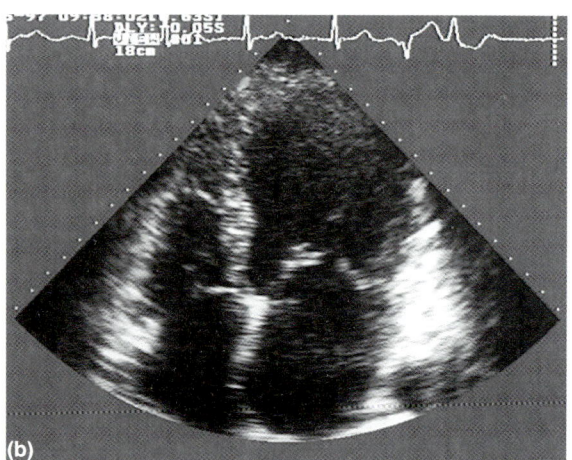

Figure 4.19 – (a) A slanted apical four chamber view not suitable for Doppler interrogation and (b) a vertical image obtained by moving the transducer laterally.

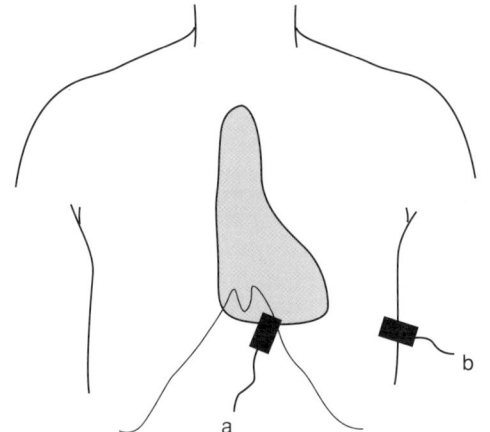

Figure 4.20 – To straighten an oblique four chamber view, (1) move the transducer further around the patient's left side and (2) tilt the transducer back towards the heart, i.e. move from position a to position b.

so that it sweeps through the entire left ventricle, so that no abnormalities, in particular masses, will be missed.

MITRAL VALVE

First assess the mitral valve and its annulus on the two-dimensional images. This will involve assessing the thickness and irregularity (masses) of the leaflets, the echogenicity (or brightness) of the leaflets and annulus, and the movement of the leaflets. Assess each leaflet during diastole. Restricted movement is due to stenosis or a low cardiac output (the M-mode trace from the parasternal view should highlight the difference), or possibly even an eccentric jet of aortic regurgitation over the anterior leaflet. Prolapse of either leaflet during systole should also be looked for.

Next, colour flow Doppler should be applied to the mitral valve. This will highlight the presence of any stenosis. If regurgitation is present it should be graded using the colour display, as described in Chapter 5.

The pulsed wave Doppler sample volume is then positioned at the mitral leaflet tips. The sample gate will need to be moved by very small amounts until a crisp spectral trace (with little or no spectral broadening) is obtained (Figure 4.21). The first peak in the biphasic flow is called the 'E wave' and corresponds to the passive filling of the left ventricle due to the pressure difference between the left atrium and left ventricle. The second peak is called the 'A wave' and corresponds to the contraction of the atrium to complete the filling of

the left ventricle. In most cases the E wave is a greater velocity than the A wave. However, in elderly people with impaired diastolic filling the A wave is larger than the E wave. Other causes of the reversal of the E/A ratio are complex, but tend to relate to the compliance of the left ventricle. The peak forward velocity should be measured on the E wave, even if the A wave is at a higher velocity.

The sweep speed of the spectral trace should now be increased and a *pressure half time measurement* performed to calculate the mitral valve area. The pressure half time of the mitral forward flow is the time it takes for the peak pressure drop to reach half its value. It is independent of both mitral regurgitation and the heart rate.[5] In the majority of patients, the pressure half time is directly related to the mitral valve area (MVA):

$$\text{MVA (cm}^2) = 220/\text{pressure half time (ms)}$$

That is, the longer the pressure half time, the smaller the mitral valve area.

Because the spectral trace plots the *velocity* of the blood flow rather than the *pressure drop*, determination of the pressure half time is not as straightforward as initially may be expected. When a spectral curve is inspected, it is easy to imagine that half the pressure difference is represented by a point half the distance from the baseline. This is not, of course, correct; the spectral trace is proportional to velocity, but (according to the Bernoulli

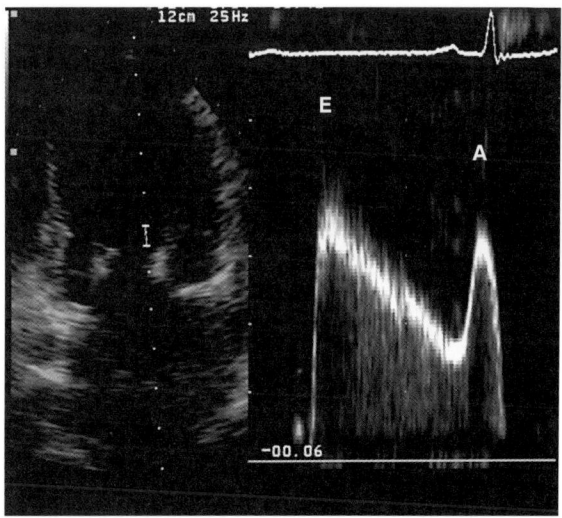

Figure 4.21 – The position of the pulsed wave Doppler sample volume at the tips of the leaflets of the mitral valve and the corresponding spectral trace. This patient has mild mitral stenosis.

principle) the pressure drop is proportional to the square of the velocity. Thus the distance on the trace should be divided by the square root of 2 to determine the point at which the pressure drop is half (Figure 4.22).

In practice, the first part of the deceleration curve should be measured. In the majority of cases the rate of deceleration remains constant. However, in some cases the rate is non-linear, and in such situations accurate placement of the measuring cursors will make a marked difference in the result. With careful technique it is often possible, to improve a non-linear trace to obtain a linear curve. If measurements are taken from a non-linear curve, use the first third of the slope only and be aware that the results may be less accurate.

The pressure half time measurement is always performed on the E wave of the spectral trace. Patients in atrial fibrillation do not have an A wave and so the pressure half time measurement can easily be measured (this is extremely useful, as most patients with mitral stenosis are in atrial fibrillation). For patients in sinus rhythm the pressure half time should be measured over three separate heart cycles and the average value quoted. Patients in atrial fibrillation have irregular heart cycle lengths; the pressure half time should be measured on five different waveforms and a range of pressure half times for the patient quoted.

The above equation can only be used to calculate the mitral valve area of native mitral valves. The area of a prosthetic valve cannot be estimated accurately using this equation. Similarly, areas calculated using pressure half time values measured immediately after valvuloplasty have also been shown to be inaccurate.[6]

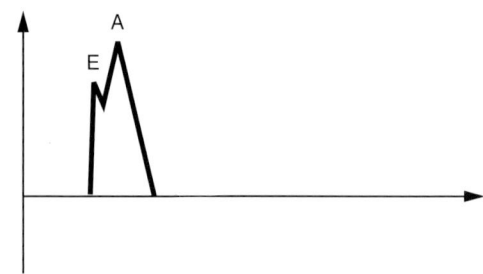

Figure 4.23 – Sketch of a short E wave.

Difficulties arise when the E wave is too short to make an accurate measurement of the pressure half time, and in such cases (e.g. in patients with a rapid heart rate) no such measurement should be made (Figure 4.23). The E-wave may be lengthened by increasing the sweep speed. However, if this is done caution should be exercised so that there is no confusion with atrial fibrillation and the slope of the A wave is mistakenly measured instead. Another problem occurs where significant aortic regurgitation is present. In cases where a strong localised jet of aortic regurgitation is directed onto the anterior mitral leaflet the pressure half time can be prolonged. In such cases, the mitral valve area calculated from the pressure half time tends to be overestimated and should not be quoted.[3]

If a clear spectral trace of forward mitral flow is difficult to obtain using pulsed wave Doppler interrogation, continuous wave Doppler interrogation can be used, ensuring that the beam is positioned through the site of maximum flow.

Continuous wave Doppler should be positioned through the mitral valve. Not only will this highlight any mitral regurgitation, but it should also bring to your attention any flow abnormalities within the left ventricular cavity (e.g. an intracavity gradient).

LEFT ATRIUM

The left atrium is now studied. First, check its size. The most accurate measurement of the atrium is made on the apical four chamber view when two dimensions are measured: one in a transverse plane and one superoinferiorly. An image should be frozen where the left atrial size is maximised to avoid underestimation.[7] The left atrium will be located in a slightly different position in every individual. When measuring the superoinferior plane, ensure that the cursor is placed at the line of the annulus of the mitral valve and not at the leaflets (Figure 4.24).

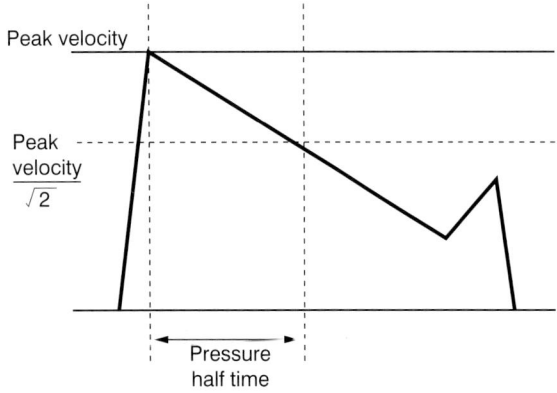

Figure 4.22 – Measurement of the pressure half time on the spectral trace of forward mitral flow.

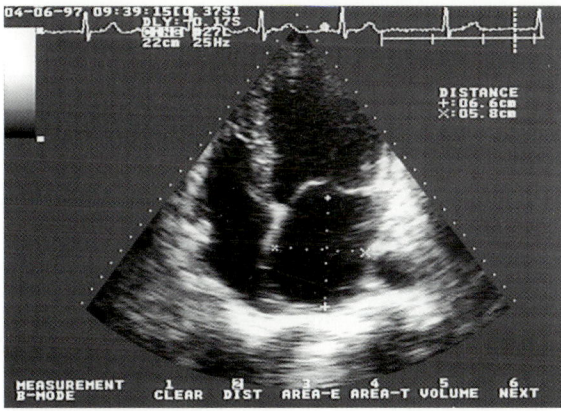

Figure 4.24 – Measurement of the left atrium. Note that the callipers are placed at the line of the annulus, not at the leaflet tips.

Masses (e.g. thrombus or tumour) need to be excluded. The pulmonary veins can be identified in the majority of patients. Inflow from the veins can usually be demonstrated on colour flow Doppler imaging. The left atrial appendage can only very occasionally be identified (Figure 4.25).

The interatrial septum can be studied for defects. However, it should be borne in mind that the four chamber view is not ideal for checking for such defects. The reasons for this are:

- the best image of a structure is obtained when the beam is perpendicular to it

- the septum thins at the foramen ovale and, because of the lateral resolution of the system, this may lead to a false-positive result

- attenuation of the beam at a distance from the transducer

- colour flow is best when the beam is parallel to the direction of flow.

RIGHT VENTRICLE

The right ventricle can now be assessed. Contractility can be observed to be normal or impaired; unlike the left ventricle, the right ventricle is not divided into segments. Search for any masses within the right ventricle. Do not confuse the moderator band at the apex with thrombus (Figure 4.26). The right ventricle can be highly trabeculated and trabeculations should also not be confused with thrombus. The diameter of the right ventricle is measured across the base, just beyond the tricuspid leaflets (Figure 4.27). This is the easiest site in which to measure the diameter and measurements are reproducible in serial studies. Ensure that the image frozen is at the end diastole point, and take care to measure between the inside edges of the endocardium. Right ventricular wall thickness should not be measured on this view. The colour flow box can be positioned over the right ventricle to include the length of the septum to highlight the presence of a ventricular septal defect.

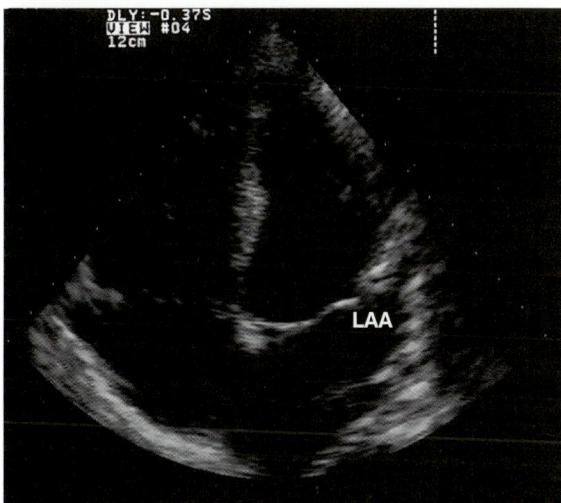

Figure 4.25 – Apical four chamber view of the left atrial appendage, LAA.

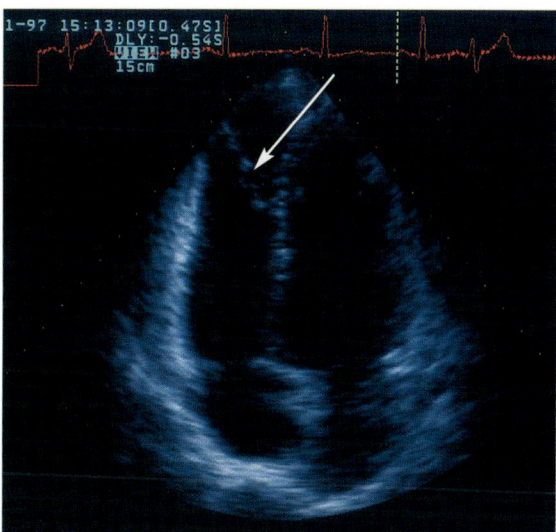

Figure 4.26 – Image of the moderator band at the apex of the right ventricle (arrow).

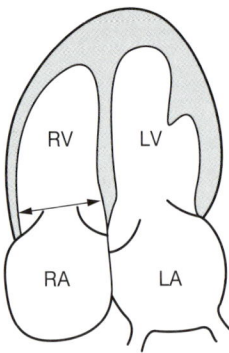

Figure 4.27 – Measurement of the diameter of the right ventricle (RV) on the apical four chamber image. LA, left atrium, LV, left ventricle; RA, right atrium.

TRICUSPID VALVE

The tricuspid valve is first assessed for its position, thickness and movement. When its position is compared with that of the mitral valve, the tricuspid annulus should be very slightly offset towards the apex. If it is much further towards the apex or lower than the mitral valve, congenital heart disease should be suspected (see Chapter 7). If there is any indication that the tricuspid valve is restricted, a pulsed wave Doppler recording of the forward flow will need to be obtained and a pressure half time calculated as for the mitral valve. Colour flow over the tricuspid valve will help to highlight fast moving jets.

Due to poorer imaging of the right heart structures, small amounts of tricuspid regurgitation are not always obvious on colour flow images. A careful search using continuous wave Doppler is important in order not to miss small jets. The pressure drop of tricuspid regurgitation is an important measurement in estimating pulmonary pressures. We suggest that a pressure drop of 25 mmHg or less is considered normal. Remember that tricuspid regurgitation and pulmonary hypertension are two completely separate items, and a patient with severe pulmonary hypertension may not have any tricuspid regurgitation.

RIGHT ATRIUM

The right atrium is measured in the same way as the left atrium. It should be assessed for the presence of any masses. The Eustachian valve which is located where the inferior vena cava (IVC) joins the right atrium, is

prominent in some people and may appear as a mass (Figure 4.28). Be careful not to identify this as thrombus. Flow from the IVC into the right atrium can be demonstrated in the majority of people; it is seen when the beam is angled towards the diaphragm. The superior vena cava (SVC) cannot be visualised in this view.

AORTIC VALVE

From the apical four chamber view the transducer is angled slightly anteriorly to obtain a section through the left ventricular outflow tract and the aortic valve. This is commonly called the five chamber view. The thickness and movement of the aortic leaflets should not be assessed from this view; it is easy to underestimate the movement as the annulus (rather than the leaflets) is quite prominent in this view and mimics immobile leaflets. The colour flow Doppler region should be positioned over the outflow tract to observe and quantify any aortic regurgitation.

When calculating the cardiac output or using the continuity equation, the pulsed wave Doppler sample volume is placed just on the ventricular side of the aortic valve. If the sample volume is not directly beside the leaflets it can be difficult to obtain a spectral trace and if it impinges on the orifice of the valve an inaccurate velocity will be recorded. It is important to be sure that the Doppler beam is well aligned with the outflow tract if results are to be accurate (Figure 4.29).

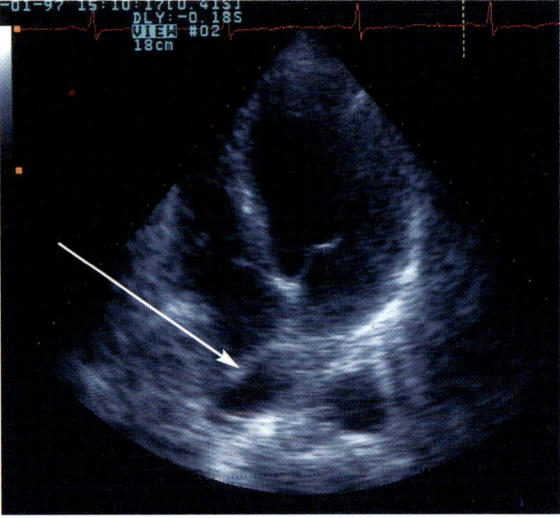

Figure 4.28 – Apical four chamber view showing the Eustachian valve at the base of the right atrium where it joins the inferior vena cava (arrow).

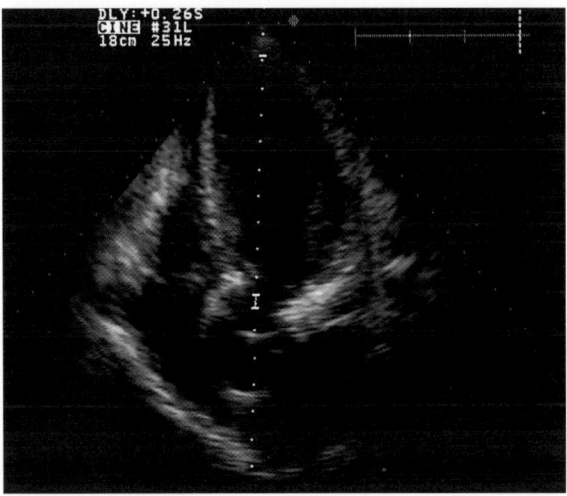

Figure 4.29 – Apical five chamber view showing the position of the pulsed wave Doppler sample volume in the left ventricular outflow tract for calculation of the cardiac output or using the continuity equation.

Continuous wave Doppler is used to ascertain the presence of stenosis. Although thin mobile leaflets may be demonstrated on the parasternal view, do not disregard the possibility of sub- or supravalvular stenosis, which may not be visible on imaging. In young patients, the valve opening and ascending aorta are vertical; in line with the long axis of the left ventricle. As a person ages, the aorta is seen to lie more horizontally (on the apical four chamber view). It is important that good alignment is achieved between the continuous wave beam and the line of the ascending aorta (in cases of severe stenosis flow may be in any direction, and therefore this position will not always be in line with the direction of flow). To achieve good alignment of the continuous wave beam with the aorta (i.e. to ensure that the Doppler trace truly reflects flow), the transducer will need to be moved further around the patient's left side to obtain an oblique apical five chamber view. This will give an image of the heart at an angle, but will give better alignment of the beam and the aorta (Figure 4.30).

A good spectral trace is identified by valve clicks on either side of the systolic flow. In a normally contracting ventricle, plug flow in the proximal ascending aorta is indicated by the outside edge of the trace being an intense white and the central part being almost echo free (Figure 4.31). The velocity of flow will increase in cases of stenosis, increased cardiac output and aortic regurgitation; it will decrease if the left ventricular function is poor.

PULMONARY VALVE

Very occasionally, when the transducer is tilted anteriorly just a fraction more from the apical five chamber view, the right ventricular outflow tract and pulmonary valve can be identified. It is wise to be aware of this, as pulmonary regurgitation on colour flow Doppler can mimic a ventricular septal defect (VSD).

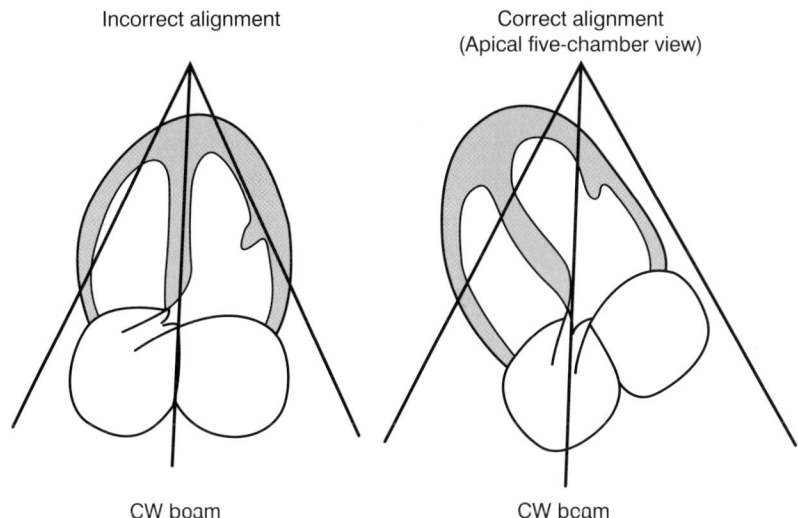

Incorrect alignment   Correct alignment (Apical five-chamber view)

CW beam   CW beam

Figure 4.30 – Alignment of the continuous wave (CW) beam with the aorta of an elderly patient.

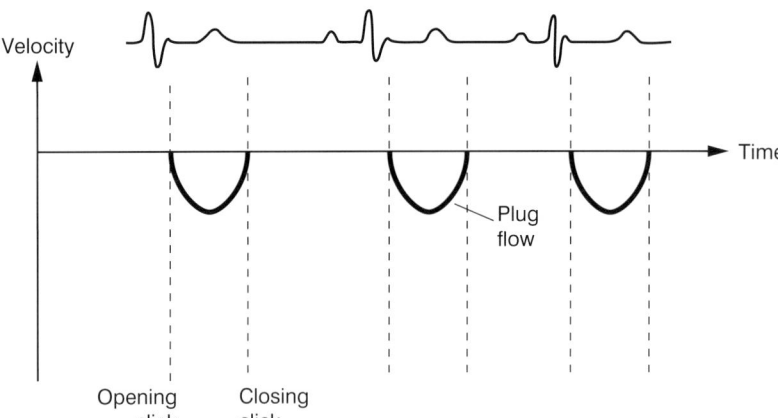

Figure 4.31 – A sketch of a good aortic valve spectral trace, showing plug flow. The valve clicks on opening and closing, and this is displayed as very thin faint lines extending across the full velocity range.

Angling the transducer posteriorly will bring the inferior wall into view. In the majority of patients, the coronary sinus can be visualised running horizontally behind the left atrium (Figure 4.32). In the same projection, the descending aorta may be visualised.

Apical long axis

By turning the transducer about 120°, so that it is oriented towards the right shoulder, the apical long axis can be viewed (Figure 4.33). This section through the heart is identical to the parasternal long axis section, but the image is rotated clockwise by almost 90°, with the transducer placed over the apex rather than over the right ventricle. If the patient has no parasternal window this view can be used to establish the amount of aortic valve opening. Colour flow Doppler applied to both the aortic and mitral valves will now give a three-dimensional impression of the degree of any regurgitation. It also gives a view at a different angle through the aortic valve, which can be used to find the highest peak forward velocity using continuous wave Doppler beam if stenosis is present.

Apical two chamber view

If the transducer is rotated 60°–80° from the apical four chamber view, the apical two chamber view is obtained

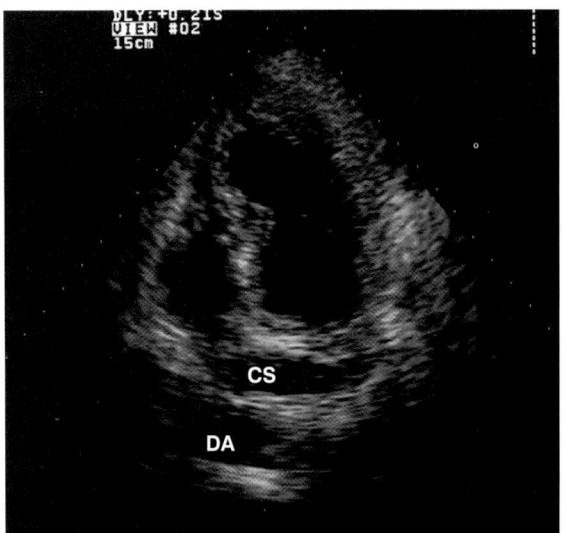

Figure 4.32 – Apical four chamber view, obtained with the transducer angled posteriorly, of the coronary sinus, CS, and descending thoracic aorta, DA. In this patient the coronary sinus is slightly more dilated than normal.

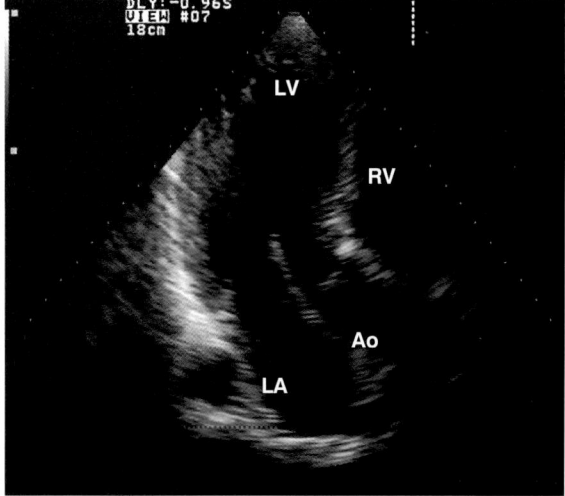

Figure 4.33 – An apical long axis view.

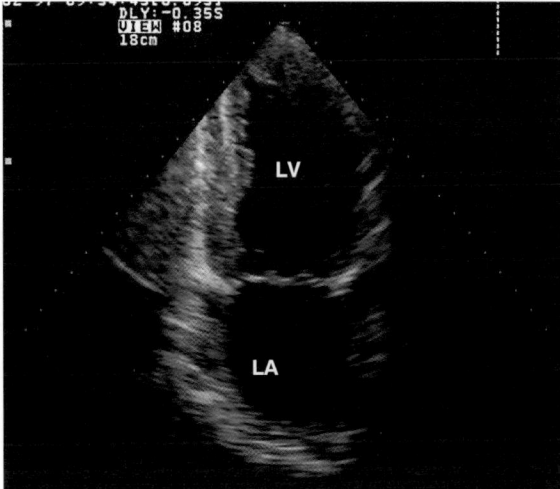

Figure 4.34 – An apical two chamber view.

It is often difficult for inexperienced echocardiographers to distinguish between the closely related long axis plane and the 'two chamber' plane. These two planes are similar, but have a slightly different orientation, the long axis view not being truly perpendicular to the four chamber plane. The long axis plane includes the aortic valve, but the two chamber plane does not (Figure 4.35). Using either of these two long axis views, the transducer can be angled medially to give a further view of the right ventricle, tricuspid valve and right atrium.

Subcostal view

The patient should be laid flat on his or her back for this view. Best results are achieved when the patient's legs are laid flat and their stomach (anterior abdominal) muscles relaxed. The transducer is placed centrally on the abdomen just below the ribs in a transverse position, orientated to the patient's left. It is necessary to push firmly on the abdomen so that as much anterior angulation as possible can be gained (Figure 4.1e). When the beating heart can be recognised, small movements towards the left of the patient and clockwise rotation will bring a four chamber view into the sector.

(Figure 4.34). The apical two chamber view is almost at right angles to the apical four chamber view and is used to assess contractility of the anterior and inferior regions of the left ventricle.

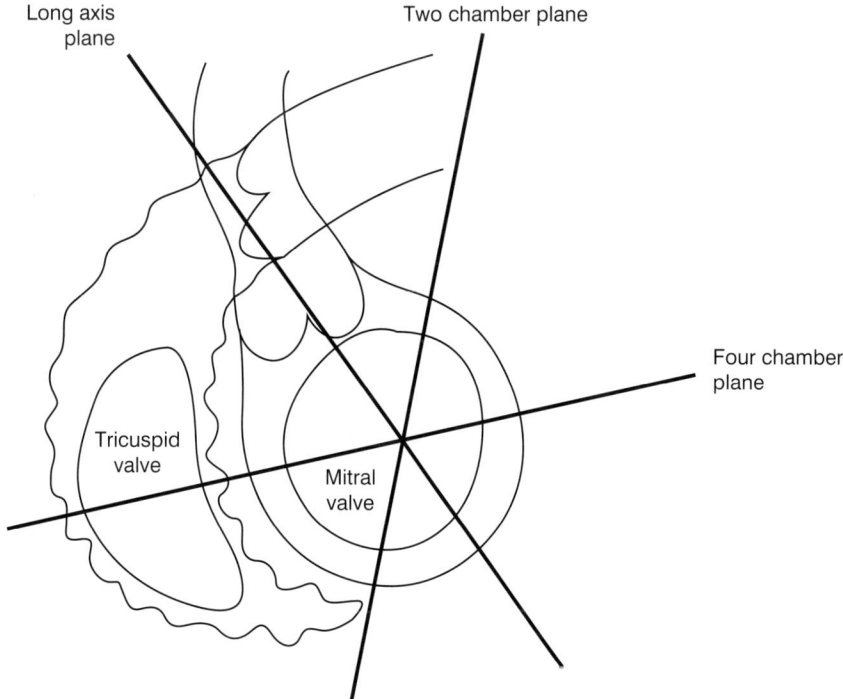

Figure 4.35 – The projections of the long axis view and the two chamber view.

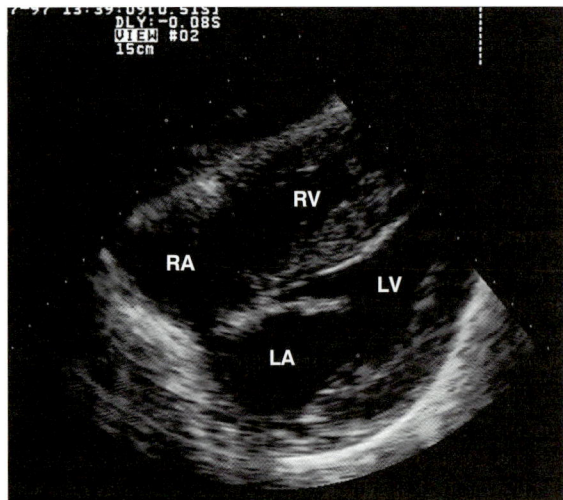

Figure 4.36 – Subcostal four chamber view in a patient with a dilated left atrium. Note that the liver lies between the transducer and the right ventricle.

The anatomy demonstrated in this view (Figure 4.36) is very similar to that seen in the apical four chamber view. Suspended deep inspiration can help to bring the heart closer to the transducer. Sometimes half a breath in is better than a full breath in, as the latter may tense the abdomen too much to allow the transducer to be pushed a little under the xiphisternum.

The right atrium and ventricle are closest to the transducer and so appear more anteriorly within the imaging sector. This view is particularly good for observing pericardial effusions, right-sided pathology and septal defects. It is also very useful if no other echo window on the chest can be found. Because the free wall of the right ventricle is almost at right angles to the beam, this view is also good for measuring wall thickness.

A colour flow Doppler image should be obtained of the interventricular septum in order to exclude any possible VSD. Because the ventricular septum is large, as the right ventricle wraps around the left, the beam will need to be swept from the very anterior aspect through to the most posterior region in order to ensure that the entire septum has been studied. A similar procedure should be performed with a continuous wave Doppler beam.

Flow through an atrial septal defect will be of low velocity and not easily demonstrated on spectral Doppler. Colour flow should be placed over the interatrial septum to exclude a septal defect in this region.

If the transducer is angled more anteriorly, the aortic valve will come into view. In cases of aortic stenosis, continuous wave Doppler should be applied to the aortic valve in this view. In some cases further anterior angulation will bring the right ventricular outflow tract and the pulmonary valve into view (Figure 4.37).

SUBCOSTAL SHORT AXIS

By turning the transducer by 90º, so that it is oriented towards the patient's head, a view of the short axis plane through the cardiac chambers is obtained. Perhaps the most useful aspect of this view is that the IVC can be seen entering the right atrium (Figure 4.38). The IVC can be seen to change diameter with respiration. This view is useful when looking for right-sided thrombus to see if the IVC is involved. Colour flow and pulsed wave Doppler studies can also be used here to look for reversal of flow in the IVC in cases of significant tricuspid regurgitation.

If the transducer is moved slightly to the patient's left, a short axis view of the right and left ventricles can be obtained. By angling the transducer slightly towards the patient's abdomen, the abdominal aorta can be visualised (Figure 4.39). The aorta lies directly over the spine and can be seen to pulsate (except when the walls are calcified). As the aorta passes through the diaphragm its maximum normal diameter is 3.0 cm. Just distal to this, to the level of the umbilicus where it divides, the maximum normal diameter is 2.5 cm.

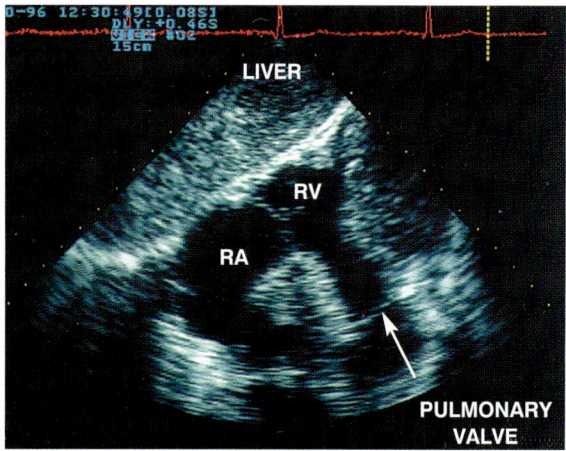

Figure 4.37 – Image obtained with very anterior angulation of the transducer in the subcostal position, showing the right ventricular outflow tract and the right ventricle. Note the liver.

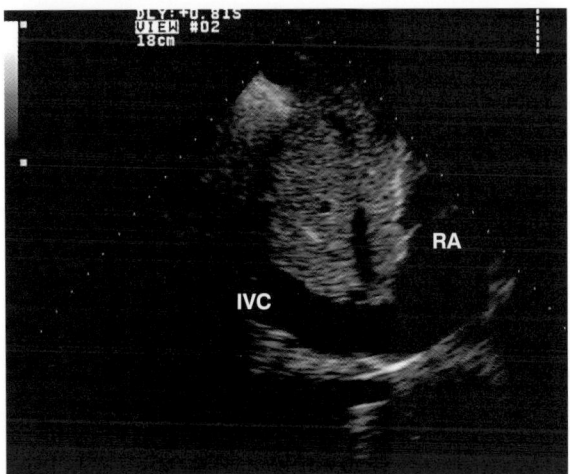

Figure 4.38 – Longitudinal section through the upper abdomen, showing the inferior vena cava entering the right atrium.

Suprasternal view

The arch of the aorta and proximal descending aorta can be seen with the transducer placed in the suprasternal notch. In patients with a particularly good window at this site, those with a dilated ascending aorta and in children, the ascending aorta can also be visualised. The patient will need to lie completely flat with their neck extended. It may be helpful to put a pillow under the shoulders so

the head can drop right back. However, do not stretch the neck so far back that the skin is pulled too taut over the sternal notch. There needs to be a bit of 'give' in the soft tissues here to be able to press the transducer gently into the notch. Do not press too firmly – this is not a comfortable window for the patient. The usual orientation (although this will vary between patients) is towards the left ear, so that the line of the scan plane is parallel with the angle of the notch (see Figure 4.1f). The transducer now needs to be tilted slowly caudally until the aortic arch is visualised. Keeping the arch in the field of view, the transducer should be rotated slowly clockwise and anticlockwise and tilted up and down until the descending aorta is visualised.

Blood flow in the descending aorta is measured using the suprasternal view. A pulsed wave Doppler sample volume can be placed in the descending aorta just distal to the head and neck vessels in order to quantify the degree of aortic regurgitation (Figure 4.40 and Chapter 5). Continuous wave Doppler studies can be used to diagnose coarctation (see Chapter 7).

The right pulmonary artery can sometimes be visualised passing under the arch of the aorta. Gently angling the transducer to the right should bring the ascending aorta into view (if it can be found).

Right parasternal view

The right parasternal view is not a commonly used window. It is used for patients with dextrocardia (heart

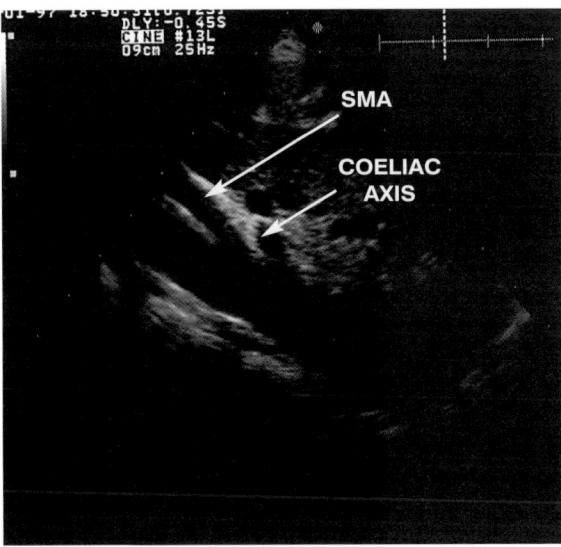

Figure 4.39 – Longitudinal section through the proximal abdominal aorta. Note the coeliac axis and the superior mesenteric artery (SMA).

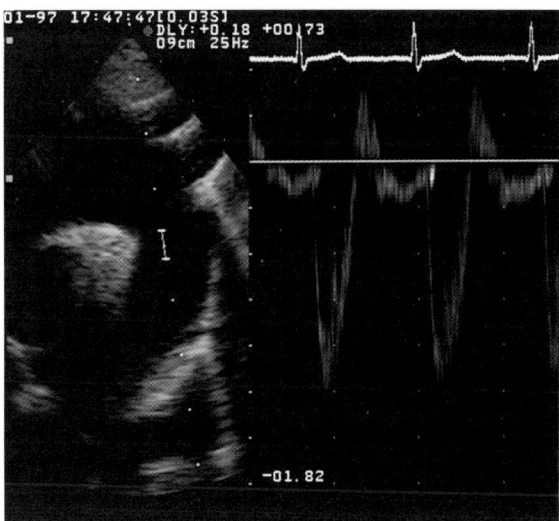

Figure 4.40 – Suprasternal view, with the pulsed wave Doppler sample volume positioned to measure the flow in the descending aorta, and the associated spectral trace.

on the right) or any case when the heart is displaced towards the right side of the chest, e.g. patients with a pneumonectomy). It is often unrecognised that the right parasternal view is a good window for examining the ascending aorta in cases of pathological enlargement (e.g. aneurysm or suspected dissection). It is also used to measure the pressure drop across an aortic valve in cases of aortic stenosis with an independent continuous wave Doppler transducer.

The patient needs to turn completely onto their right side, facing the operator. The bed should remain almost flat. The transducer is placed between the second and third (or third and fourth) ribs and angled centrally and caudally towards the heart (see Figure 4.1a)

Lungs and pleura

Echocardiographers are sometimes asked to comment on the presence, or absence, of pleural effusions. When a patient lies flat on his or her back, or sits upright, any fluid typically collects at the base of the lungs. Normal lung will not give an image, due to amount of reflection of the ultrasound at its surface. Fluid at the base of the lungs, however, will show up as an echo-free area just above the diaphragm.

Place the transducer halfway back on the patient's side at the level of the diaphragm (the transducer is placed in similar positions for both the left and the right diaphragm). Obviously this level differs between patients and also in one patient with respiration, but as a general rule is higher in the chest than you would expect and further towards the spine (Figure 4.41). It may be helpful to raise the patient's arm to rest over his or her head.

The diaphragm is a large smooth surface that reflects ultrasound well and hence can be seen as a bright white curved line (Figure 4.42). The transducer can be moved posteriorly and anteriorly to check along the length of the diaphragm. On the right side of the abdomen the liver can be seen below the diaphragm and is a good indicator of the level of the diaphragm. The spleen lies below the diaphragm on the left side of the abdomen and is often small and difficult to visualise. The presence of a left pleural effusion will enable the spleen to be visualised more clearly.

Do not attempt to diagnose extracardiac abnormalities unless you are trained and experienced in this area. It is too easy to make mistakes in unfamiliar territory. Your radiology department will have someone skilled in interpreting extracardiac findings, who can help in such cases.

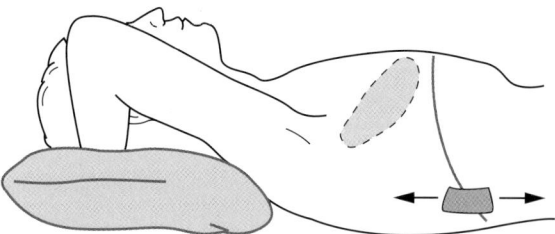

Figure 4.41 – The position of the transducer on the lateral chest wall to scan the base of the lungs and look for pleural effusion.

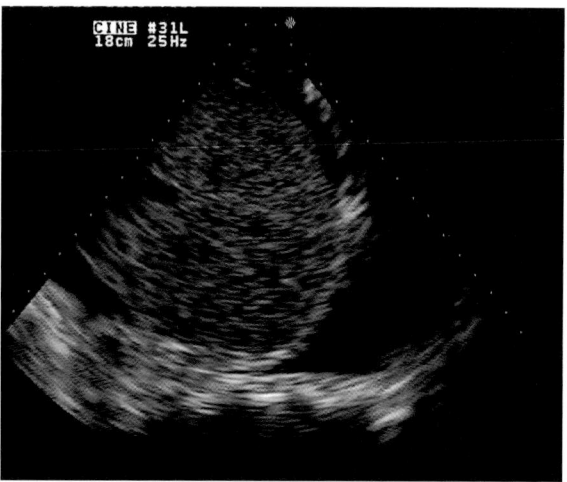

Figure 4.42 – Image showing a right pleural effusion. Note the smooth, curved diaphragm, with the liver lying inferiorly.

Tables of normal measurements

Table 4.2 – Ranges of the normal diameters of the cardiac chambers and great vessels in adults

Chamber/artery	Diameter	Range (cm)
Left ventricle	EDD	4.8 ± 0.4
	ESD[8]	3.0 ± 0.4
Right ventricle	Four chamber at base[9]	1.5 – 3.0
Left ventricular wall thickness	M-mode or two-dimensional[10]	0.6 – 1.1
Right ventricular wall thickness	Parasternal or subcostal[9]	0.2 – 0.7
Left atrium	M-mode parasternal	2.4 – 3.8
	Four chamber:	
	Mediolateral	2.9 – 4.4
	Superoinferior	3.3 – 5.2
	Area[11]	10.2 – 17.8 cm²
Right atrium	Four chamber:	3.1 – 4.5
	Mediolateral	3.4 – 4.9
	Superoinferior	11.3 – 16.7 cm²
	Area[11]	
Aorta	Aortic annulus	1.6 – 2.6
	Sinus of valsalva	2.4 – 3.9
	Ascending aorta	2.2 – 3.4
	Aortic arch[11]	2.2 – 2.7
	Proximal abdominal (diaphragm)	<3.0
Main pulmonary artery	Just distal to pulmonary valve[11]	1.5 – 2.5

Table 4.3 – Left ventricular measurements in normal children*.

Age (years)	EDD (cm)	ESD (cm)	End diastolic wall thickness (cm)
1.5 – 3	3.2 ± 0.2	2.2 ± 0.1	0.4 ± 0.1
3 – 5	3.3 ± 0.2	2.2 ± 0.2	0.5 ± 0.1
5 – 7	3.6 ± 0.3	2.4 ± 0.3	0.5 ± 0.1
7 – 9	3.9 ± 0.3	2.6 ± 0.3	0.6 ± 0.1
9 – 11	4.2 ± 0.4	2.8 ± 0.3	0.6 ± 0.1
11 – 13	4.2 ± 0.3	2.8 ± 0.3	0.6 ± 0.1

* Reproduced with permission from Sutton *et al*[12]

Table 4.4 – Ranges of normal peak blood flow velocities through the cardiac valves in adults and children

Valve	Velocity range (m/s)
Aortic	
Adults	1.0 – 1.7
Children[3]	1.2 – 1.8
Mitral	
Adults	0.6 – 1.3
Children[3]	0.8 – 1.3
Tricuspid	
Adults	0.3 – 0.7
Children[3]	0.5 – 0.8
Pulmonary	
Adults[3]	0.6 – 0.9

References

1. Schabelman S, Schiller NB, Silverman NH, Potts TA. Left atrial estimation by two-dimensional echocardiography. *Catheterisation Cardiovasc Diagnosis* 1981; **7**(2): 165–178.

2. Abramson SV, Burke JB, Pauletto FJ, Kelly JJ. Use of multiple views in the echocardographic assessment of pulmonary artery systolic pressure. *J Am Soc Echocardiog* 1995; **8**(1): 55–60.

3. Hatle L, Angelsen B. *Doppler Ultrasound in Cardiology*, 2nd edn. Lea & Febiger, Philadelphia, 1985.

4. Wilde P (Ed). *Cardiac Ultrasound*. Churchill Livingstone, Edinburgh, 1993.

5. Bryg RJ, Williams GA, Labortiz AJ *et al*. Effect of atrial fibrillation and mitral regurgitation on calculated mitral valve area in mitral stenosis. *Am J Cardiol* 1986; **57**: 634–638.

6. Reid CL, McKay CR, Chandrartna PAN *et al*. Mechanisms of increase in mitral valve area and influence of anatomic features in double-balloon, catheter balloon valvuloplasty in adults with rheumatic mitral stenosis: a Doppler and two-dimensional echocardiographic study. *Circulation*. 1987; **76**: 628–636.

7. Kircher B, Abbott JA, Pau S *et al*. Left atrial volume determination by biplane two-dimensional echocardiography: validation by cine computed tomography. *Am Heart J* 1991; **1213**(1): 864–871.

8. St John Sutton M, Reichek N, Lovett J, Kastor JA, Giuliani ER. Effects of age, body size and blood pressure on the normal human left ventricle. *Circulation* 1980; **62**(Suppl III): 305.

9. Foale R, Nihoyannopoulos P, McKenna W *et al*. Echocardiographic measurement of the normal adult right ventricle. *Br Heart J* 1986. **56**: 33–34.

10. Feigenbaum H. *Echocardiography* 3rd edn. Lea & Febiger, Philadelphia, 1981.

11. Weyman AE. *Cross-sectional Echocardiography*. Lea & Febiger, Philadelphia, 1982

12. St John Sutton MG, Marier DL, Oldershaw PJ, Sacchetti R, Gibson DG. Effect of age related changes in chamber size, wall thickness and heart rate on left ventricular function in normal children. *Br Heart J* 1982; **48**: 342–351.

5

ACQUIRED VALVE DISEASE

Stenosis
Regurgitation
Mitral valve disease
Aortic valve disease
Tricuspid valve disease
Pulmonary valve disease
Pulmonary hypertension
Infective andocarditis
Prosthetic valves

Stenosis

In the past, the most common cause of valvular stenosis was a medical history of rheumatic fever. This disease has now been almost eradicated from the Western world, and is seen only in the middle aged or elderly or in immigrants. It is most frequently seen in the mitral valve and secondly in the aortic valve (often, both valves are affected) but can also be seen, albeit very rarely, in the tricuspid and pulmonary valves. Today, valve degeneration (especially of a bicuspid aortic valve) has overtaken rheumatic disease as the main cause of stenosis. Congenital heart disease is also a major contributor to valve stenosis (see Chapter 7).

In all cases of stenosis the orifice area of the valve is restricted. In the majority of cases, the reduction in area will be due to thickened leaflets, the opening of which is thus restricted. The reduction in area of the open valve will increase the forward velocity of the blood through the valve (imagine placing your thumb over the end of a hose; the velocity of the water increases, it becomes turbulent and travels further).

Quantifying stenosis is a complex procedure and is different for each valve. Here, we consider each valve in turn, and explain the different methods used.

Regurgitation

Regurgitation (sometimes called insufficiency or incompetence) through a closed valve may be due to a number of causes:

- A trivial amount of regurgitation is often seen just as the leaflets are closing, and this is normal.

- Functional regurgitation will occur if the annulus of a valve is stretched such that the leaflets have difficulty in coapting (coming together). This occurs in cases of ventricular, aortic root or pulmonary artery dilatation.

- Prolapse of a leaflet is a condition where the closed leaflets of a valve fall back further than normal, usually behind the level of the valve ring at which the leaflets are hinged. This can be due to abnormally floppy valve tissue, elongated chordae, or disruption of the leaflet itself. This typically results in imperfect coaptation, and often in an eccentric jet of regurgitation. Prolapse is most commonly associated with regurgitation, but not always.

- Regurgitation may also be due to degeneration of the valve leaflets, and is commonly seen in the elderly.

- Infective endocarditis can also make the valve leaflets incompetent, and in some cases can perforate the leaflet.

- A flail leaflet occurs when there are ruptured chordae, affecting the mitral or tricuspid valves, resulting in eccentric regurgitation. In this case, unrestrained by chordae, the free edge of the leaflet itself flips back into the atrium.

- Regurgitation can associated with balloon valvuloplasty or previous surgical valvotomy, and needs to be assessed both before and after such procedures.

With experience, the audio signal from the Doppler trace can help to identify regurgitation.

Quantifying regurgitation is particularly difficult and presents a major clinical and echocardiographic challenge. One of the commonest approaches is the use of colour flow Doppler mapping in the assessment of valve regurgitation. This is achieved by observing the size, site, intensity and duration of the regurgitant jet. It is therefore essential to set the gain of the colour flow correctly, otherwise it is easy to underestimate the regurgitation (see Chapter 3 for optimum colour flow Doppler settings). When first learning echocardiography, it can be difficult to pick up regurgitation on real-time scanning using colour flow due to the fast heart rate. It is very useful to freeze an image and then to use the cine loop to review one or two of the heart cycles slowly. Other signs can also be used to help in quantifying regurgitation (these will be covered in the relevant sections); for example, in cases of significant mitral or aortic regurgitation, the left ventricle will show volume overload. This is indicated by hyperkinetic myocardium with a normal end systolic diameter, but an end diastolic diameter outside the normal range.

The velocity of regurgitation is *only* measured for tricuspid regurgitation, where it can be used to estimate the right-sided pressures (for more detail, see the section on tricuspid regurgitation). The velocity of the regurgitant jet will help in assessing intracardiac pressure differences, but will not generally allow quantitation of regurgitant volumes.

In the following sections, each valve is considered in turn, and in each valve section, discasos inherent to each valve that cause regurgitation are described

Diseases that affect all valves, (e.g. infective endocarditis) are dealt with in separate sections.

Mitral valve disease

Mitral stenosis

It is very common for patients with mitral stenosis to be in atrial fibrillation, although this is not always the case.

CAUSES OF MITRAL STENOSIS
Rheumatic disease – common
Degenerative disease – rare
Thickened mitral annulus – rare
Obstruction due to atrial myxoma – rare

The mitral valve is first visualised using the parasternal long-axis view. It should be immediately obvious that the tips of the leaflets are not separating. In many cases, the bodies of the leaflets are mobile but the tips are fixed, causing a doming motion of the leaflets upon opening. The edges of the leaflets are usually more thickened than the remainder of the valve, but in severe chronic cases the entire valve shows thickening, shortening and irregularity of the leaflets, often with a highly echogenic appearance, indicating fibrosis or calcification. The subvalvar apparatus (papillary muscles and chordae) is often also affected, being thickened, echogenic and shortened.

The M-mode trace typically shows the following signs (Figure. 5.1)

- thickening of the leaflet tips
- reduced diastolic closure rate in early diastole (traditionally called a 'flat' EF slope, i.e. the valve opening is prolonged)
- reduced separation of the anterior and posterior leaflets
- parallel movement of leaflets (the posterior leaflet moving up towards the anterior leaflet during diastole rather than down and away from it)
- large left atrium
- slow left ventricular filling.

If the M-mode beam is mistakenly placed through a mobile part of a leaflet, it will not give the typical telltale trace of mitral stenosis. It is therefore important that the beam is carefully placed through the leaflet tips. The resultant trace will commonly have a long downward slope without the second the biphasic movement (due to atrial fibrillation) (Figure 5.2).

The parasternal short axis view will also show obviously restricted movement of the leaflets. If the leaflet tips can be seen clearly, a planimetry measurement can be made (Figure 5.3). An image of the leaflets open to their fullest extent should be frozen and the *inside* edge carefully traced around. From this the valve area is calculated (by the machine). This measurement can be fraught with error. It can be difficult to determine when the leaflets are open to their maximum, and hence an underestimate of valve area can be made. Commonly, the commisures are not clearly visualised (due to 'drop out' of the beam parallel with the imaging

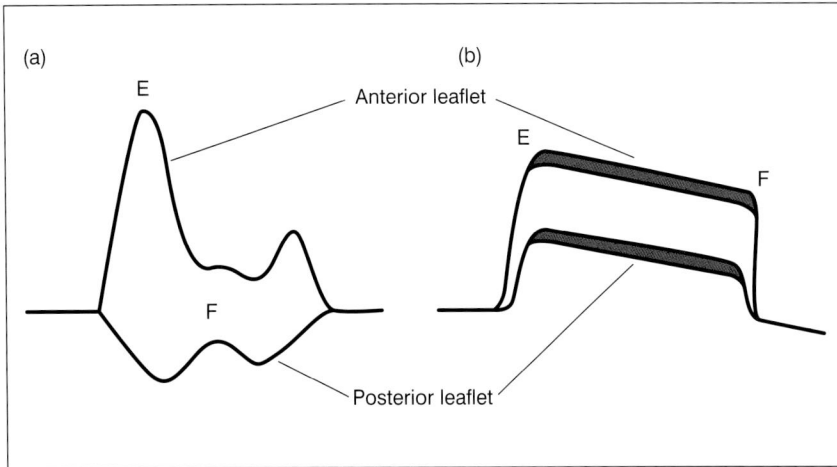

Figure 5.1 – (a) A normal mitral M-mode trace and (b) the M-mode trace seen in mitral stenosis. The maximum amplitude of diastolic opening of the anterior leaflet is the E point, and the end of the first diastolic closure period is the F point.

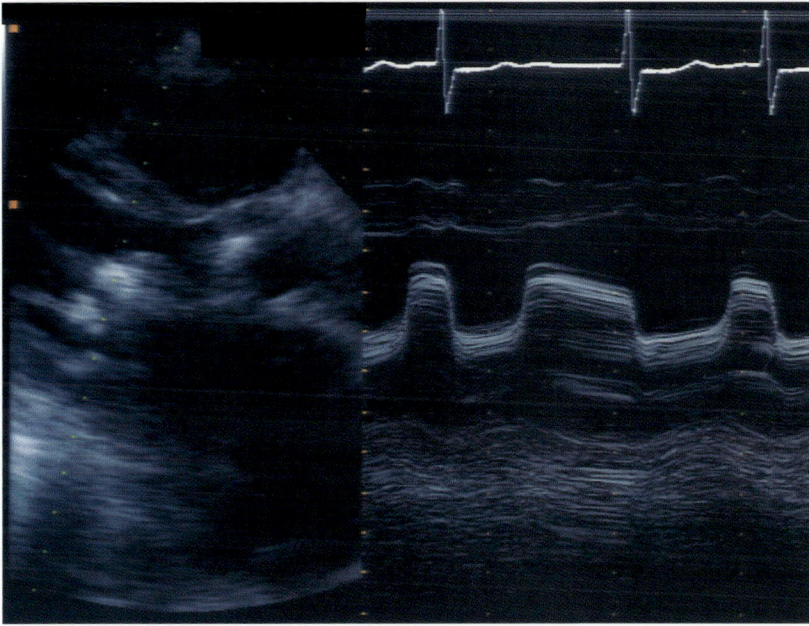

Figure 5.2 – M-mode trace of a stenotic mitral valve. Note the 'flat top' of the EF slope and the absence of the A wave.

plane) and so accurate tracing cannot be made; in these cases, the valve area should not be calculated. Three planimetry measurements should be made and the average taken. If a good trace is obtained, the area by planimetry can then be used to confirm the valve area calculated from the pressure half time measurement.

The mitral valve can now be assessed using the apical four chamber view. Again the leaflets are assessed for

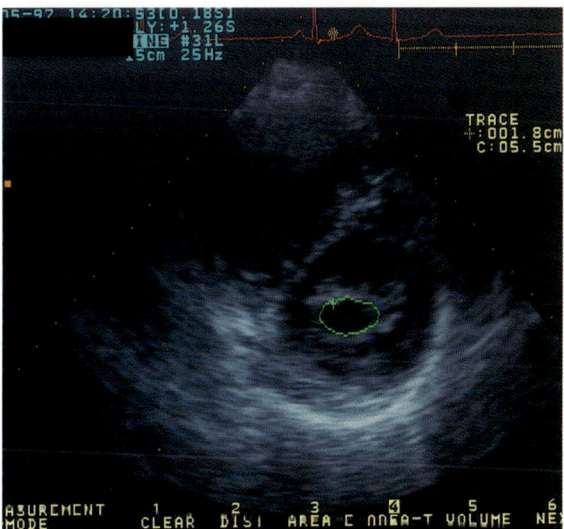

Figure 5.3 – A planimetry measurement of the mitral valve area is made by tracing around the inside edge of the mitral leaflets when they are open to their maximum.

their mobility and the doming motion can be visualised (Figure 5.4a). Colour flow Doppler placed over the mitral valve will show high velocity aliasing flow though the narrow opening of the valve. The colour will be seen to extend a long way into the left ventricle (Figure 5.4b). Acceleration of flow on the atrial side of the valve can also be observed on colour flow. This is seen as a small arc of colour below the leaflets during diastole.

At this stage any mitral regurgitation should be assessed and kept in mind when measuring the forward velocity through the valve. The forward velocity through a mitral valve increases as the valve becomes narrower. However, a significant amount of mitral regurgitation (moderate or greater) will also increase the forward velocity through the valve, because additional flow must occur through the valve to maintain cardiac output. Colour flow will obscure the valve and should be removed before positioning the pulsed wave cursor.

The pulsed wave sample volume is placed just at the leaflet tips. With a stenosed valve it is very easy to position the cursor correctly as there is no ambiguity about where to place it. If a crisp spectral trace is not obtained, it may be necessary to reapply colour flow to fine tune the position of the cursor at the most aliasing part of the flow. When a crisp trace has been obtained, the peak velocity, mean velocity and pressure half time measurements should be made (see Chapter 4). These mea-

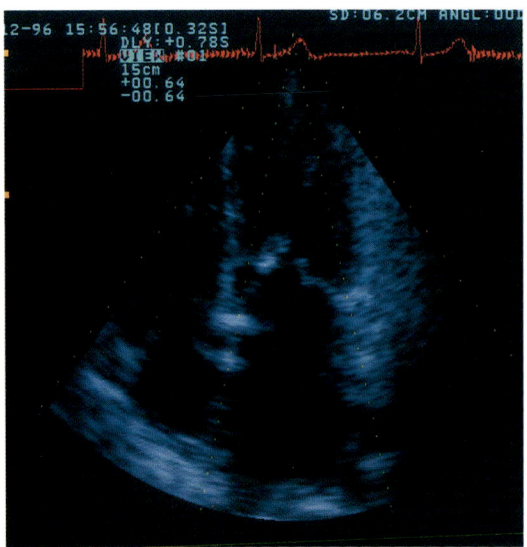 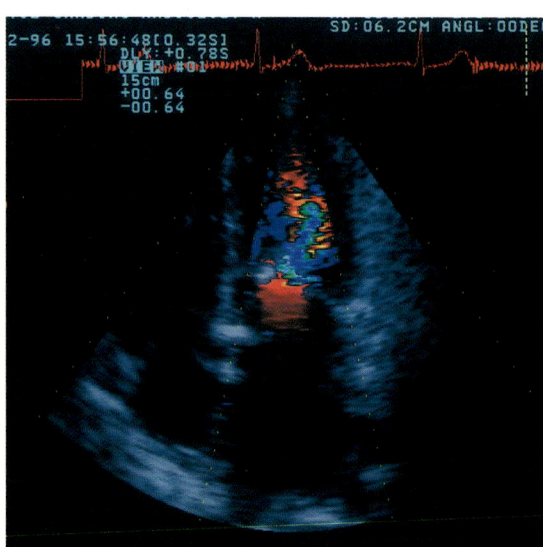

Figure 5.4 – (a) Apical four chamber view illustrating restricted opening of the mitral valve. (b) Colour flow Doppler applied to the stenosed mitral valve in (a). Note the highly aliased forward flow extending towards the apex, and the 'pool' of red below the valve in the left atrium, which indicates flow acceleration.

surements should be repeated twice more and a range quoted. A range is used because a patient in atrial fibrillation will have irregular beats and one measurement would not be representative of the mitral valve function over time.

The forward velocity through a normal mitral valve is low, about 1 m/s. A stenosed valve will have a raised forward velocity, usually between 1.5 and 2.0 m/s. Be aware that this velocity will be raised if there is significant mitral regurgitation even in a valve that is not stenosed. The pressure half time measurement will give a much more accurate estimate of the degree of stenosis (Table 5.1).

MITRAL STENOSIS DUE TO ANNULAR THICKENING

It is common to see posterior annular thickening in the elderly (Figure 5.5). If anterior annular thickening is also present, the valve should be assessed for stenosis. The mitral leaflets are usually thin and mobile and a normal M-mode trace can be obtained. In such cases, the forward flow through the valve can be eccentric, making placement of the pulsed wave sample volume difficult, and colour flow may be used to help position the sample volume. The stenosis should be assessed and graded in the same way as described above. However, annular thickening is relatively rare and is usually seen only in elderly patients. It rarely produces more than mild stenosis.

Table 5.1 – Suggested measurements for quantifying mitral stenosis

Degree of stenosis	Pressure half time (ms)	Calculated valve area (cm^2)
Normal	40 – 70	4.0 – 5.0
Very mild	70 – 110	2.0 – 4.0
Mild	110 – 140	1.5 – 2.0
Moderate	140 – 220	1.1 – 1.5
Severe	> 220	≤ 1.0

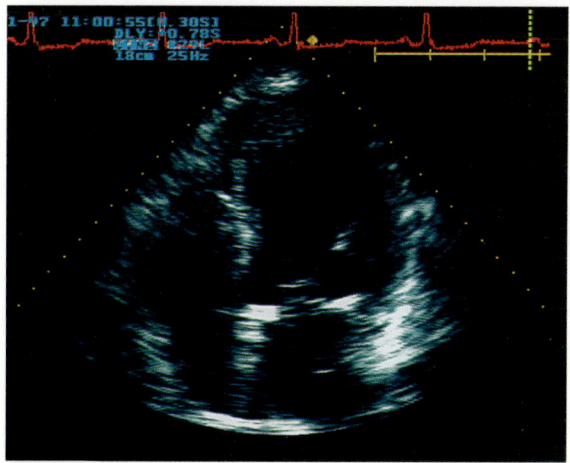

Figure 5.5 – Image showing thickening of both the anterior and posterior mitral annulus.

LEFT ATRIAL DILATATION

The left atrium is commonly dilated in patients with mitral stenosis due to the increase in loading pressure. This means there can be stasis of blood in the atrium, especially as patients are often in atrial fibrillation, and thrombus can form. In patients in whom mitral stenosis was previously unknown, the left atrium should be particularly carefully investigated. However, it should not be assumed that patients who are already on anticoagulants will have no thrombus, as the level of anticoagulant is not always constant and thrombus may still form. Thrombus cannot be totally excluded from the left atrium on transthoracic echocardiography as the atrial appendage cannot generally be visualised (a transoesophageal echo image is needed to exclude thrombus with confidence). Measurements of the left atrium should be made as explained in Chapter 4.

RIGHT-SIDED FINDINGS

Severe chronic mitral valve disease will raise pulmonary pressures and will often show secondary effects on right-heart structures. The most common findings are dilatation of the right ventricle and tricuspid regurgitation. The tricuspid regurgitant jet velocity should be measured in order to estimate the right ventricular (and pulmonary) pressure. In addition, do not forget organic disease of the tricuspid valve. Tricuspid stenosis occasionally accompanies mitral stenosis and has a similar morphological appearance. Take care, however, because tricuspid stenosis can look less severe but still be important.

SUMMARY OF SIGNS OF MITRAL STENOSIS
Tethered and echogenic leaflet tips, small obstructing orifice
Shallow slope on M-mode trace
Pressure half time $\geqslant$ 0.11sec (Valve area $\leqslant$ 2.0cm^2)
Mosaic forward mitral flow on colour mapping
Increased forward velocity through mitral valve (may be due in part to mitral regurgitation)
Dilated left atrium
Raised pressure drop of tricuspid regurgitation (secondary pulmonary hypertension)

Mitral regurgitation

The two main observations that need to be made in assessing mitral regurgitation are the cause and the amount of regurgitation. The amount of regurgitation will determine at what stage surgical interventions will be needed, and the cause will determine what type of surgery will be planned (e.g. a prolapsing leaflet can be repaired, but a leaflet that has vegetations on it will need to be replaced). Of course surgery may not be needed in many patients, but monitoring of medical therapy is also very important. Spectral Doppler can be useful in detecting trivial amounts of regurgitation that may not be picked up on colour flow imaging. Such trivial amounts will not be haemodynamically significant, but may account for a murmur.

CAUSES OF MITRAL REGURGITATION
Functional – left ventricular dilatation
Rheumatic (with or without stenosis)
Degenerative (prolapse)
Chordal rupture (flail leaflet)
Infective endocarditis
Papillary muscle rupture (secondary to myocardial infarction)

QUANTIFYING MITRAL REGURGITATION

Mitral regurgitation is primarily quantified by observation of colour flow Doppler patterns. This is usually done using the apical four chamber and two chamber views when flow is parallel with the ultrasound beam (Figure 5.6), but other views are also useful. The colour flow area should be placed such that it covers the area from a couple of centimetres of the base of the left ven-

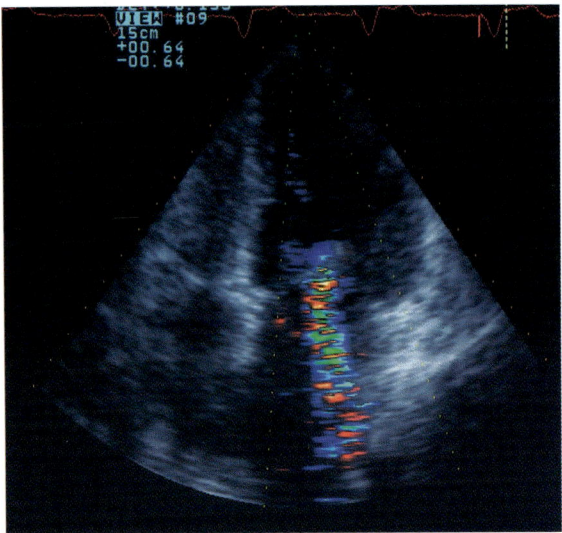

Figure 5.6 – Colour flow Doppler representation of mitral regurgitation. Areas that are mainly blue indicate flow away from the transducer, which occurs during systole. Due to the high velocity of the flow, the colour has aliased and also includes green, indicating turbulence.

tricle above the mitral valve and all of the left atrium. If the regurgitation is central into the left atrium, quantification is much easier.

First, the colour flow jet is assessed for how far it streams into the left atrium:

- A *trivial amount of mitral regurgitation* will be displayed as a tiny signal of blue between the leaflets and possibly about a centimetre into the left atrium. The duration of flow may be less than that of systole.

- *Mild regurgitation* will be seen as flow about half-way back into a normal sized left atrium; the jet will remain narrow. The stream will be present for the duration of systole. As *regurgitation increases above mild*, colour proximal to the mitral valve (on the ventricular side of the leaflets) can be seen. This is indicated on colour flow as a blue arc above the leaflets as the blood starts to accelerate in order to pass through the incompetent area and is produced by the acceleration of blood proximal to the regurgitant orifice.

- *Moderate regurgitation* will be demonstrated as the colour flow jet reaching the back of a normal sized atrium. The flow will show obvious aliasing. The diameter of the jet is increased. The intensity of the spectral Doppler signal is greater.

- *Severe regurgitation* will be seen as the regurgitant jet spraying into and filling the whole of a normal sized left atrium. Much turbulence will be demonstrated if variance is used and the intensity of the spectral Doppler signal will be very high.

Problems arise in quantifying mitral regurgitation if there is an eccentric jet or if the left atrium is dilated.

An eccentric jet of mitral regurgitation will track along one of the walls of the left atrium. Although it can be visualised in two dimensions, the size of the third dimension of the flow cannot be seen from one view. It is therefore necessary to be wary when quantifying such regurgitation, as it can be very easy to underestimate it. The left atrium needs to be visualised in all planes with colour flow to obtain the best idea of the size of the jet. If an eccentric jet is severe, it can be seen to track along one wall to the back of the left atrium before swirling around and heading upwards again, and so now is coded blue. Jets adherent to a wall will also entrain or induce less movement of surrounding blood whereas a free jet in the centre of a cavity will cause more turbulence in the surrounding blood. Thus adherent jets tend to be underestimated and free jets tend to be overestimated.

Other associated factors of mitral regurgitation on the heart should also be looked for (see the box listing signs of mitral regurgitation). In particular, left ventricular function should be assessed. A very volume overloaded ventricle will suggest a severe leak (if no other cause for volume overload is present) and a small normally contracting ventricle will tend to exclude severe regurgitation. Use of left ventricular function is much more unreliable in the presence of myocardial disease, so great care must be taken not to rely too much on this method in patients with ischaemic heart disease or other cardiomyopathy.

Left atrial dilatation will also cause problems in quantifying mitral regurgitation, and in long-standing moderate or severe regurgitation, the left atrium will inevitably dilate. What may appear in a dilated atrium as mild regurgitation may really be moderate if the same amount were to be viewed in a normal atrium. Unfortunately, there is no method for absolutely quantifying regurgitation from volume-flow measurements, but this is currently being researched.

QUANTIFYING MITRAL REGURGITATION FROM THE SPECTRAL DOPPLER TRACE

Mitral regurgitation may be estimated semi-quantitatively by using the spectral trace (Figure 5.7). These

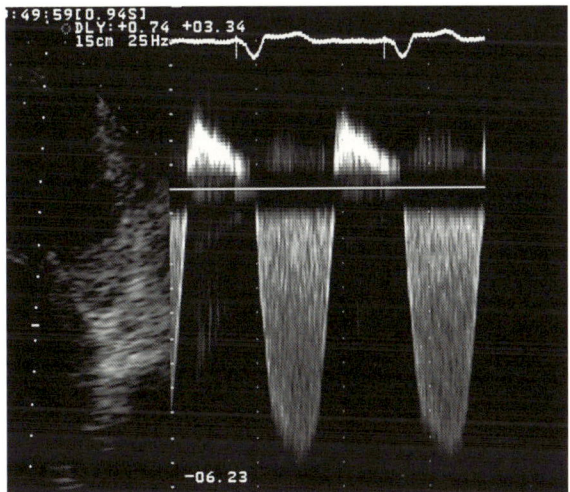

Figure 5.7 – Continuous wave spectral trace of moderate mitral regurgitation.

guidelines should only be used when there is a good forward mitral trace, indicating that the reverse flow will be of equal quality. The brightness of the spectral trace increases as the amount of regurgitation increases as there is increased blood flow at all velocities.[1] Trivial regurgitation will be displayed as an incomplete envelope of very low intensity; commonly, it is not pansystolic. Mild regurgitation will be displayed as a complete envelope, still of low intensity; but of high-velocity. Moderate regurgitation will have a similar appearance to that of mild regurgitation, but will be of higher intensity. Severe regurgitation will be of equal intensity to the forward mitral flow. It will be of a lower velocity, and results in a noisy trace as the flow is typically extremely turbulent. These signs are 'semi-quantitative' and should not be relied upon in isolation.

Mitral valve prolapse

Mitral prolapse is indicated when one or both of the mitral leaflets buckle back into the left atrium when closing. The line of closure of a leaflet must be below the hinge points of the valve for this to be described technically. If both leaflets technically prolapse but there is no regurgitation, some echocardiographers would call this 'billowing' of the valve (but this term is not recognised universally). If both leaflets prolapse to the same degree and there is regurgitation, the regurgitation will be central. More commonly, only one of the leaflets will prolapse. In this case the resultant jet of regurgitation will pass under whichever leaflet does not

prolapse (Figure 5.8). Therefore, even in a patient with poor echo windows, it can be possible to determine if prolapse is present, and which leaflet is prolapsing. From the surgeon's point of view, it is important to know if regurgitation is due to prolapse because a prolapsing leaflet can be repaired, rather than replaced. It is also surgically much easier to repair a prolapsing posterior leaflet than an anterior one.

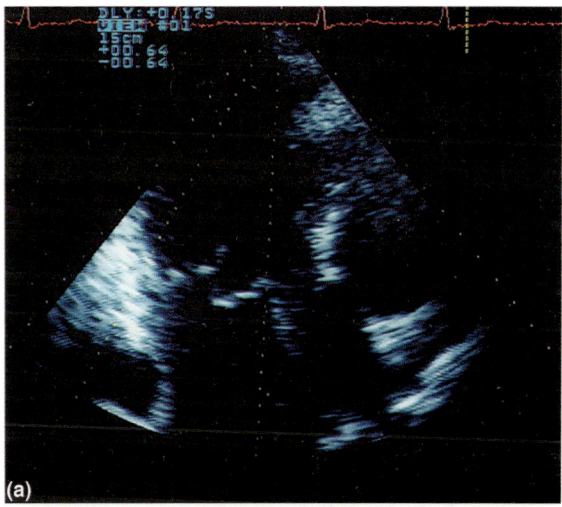

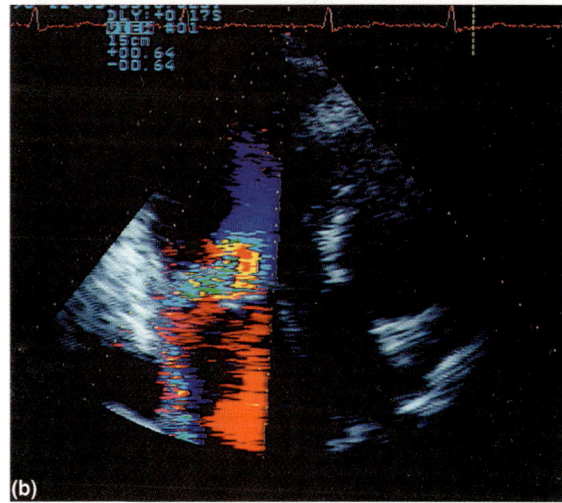

Figure 5.8 – (a) Apical long axis view of anterior mitral leaflet prolapse. (b) The same image as in (a), but with colour display, illustrating an eccentric jet of regurgitation under the posterior leaflet. Note the acceleration of flow on the ventricular side of the valve and the flow (in red) in the anterior half of the left atrium as the regurgitation hits the back of the atrium and swirls back up again.

A prolapsing leaflet should be investigated carefully, as vegetations caused by infective endocarditis can cause a leaflet to prolapse, even if they are tiny. A ruptured chord will result in similar appearances to a prolapsing leaflet with a suggestion of something attached to the leaflet. It is not possible to distinguish between thread-like vegetations and a ruptured chord on echocardiography (this is a clinical judgement) (Figure 5.9).

As mentioned previously, care must be taken when quantifying an eccentric jet of regurgitation as it can easily be underestimated.

The continuous wave Doppler spectral trace can be helpful in detecting late systolic regurgitation which, although usually trivial, is most likely to be due to slight prolapse of one of the leaflets. The prolapse cannot be detected easily on two-dimensional imaging as it is so slight, and thus the diagnosis relies on the spectral trace.

Flail leaflet

A mitral leaflet is described as 'flail' when it is seen to arc freely between the left atrium and the left ventricle. Flail is due to rupture of the chordae. This results in the leaflet, or a part of it, having no anchorage during systole. The ruptured chordae may be visualised in patients with good imaging windows as thin strands attached to the tip of the leaflet. Rupture of a papillary muscle has a similar effect (see the section on ruptured chordae later in this chapter).

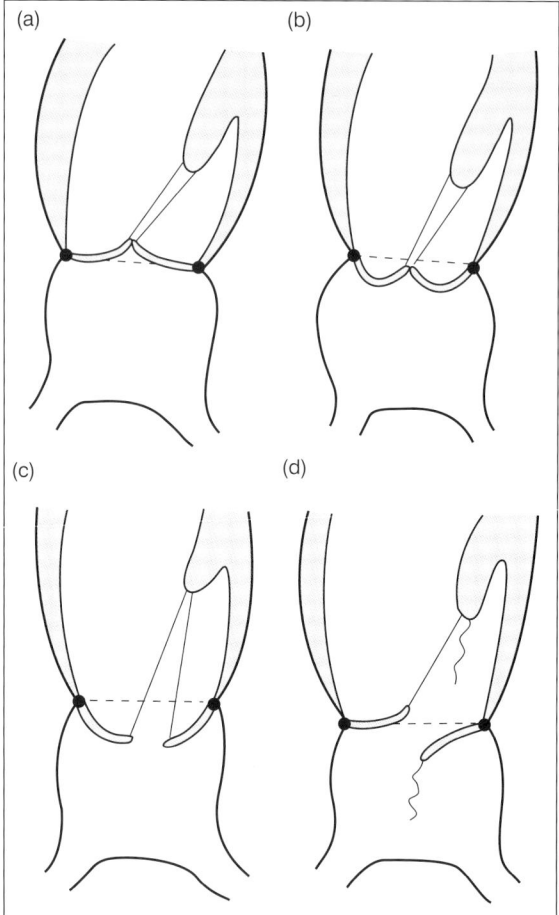

Figure 5.9 – Closure movements of the mitral valve. (a) Normal closure – the leaflets do not move behind the plane of the annulus. (b) Mild prolapse – the closed leaflets lie behind the plane of the annulus, but the tips still make contact; there may not be any regurgitation. (c) Severe prolapse of both leaflets – the leaflets are well behind the annular plane and their tips do not meet; there will be significant regurgitation. (d) Flail leaflet – a ruptured chord allows the free edge of a leaflet (or part of a leaflet) to move into the left atrium; there will be significant regurgitation.

SIGNS OF MITRAL REGURGITATION

Colour flow Doppler displaying reverse flow through the valve in systole

Flow demonstrated below the baseline on spectral Doppler

Raised forward velocity through the valve (in the absence of mitral stenosis)

Left ventricular volume overload for significant regurgitation

Left atrial dilatation for significant regurgitation

Aortic valve disease

Aortic stenosis

Acquired stenosis of the aortic valve is characterised by leaflets of increased echogenicity that have a reduced opening area. It can often be found in the elderly with no presenting clinical signs. Most severe aortic stenosis presenting in the elderly has its origin in a mild congenital abnormality of the valve, usually bicuspid leaflets. Rheumatic aortic stenosis is rarely found without accompanying mitral stenosis.

The aortic valve is first visualised on the parasternal long axis view. The first indication of stenosis is that the leaflets appear shorter and thickened. Rather than the leaflets opening to the walls of the aorta, restricted

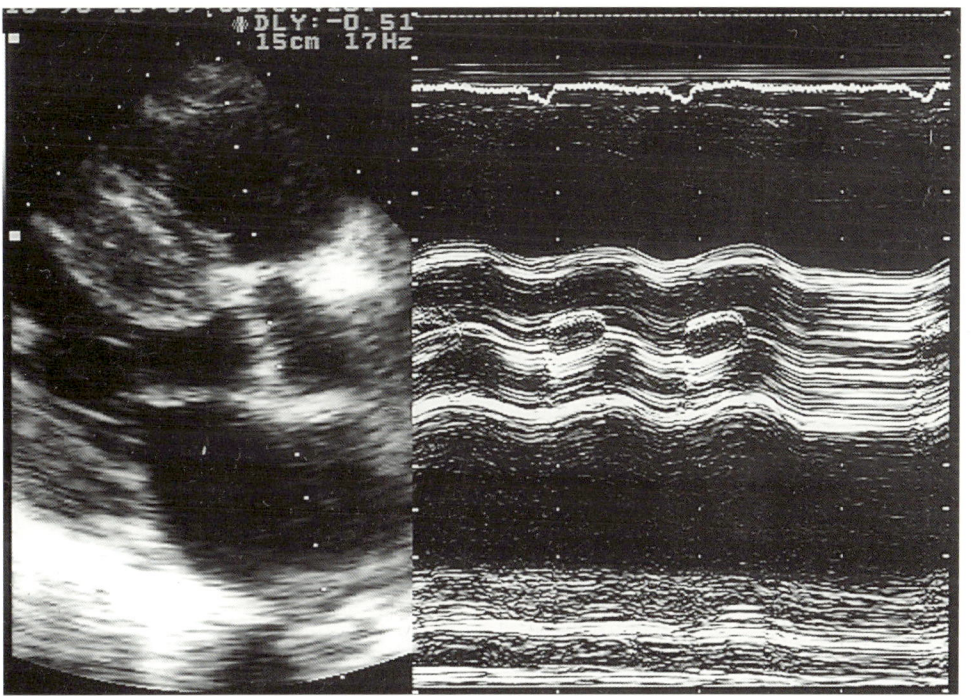

Figure 5.10 – M-mode image through a stenotic aortic valve. Instead of the leaflets opening to the walls of the aorta to form a box shape, they are restricted and form a rectangular shape.

movement can be noted. This is displayed well on M-mode image, with by the usual 'box' shaped trace being replaced by a thick rectangle (Figure 5.10); alternatively in cases of very severe stenosis, no movement may be detected at all. Sometimes the lesion is so severe it is difficult to see the leaflet morphology clearly on the two-dimensional image, and a mass of echogenic structures in the valve orifice is all that can be seen. It is essential to have a well positioned image in order to avoid confusion with the echogenic pattern of a tangentially sectioned aortic wall. If colour flow is applied at this stage, it may be possible to visualise a very aliased stream passing through the leaflets (Figure 5.11).

Because the leaflets are thickened, it makes them more visible on the parasternal short axis view. In many cases the number of leaflets can be counted. The mobility of all three leaflets should now be assessed. If just one leaflet remains thin and mobile, no significant aortic stenosis will be present. If all three leaflets are restricted, an idea can be formed as to the degree of stenosis. If this judgement does not match the maximum velocity recorded across the valve, a higher value should be sought. Planimetry should not be used on a

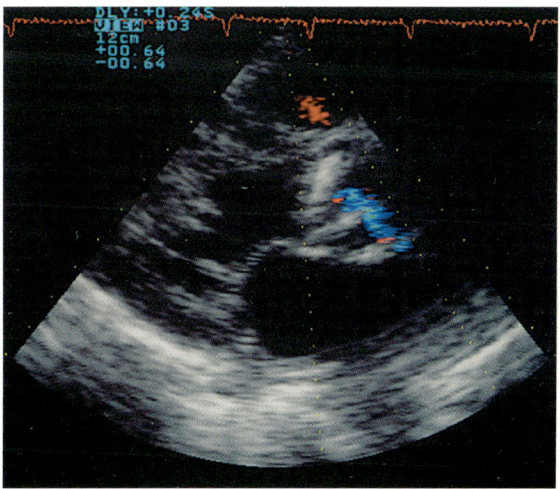

Figure 5.11 – Colour flow Doppler applied to a severely stenotic aortic valve. Note the very narrow jet and the direction of flow, which is not aligned with the angle of the ascending aorta. (For this reason, it is important to apply continuous wave Doppler to the aortic valve from as many different angles as possible, in order to record the maximum forward velocity.)

stenotic aortic valve, except in cases where there is exceptionally clear imaging.

The degree of aortic stenosis is most accurately graded by means of the peak velocity or the pressure drop across the valve. The direction of the maximal jet varies greatly from patient to patient, so it is essential to use all possible windows to measure pressure drops (parasternal, apical, subcostal, right parasternal and suprasternal). This ensures the closest alignment of the beam with the flow direction. Poor alignment will seriously underestimate pressure differences across the aortic valve.

To obtain good alignment it will often be necessary to move transducer down a rib space in order to angle more superiorly into the valve and more parallel with the flow. The resultant image may be of poorer quality, but often the velocity reading will be higher. In an elderly patient it will be necessary to scan from further around the left side to make the aorta as vertical to the beam as possible (see Chapter 4). A non-imaging continuous wave transducer is very sensitive and, with practice, should yield the highest velocity, which is typically found at the right parasternal window. Care should be taken in patients with a dilated left atrium. In an apical four chamber view the continuous wave cursor will pass through the left atrium as well as the aortic valve. This means that mitral regurgitation can be detected on the same spectral trace at almost the same instant as the aortic stenosis trace (Figure 5.12). The valve clicks from the aortic valve are helpful in separating the two traces. (see Chapter 2)

Aortic stenosis will usually result in a strong spectral trace. The Doppler filter should be increased to give a clean trace. In cases where the jet is difficult, increasing the Doppler filter can make the trace more obvious. Increasing the Doppler gain may also be of use in such cases. Increasing the rejection and compression can help to highlight a faint trace. Once the continuous wave trace has been obtained the transducer should be moved 'blind' by tiny amounts to see if a higher velocity can be found.

When the highest velocity has been found, the trace is frozen and a peak velocity/pressure measurement made. This should be repeated twice more to ensure that the maximum velocity has been recorded. An occasional longer diastole will be followed by an increased maximum velocity. These peaks should be ignored as they do not accurately reflect the function of the valve. Instead, the maximum velocity of the average peak should be measured (Figure 5.13).

The sweep speed of the spectral trace should now be increased. On some machines, this is possible on the already frozen Doppler trace, while on others it is necessary to obtain another trace. In the latter case, the peak velocity found from the new trace will need to be compared with that from the original trace in order to ensure that the maximum velocity is again recorded (on a faster sweep speed the spectral trace appears to have a

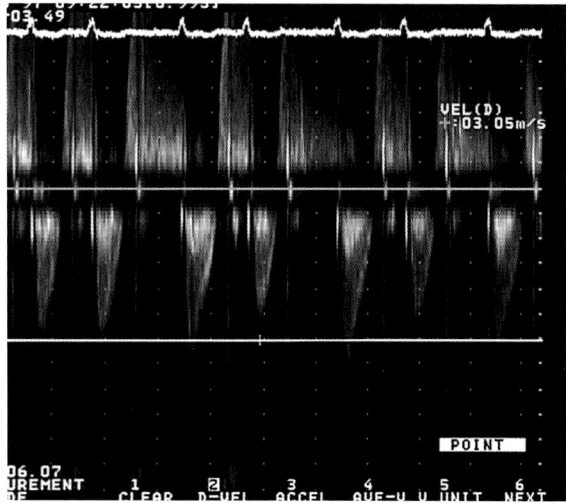

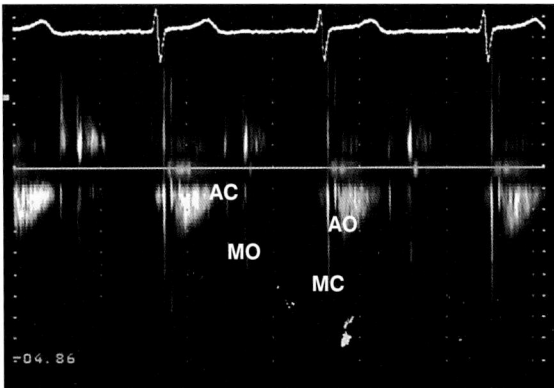

Figure 5.12 – An apical recording from a patient with a mitral prosthesis and thickened aortic leaflets, showing the timing of valve opening and closing by the click artefacts. AC, aortic closure; AO, aortic opening; MC, mitral closure; MO, mitral opening.

Figure 5.13 – Patients with an irregular heart rate (e.g. those in atrial fibrillation) will have a different peak velocity at each beat. The average of the peak values should be measured, rather than the highest or lowest. This requires watching the spectral trace over some period of time and making multiple measurements. This image was recorded using a slow scroll speed so that multiple peaks could be compared on one screen.

lower velocity until measured). On the stretched out trace, a mean velocity is calculated. This is achieved by tracing around the curve. Both the peak and the mean velocity/pressure drop should be quoted in the report.

The peak pressure drop is not the same as the catheter 'pull-back gradient' familiar to cardiologists, and these two values should not be used interchangeably. The peak Doppler pressure drop is an instantaneous value and is usually higher than the catheter pull-back value. The mean pressure difference is also different from the pull-back pressure drop at the catheter, but the values are often closer. Some people tend to equate the two measurements but this can be misleading. There is no substitute for becoming familiar with the Doppler-derived pressure drop values themselves and learning their clinical context (Table 5.2).

The values given in Table 5.2 are a true indication of aortic valve function if the left ventricle is of normal contractility and there is no, or mild, aortic regurgitation. If the left ventricle is reduced in its function, the resultant peak velocity through a stenosed aortic valve will be lower, and the degree of stenosis will be underestimated. If there is a significant amount of aortic regurgitation (moderate or more), there will be increased forward flow through the aortic valve and hence the aortic stenosis will be overestimated. In both these cases the continuity equation will need to be used to accurately determine the amount of stenosis.

CONTINUITY EQUATION

The theory behind this equation states that the volume flow in a closed system remains constant. The equation is used to calculate the area of the aortic valve. In Figure 5.14, A_1 is the cross-sectional area of the left ventricular outflow tract, V_1 is the mean velocity in the outflow

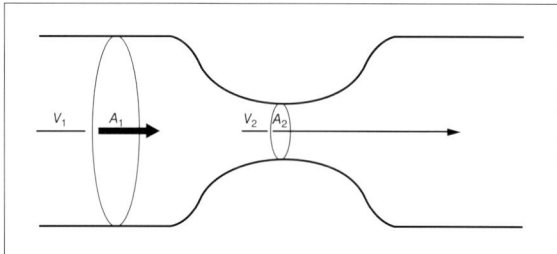

Figure 5.14 – Measurements for use in the continuity equation. Refer to text for description.

tract, A_2 is the area of the aortic valve (to be calculated) and V_2 is the mean velocity through the aortic valve:

$$V_1 A_1 = V_2 A_2$$

The cross-sectional area of the left ventricular outflow tract A_1 is calculated by measuring the diameter of the outflow tract on the parasternal long axis view (see Chapter 4), and using the formula for the area of a circle:

$$A_1 = \pi \left(\frac{D}{2}\right)^2$$

Where D is the diameter of the left ventricular outflow tract.

The velocity in the left ventricular outflow tract V_1 is measured on the apical four chamber view where a pulsed wave cursor is placed in the outflow tract just on the ventricular side of the valve (see chapter 4). The *mean* velocity of this spectral trace is used; with slight loss of accuracy, the peak values can be used instead.

It is assumed that the maximum velocity recorded on the continuous wave Doppler trace through the aortic valve will occur actually in the valve. The *mean* velocity of the continuous wave trace is used to obtain V_2.

$$A_2 = A_1 \times V_1 / V_2$$

An aortic valve area of less than 1.0 cm^2, indicates severe stenosis.

The diameter of the outflow tract is difficult to measure accurately and, as this measurement is squared, errors can be large. It is therefore suggested that the technique is only used in cases with normal outflow anatomy and good quality recordings with good alignment. The derived values should be used as a guide only.[2]

Aortic regurgitation

Aortic regurgitation is detected and quantified on both colour flow and continuous wave Doppler. A regurgi-

Table 5.2 – Typical guideline clinical values in aortic stenosis (all values are approximations)

Degree of stenosis	Peak Velocity (m/s)	Peak Doppler Pressure drop (mmHg)	Valve area★ (cm²)
Normal	1.4 – 2.2	8 – 20	> 3
Trivial	2.2 – 2.5	20 – 25	2.0 – 3.0
Mild	2.5 – 3.2	25 – 40	1.5 – 2.0
Moderate	3.2 – 4.2	40 – 70	1.0 – 1.5
Severe	> 4.2	> 70	< 1.0

★ Calculated using the continuity equation.

ASSOCIATED SIGNS OF AORTIC STENOSIS

Left ventricular hypertrophy – usually only present in cases of severe aortic stenosis

Dilatation of the ascending aorta

Long-term aortic stenosis will result in a dilated, failing left ventricle

tant jet can usually be detected by colour flow on the parasternal long axis view. In this case flow is usually in the direction away from the transducer and so is coded blue. The degree of regurgitation may be underestimated on this view, however, as the general angle of flow is close to 90° to the beam. Thus, although the presence of regurgitation may be identified on the parasternal long axis view, quantification should be made on the apical four chamber view when flow is almost parallel with the beam.

CAUSES OF AORTIC REGURGITATION

Degenerative

Dilated aortic root – annuloaortic ectasia or Marfan's syndrome

Congenital (e.g. bicuspid valve)

Rheumatic disease

Infective endocarditis

Dissection of aorta involving the aortic valve

It is possible to determine from which cusps the regurgitation originates from by placing the colour flow box over the aortic valve on the parasternal short axis view. Most commonly the jet is central, but in some cases it may originate from between just two cusps, or even a perforation in one of the leaflets.

On the apical four chamber view, the direction of aortic regurgitation is towards the transducer and so will be coded red. However, if the regurgitation is greater than mild, the velocity of the regurgitant jet increases, and the colour flow will be aliased.

The amount of regurgitation is quantified on the colour flow by the width of the regurgitant jet at its base and also by how far the jet extends into the left ventricle. Obviously, the size of the left ventricle must be kept in mind when making this assessment.

Although regurgitation is in the opposite direction to forward aortic flow, the actual direction of the reverse flow is not always directly in line with the maximum forward flow.[3] Therefore it is much easier to locate the

regurgitation on continuous wave Doppler by using colour flow to position the beam. The angle of the downward slope of the continuous wave spectral Doppler trace is used to quantify the aortic regurgitation. At the end of systole, the pressure in the aorta is greater than that of the left ventricle. The greater the amount of regurgitation, the faster the pressures between the aorta and left ventricle will equalise. This occurs not only because the aortic pressure drops rapidly, but also because the left ventricular filling pressure rises. This is illustrated on the continuous wave Doppler spectral trace by an increased angle of the slope of the regurgitant jet. However, this increase in slope does not change linearly with the increase in regurgitation, and often it is difficult to differentiate between mild and moderate regurgitation on the spectral trace[4] and other methods will need to be used.

Regurgitation can also be detected at a distance from the aortic valve by observing the amount of reverse flow in the descending aorta. This is achieved by placing a pulsed wave Doppler cursor in the descending aorta as vertically as possible (from the parasternal notch), making sure that it is well clear of the head and neck branches (see Fig. 4.40) This is a particularly useful method for quantifying regurgitation when other methods produce questionable results (see the section on pitfalls, below).

As with mitral regurgitation, left ventricular volume overload is an important sign of severity of regurgitation.

QUANTIFYING AORTIC REGURGITATION

Aortic regurgitation can be quantified by four main methods:

1. Colour flow Doppler
2. Continuous wave spectral Doppler trace of regurgitant jet
3. Pulsed wave spectral Doppler trace of flow in the descending aorta
4. Left ventricular volume overload.

Mild aortic regurgitation

1. The colour flow trace shows a small red flame that lasts for the entire length of diastole. The trace is thin at the base (at aortic valve) and will not extend much further than the left ventricular outflow tract (Figure 5.15).
2. 'Flat-topped' continuous wave trace (Figure 5.16).
3. Flow in the descending aorta displays a small transient amount of reverse flow in early diastole (a normal appearance) (Figure 5.17).
4. Normal left ventricular function.

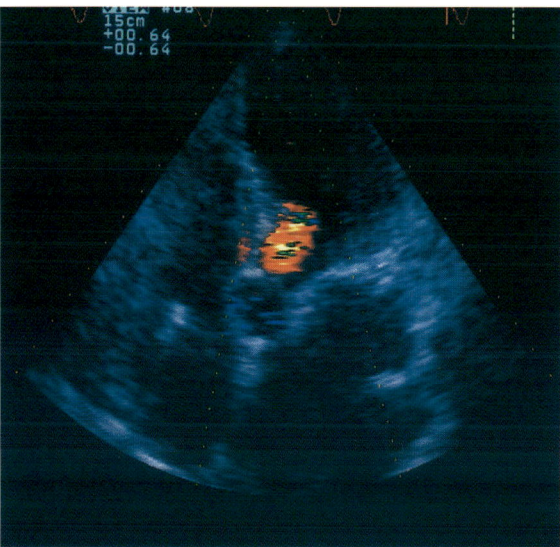

Figure 5.15 – Mild aortic regurgitation: colour flow Doppler image. Note the narrow base of the trace, which extends only for the length of the left ventricular outflow tract.

Moderate aortic regurgitation

1. The base of the colour jet is wider and extends at least half-way into the left ventricle.
2. Increased angle on the continuous wave trace (see Figure 3.12).
3. Increased reverse flow in descending aorta, persisting throughout diastole.
4. Mild left ventricular volume overload.

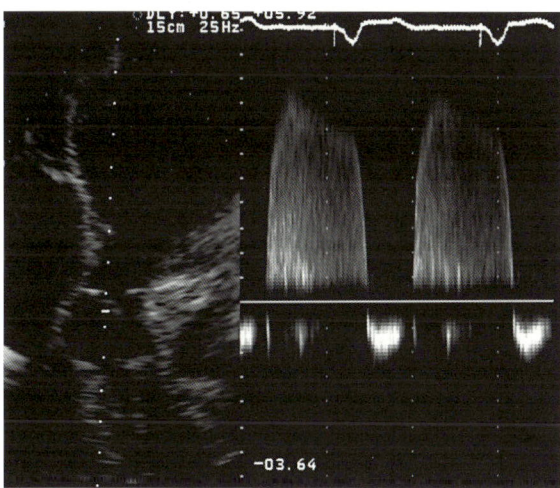

Figure 5.16 – Mild aortic regurgitation: continuous wave Doppler spectral trace through the aortic valve.

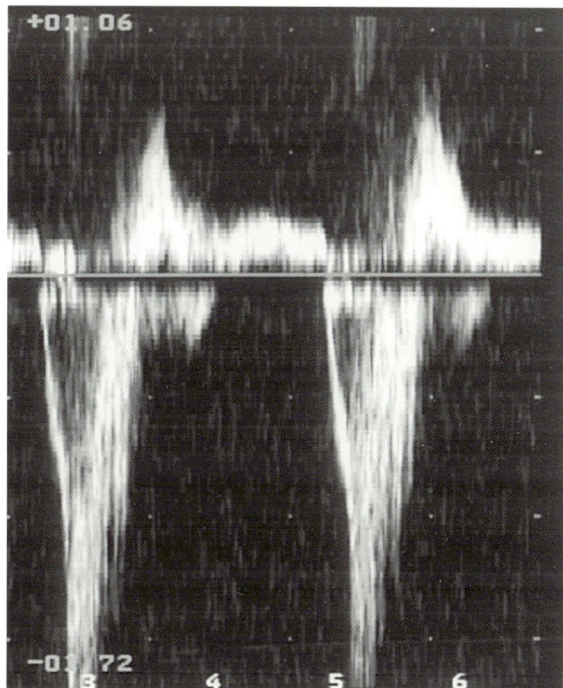

Figure 5.17 – Mild aortic regurgitation: pulsed wave Doppler spectral trace of the reversal of flow in the descending aorta. Reversed flow is above the zero line.

Severe aortic regurgitation

1. Colour flow fills the left ventricular outflow tract and extends to the apex, filling most of the cavity of the left ventricle (Figure 5.18).
2. Pressure between the aorta and the left ventricle equalises quickly, resulting in a steep slope on the continuous wave spectral trace (Figure 5.19).
3. Major reverse flow in the descending aorta occurs at a similar velocity to the forward flow (Figure 5.20).
4. Marked left ventricular volume overload, and dilatation in cases of chronic significant regurgitation.
5. Increase in forward aortic velocity.

The shapes of the continuous wave and pulsed wave Doppler traces for the different grades of aortic regurgitation are shown in Figures 5.21 and 5.22 respectively.

PITFALLS

Most commonly the regurgitation is centrally into the left ventricle. Difficulties arise in quantifying the jet when it is eccentric over the anterior mitral valve leaflet. On colour flow the diastolic jet of aortic regurgitation mixes with the forward mitral flow, and there

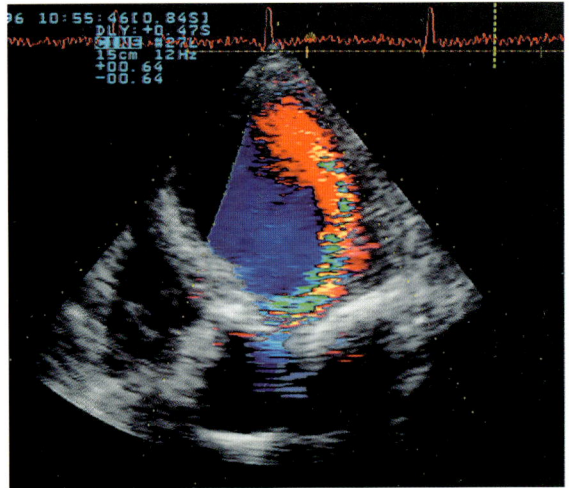

Figure 5.18 – Severe aortic regurgitation: colour flow Doppler image. The flow accelerates in the aorta before entering the ventricle. Colour fills the outflow tract, with an eccentric jet moving along the lateral wall of the left ventricle to the apex, before swirling around, where the colour changes to blue.

is difficulty in separating the two flows and hence in quantification.

Placement of the continuous wave beam parallel with the flow is almost impossible and a clear trace cannot be obtained. In such a situation the continuous wave beam may be positioned on the parasternal long axis view or subcostal four chamber view in an attempt to achieve good alignment. However, in most cases good alignment is still impossible to achieve, and the amount of regurgitation will have to be estimated by other means.

In a normally functioning left ventricle, moderate to severe aortic regurgitation will result in a volume overload. Consequently, forward flow through the aortic valve will be increased, and this should not be confused with aortic stenosis.

Tricuspid valve disease

It is rare for the tricuspid valve to be affected by significant disease. By far the most common tricuspid valve finding is tricuspid regurgitation. However, mild tricuspid regurgitation is found in the majority of the nor-

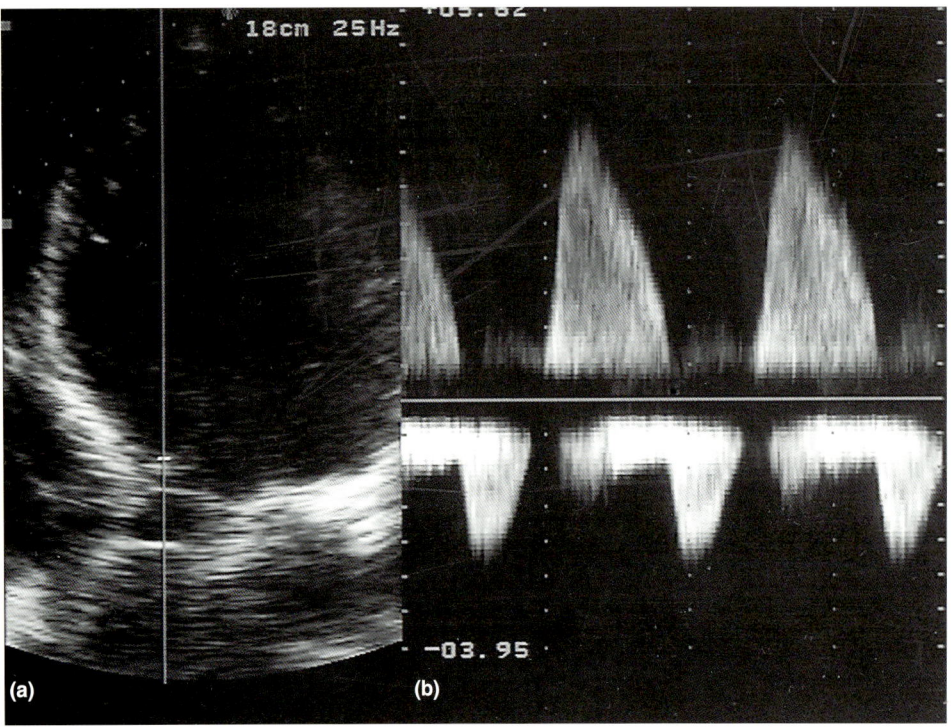

Figure 5.19 – Severe aortic regurgitation: (a) apical four chamber view showing the position of the continuous wave beam; (b) apical four chamber continuous wave Doppler spectral trace.

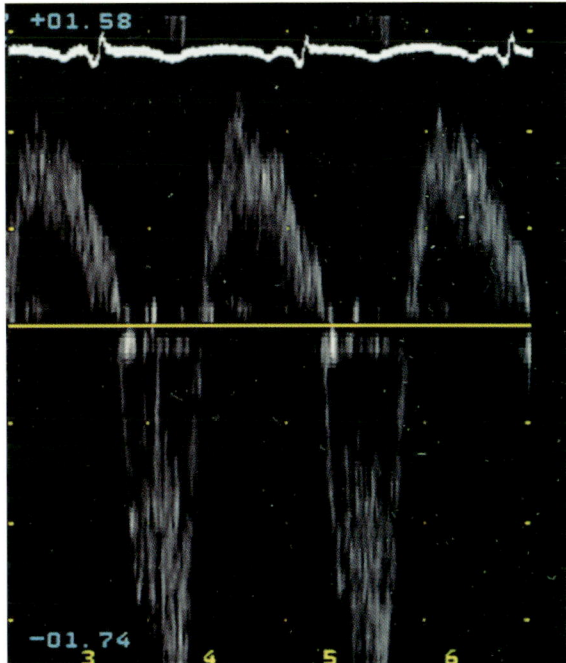

Figure 5.20 – Severe aortic regurgitation: pulsed wave Doppler spectral trace from the descending aorta. Forward flow is below the zero line.

mal population[5] It is actually a very useful finding, as pulmonary pressures can be estimated from the regurgitation.[6] Tricuspid stenosis is rare, but can result from rheumatic disease. Infective endocarditis is also a rare finding on the right side of the heart, but may occur in drug abusers or in patients with right-sided lines (e.g. a pacemaker).

Tricuspid stenosis

Tricuspid stenosis is often associated with tethered leaflets rather than thickened leaflets. Thin tricuspid valve leaflets are not easy to visualise. For this reason, it is not always easy to detect tricuspid stenosis in a previously undiagnosed patient. Therefore, in patients presenting with a stenosis of the aortic and/or mitral valve, the tricuspid valve should be carefully examined, as this valve is not usually examined in such detail.

Forward flow through a normal tricuspid valve does not give rise to a significant colour flow image as the velocity is low. Therefore, if aliased flow is seen, this should prompt a more detailed examination at the valve.

CAUSES OF TRICUSPID STENOSIS
Rheumatic disease
Carcinoid disease (thickened leaflets) – rare
Obstruction by right atrial myxoma – rare
Congenital (see Chapter 7) – rare

The tricuspid valve can be visualised, in patients with a good parasternal window, on the parasternal long axis view. This helps to show all three leaflets if the beam is swept over the entirety of the valve. The valve can be seen in the majority of patients on the parasternal short axis view. Because the valve is closer to the transducer in this view than in the apical four chamber view, it can often be seen in good detail, and hence the results of colour-flow mapping are also better.

Although calculation of valve area using the pressure half time measurement is only accurate for native mitral valves, this is the only measurement available for estimating tricuspid valve function. The pulsed wave cursor is placed at the leaflet tips in the right ventricle on the apical four chamber view so that a crisp spectral trace is achieved. Certainly, the pressure half time measurement is accurate and can be compared at serial scans. The valve area cannot reliably be calculated for tricuspid stenosis.

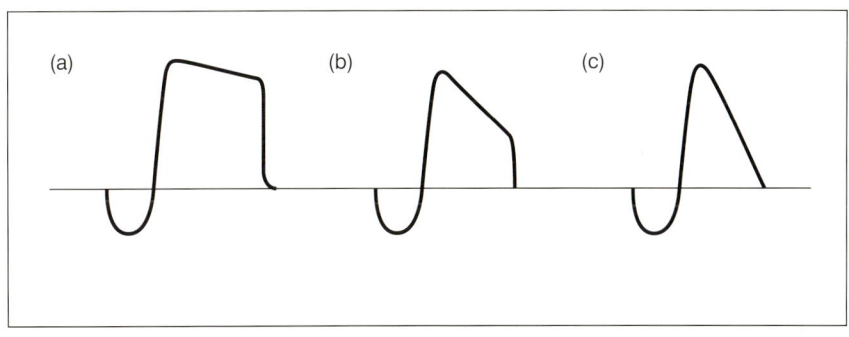

Figure 5.21 – The shape of the continuous wave Doppler trace in (a) mild, (b) moderate and (c) severe aortic regurgitation.

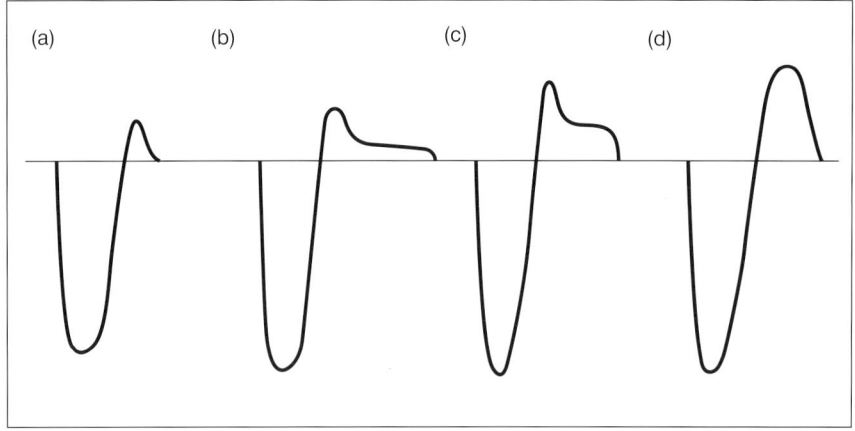

Figure 5.22 – The shape of the pulsed wave Doppler spectral trace in (a) normal, (b) mild, (c) moderate and (d) severe aortic regurgitation (descending aorta).

ASSOCIATED SIGNS OF TRICUSPID STENOSIS
Dilated inferior vena cava and hepatic veins
Dilated right atrium

Tricuspid regurgitation

CAUSES OF TRICUSPID REGURGITATION
Normal (trivial/mild)
Raised pulmonary pressure (lung disease)
Dilated right ventricle and/or right atrium
Pacing wire or other line preventing complete closure
Infective endocarditis
Post mitral valve replacement
Congenital

Mild tricuspid regurgitation can be demonstrated in most patients by means of a continuous wave Doppler examination. Colour flow images often will not demonstrate this small amount of regurgitation. It is good practice to examine the tricuspid valve on the parasternal short axis view with colour flow and continuous wave Doppler as this view will often yield a higher quality Doppler recording.

Although tricuspid regurgitation is not considered clinically significant unless it is severe, it can be useful for estimating right-sided pressures when pulmonary hypertension is suggested[6]. The peak pressure of the regurgitant jet on the continuous wave spectral trace can be measured and converted into a right ventricular systolic pressure. It is assumed that the right atrial pressure is 10 mmHg or less. Bearing this in mind, a peak pressure drop between the right ventricle and atrium of less than 25 mmHg indicates that there is no pulmonary hypertension (Table 5.3). However, it must be noted that this is only an *estimate* of the degree of hypertension and does not given an absolute value, as the pressure in an individual's right atrium is not actually known. In cases where the right atrial pressure is high, the right ventricular pressure might be underestimated.[7]

It is possible that a cor pulmonale (primary lung disease) may be diagnosed from the measurement if no other causes of a high right-sided pressure (e.g. significant mitral stenosis or regurgitation, pulmonary valve stenosis, ventricular septal defect) can be identified.

Tricuspid regurgitation is actually quantified using colour flow Doppler. The amount of regurgitation is not related to right-sided pressures, and a high pressure drop observed on the spectral trace does not indicate a large amount of regurgitation. It is beneficial to use colour flow on both the parasternal short axis and apical four chamber view when quantifying tricuspid regurgitation (and for placement of the continuous wave beam). On good colour flow images it may be possible to detect more than one regurgitant jet.

Table 5.3 – Suggested peak pressure drop values for grading pulmonary hypertension

Degree of pulmonary hypertension	Peak pressure drop★ (mmHg)
Normal	25
Mild	25 – 40
Moderate	40 – 60
Severe	> 60

★ Measured on the tricuspid regurgitant jet.

Quantifying tricuspid regurgitation is performed in a similar way to that of mitral regurgitation, i.e. by assessing the:

- width of the colour jet at its base (Figure 5.23a)

- extent of colour flow within the right atrium (Figure 5.23a)

- acceleration of flow on ventricular side of valve (Figure 5.23a)

- presence of reversal of flow in the inferior vena cava/hepatic veins.

Severe tricuspid regurgitation may occur following mitral valve replacement surgery.[8]

ASSOCIATED SIGNS OF SIGNIFICANT TRICUSPID REGURGITATION
Dilated right atrium
Reversal of flow in the inferior vena cava
Volume overloaded or hyperdynamic RV

Pulmonary valve disease

Acquired pulmonary valve disease is extremely rare. The main hurdle in assessing the pulmonary valve is the difficulty in being able to visualise the valve. It can really only be imaged on the parasternal views (long and short axis), and is often obscured by lung (see Chapter 4 on how to best visualise the pulmonary valve).

Pulmonary stenosis

CAUSES OF PULMONARY STENOSIS
Rheumatic disease
Carcinoid disease
Congenital (see Chapter 7)

The leaflets of the pulmonary valve may or may not be thickened. If the leaflets can be visualised, they will be seen to dome on opening. Simply passing a continuous wave Doppler cursor through the valve and measuring the maximum resultant pressure drop does not given an accurate representation of the valve function, because flow in the right ventricular outflow tract already has significantly increased velocity. The modified Bernoulli equation ($P = 4V^2$) assumes that flow before a valve is negligible. Forward velocity through a normal pul-

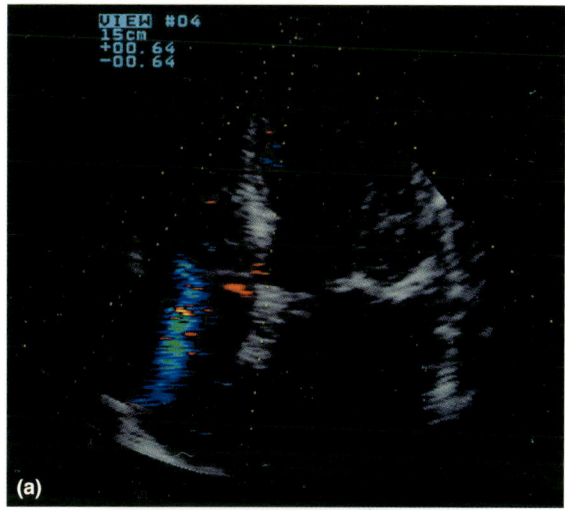

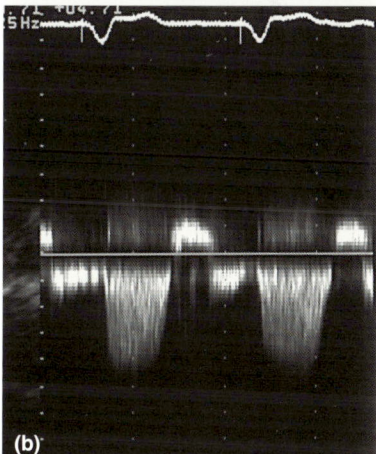

Figure 5.23 – (a) Apical four chamber colour flow image, showing mild tricuspid regurgitation. (b) A continuous wave Doppler spectral trace of tricuspid regurgitation, showing the characteristic envelope shape, caused by fast acceleration and deceleration of flow, with a flat-topped peak.

monary valve will be increased if there is right ventricular volume overload (e.g. significant pulmonary regurgitation or a septal defect). To obtain a representative pressure drop across the pulmonary valve, pulsed wave Doppler must be used. The velocity of flow both just proximal and just distal to the valve needs to be measured, and a slightly more complex version of the Bernoulli equation applied:

$$P = 4(V_2^2 - V_1^2)$$

where V_1 and V_2 are the velocities just proximal to and just distal to the pulmonary valve, respectively.

> **ASSOCIATED SIGNS OF SIGNIFICANT PULMONARY STENOSIS**
> Right ventricular hypertrophy
> Turbulent aliased colour flow in pulmonary artery
> Post-stenotic dilatation of pulmonary artery

Pulmonary regurgitation

> **CAUSES OF PULMONARY REGURGITATION**
> Normal (mild)
> Functional (dilated pulmonary artery and/or right ventricular outflow tract)
> Raised pulmonary pressure
> Rheumatic disease
> Degenerative disease
> Infective endocarditis
> Carcinoid disease
> Congenital (see Chapter 7)

A small amount of pulmonary regurgitation can be detected in the majority of patients. It can be visualised on colour flow as a small red flame extending for a centimetre or two into the right ventricular outflow tract (Figure 5.24a). The greater the amount of regurgitation, the wider the flame will appear on colour flow and the further it will extend into the right ventricular outflow tract and the right ventricle. Continuous wave Doppler is quite sensitive in detecting pulmonary regurgitation, even in patients with a poor two-dimensional image. The resultant spectral trace is similar to that of aortic regurgitation (Figure 5.24b).

> **ASSOCIATED SIGNS OF SIGNIFICANT PULMONARY REGURGITATION**
> Right ventricular volume overload
> Right ventricular dilatation

Pulmonary hypertension

> **CAUSES OF PULMONARY HYPERTENSION**
> Mitral valve or other left heart disease
> Respiratory disease   – primary
>   – secondary (eg embolic, chronic lung disease)
> Congenital   – secondary to increased flow or pressure

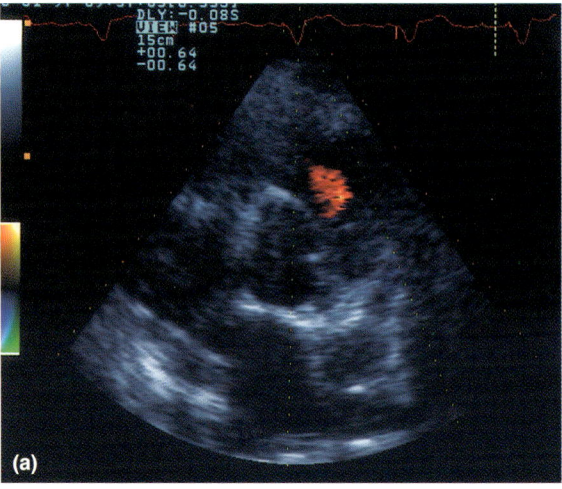

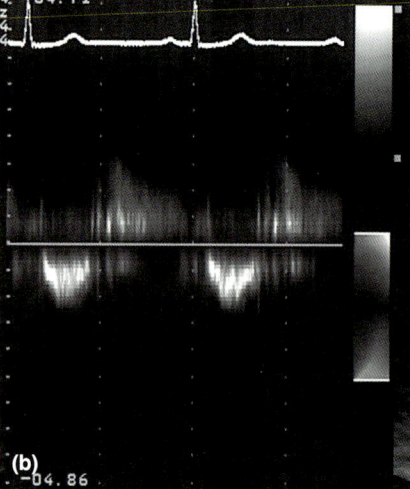

Figure 5.24 – Mild pulmonary regurgitation: (a) parasternal short axis colour flow Doppler image; (b) the corresponding continuous wave Doppler spectral trace.

In the absence of pulmonary stenosis, pulmonary pressures can be estimated reasonably accurately by measuring the maximum velocity of tricuspid regurgitation (see the section on tricuspid regurgitation earlier in this chapter). If no tricuspid regurgitation can be detected in a patient, another method of assessing the presence of pulmonary hypertension is to measure the pulmonary acceleration time as described in Chapter 4.

Patients without pulmonary hypertension have a pulmonary acceleration time above 100 ms. In patients that have significant pulmonary hypertension the peak velocity will occur sooner, and the acceleration time will be less than 100 ms. This measurement does not grade the degree of hypertension, as does the peak pressure drop of tricuspid regurgitation, but only indicates the presence or absence of it.

Infective endocarditis

Infective endocarditis is a bacterial infection of the heart. It may involve one or more of the four heart valves. It may also involve pacing wires or other indwelling catheters in the right heart. In very rare instances it can affect the myocardium. Infective endocarditis commonly occurs on a valve that is previously diseased (e.g. congenital heart disease, prolapsing leaflet). However, this is not always the case, and normal valves may also be affected.[9]

Left-sided valves are more commonly infected in cases of bacteraemia. Right-sided infective endocarditis is much rarer but is becoming more frequent. It is found in intravenous drug abusers and patients with right-sided lines (e.g. a pacing wire). The pulmonary valve is very rarely involved but needs to be investigated if the patient has a right-sided risk. If the patient has a septal defect, the infection can spread from one side of the heart to the other. Prosthetic heart valves and other material are strong predisposing causes of infective endocarditis (see the section on prosthetic valves later in this chapter).

It is important that infective endocarditis is diagnosed quickly because of the risks of sepsis, haemodynamic consequences and embolisms. Hence referrals with a clinical indication of infective endocarditis should be dealt with urgently. As it takes 48 hours to obtain the results of blood cultures (microbiological diagnosis), an echocardiogram may provide the first diagnosis of infective endocarditis.

CLINICAL SIGNS OF INFECTIVE ENDOCARDITIS
Pyrexia
New murmur
± positive blood cultures
± splinter haemorrhages
± signs of CVA or pulmonary embolus.

In its active state, infective endocarditis can affect heart valves in one or more of the following ways:

- vegetations (infected thrombotic masses on or near valves)
- tears or perforations of the valve leaflets

- ruptured chordae
- valve ring abscesses.

Vegetations

Vegetations are composed of fibrin and platelets encasing the bacteria. They have varied echocardiographic appearances (Figures 5.25 and 5.26).

(i) Mobile (pedunculated) mass(es) of increased echogenicity attached to a valve leaflet will be seen on

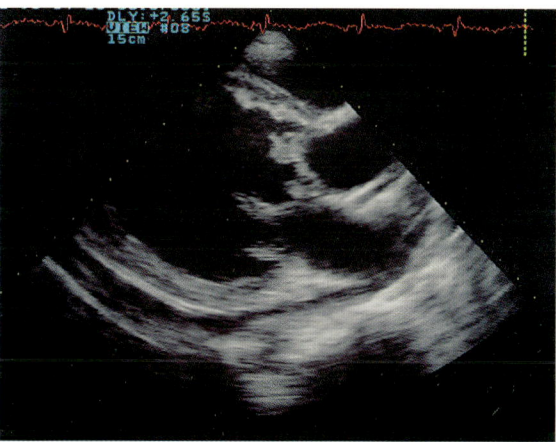

Figure 5.25 – Parasternal long axis view of two irregular, mobile masses on the aortic valve, which on surgery proved to be vegetations on a bicuspid valve. Note also the small amount of pericardial effusion. The patient also had associated severe aortic regurgitation, which accounts for the dilated left ventricle.

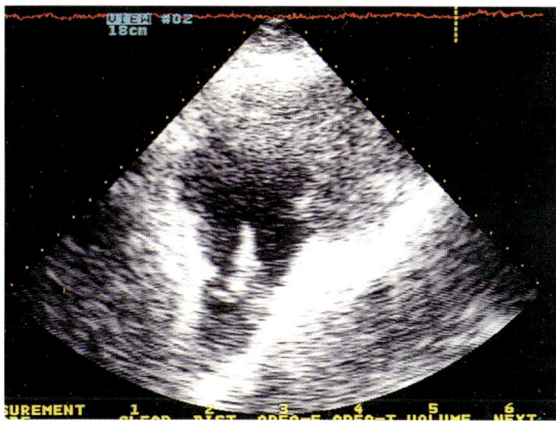

Figure 5.26 – Modified short axis parasternal projection of a vegetation on the pulmonary valve. This is a rare finding, but the pulmonary valve should always be checked in cases of suspected infective endocarditis.

real-time scanning to flick through the valve orifice during the cardiac cycle. They may be large and obvious (vegetations on the right side of the heart tend to be larger[9] or very small and difficult to detect in patients with poor echo windows. Transthoracic scanning is not sufficiently sensitive to demonstrate vegetations less than 2 mm (the resolution of the ultrasound) in size, and consequently vegetations can never be completely excluded. Transoesophageal studies may be indicated.

(ii) Thin mobile strands that can easily be confused with flail chordae. It is not possible to differentiate between the two on the basis of their echocardiographic appearances. The fine strands can be seen to pass through the valve orifice during the cardiac cycle.

(iii) Vegetations may adhere along the surface of a leaflet making it appear thickened. The leaflet will show an increased echogenicity. The appearance on the image is very similar to that of degenerative valve disease, and it is not possible to differentiate between the two diseases on the echocardiogram.

Tears and perforations

Infective endocarditis can erode a valve cusp. This is best demonstrated on colour flow Doppler, where a regurgitant jet can be demonstrated at some distance from the coaptation site. There can be multiple perforations on one leaflet, which appear on the images as many colour flow regurgitant jets. If this occurs on a mitral valve, flow convergence on the ventricular side of the valve will help to pinpoint the site(s) of perforation. Short axis views with colour flow will help to determine if the regurgitation is through the body of a leaflet or through an incompetent orifice.

If a leaflet is infected, it will become weakened and may tear. This typically results in significant regurgitation. The short axis view will help decide which leaflet is affected.

Ruptured chordae

Ruptured chordae can be due to factors other than infective endocarditis. Thus, although the presence of ruptured chordae can be confirmed, this does not implicate infective endocarditis as the cause. Flail chordae can mimic strand-like vegetations, and other clinical data are needed to make the diagnosis of infective endocarditis.

Valve ring abscesses

Abscesses are often difficult to visualise transthoracically. The site of an abscess will demonstrate thickening of the surrounding tissue, but the tissue involved retains the same echogenicity and is not always obvious. The abscess may contain blood flow and/or cystic areas. Colour flow can help delineate the abscess if it contains flow. Most typically, abscesses occur around the annulus of a valve and will demonstrate regurgitation. The aortic valve annulus is the most common site. Abscesses may also occur in the aortic root or within the myocardium. These are very difficult to detect unless they perforate, in which case colour flow Doppler should help identify the area. The best way to assess abscesses is by transoesophageal echocardiography.

Differential diagnoses

- Thrombus can form on valve leaflets and pacing wires and has similar appearances to pedunculated vegetations.

- Degeneration of valve leaflets, especially if irregular, can mimic laminar vegetations.

- A previous echo can act as a baseline and may prove very useful in cases of questionable results.

Because of the difficulty in detecting very small vegetations and in imaging abscesses, infective endocarditis can never be completely excluded by echocardiography, and this fact should be stated on the report if no obvious sign of infective endocarditis can be found. Although transoesophageal echo may help with better resolution, active infective endocarditis can really only be excluded by blood cultures.

Valve replacements

Infective endocarditis on a prosthetic valve is very difficult to detect, especially on mechanical valves, due to poor visibility of the valve. Unless there is a large obvious vegetation or dehiscence, transoesophageal echocardiography is the examination of choice. Abscess formation around an aortic valve replacement is a typical finding. However, even transoesophageal imaging is not definitive, and the final diagnosis must rely on microbiological findings and clinical symptoms.

Follow-up

After a course of antibiotics, most patients are referred for a follow-up echocardiographic examination. This may show a reduction in size of a vegetation or, as occurs in many cases, no change at all. It is not possible to determine by echocardiography if a vegetation is from a previous episode or active infective endocarditis.

If a valve becomes perforated or torn by the infective endocarditis, valve replacement is the normal treatment. Infected prostheses must be replaced. Abscesses are very difficult to treat, and therapy can last for many months.

Prosthetic valves

Prosthetic valves come in a variety of different forms (Figure 5.27), but they are basically of two types: bioprostheses or mechanical prostheses. Bioprostheses are most commonly porcine (pig valve). Other forms of bioprostheses include valves crafted from pericardium and more recently, homografts (treated human heart valves). All bioprostheses have three leaflets attached to a sewing ring (of man-made material). The leaflets are suspended from three stents, or pillars, projecting from the valve sewing ring in the direction of flow. The leaflets open in a physiological manner and on closure there should be no significant regurgitation (Figure 5.28).

The advantage of a bioprosthesis over a mechanical prosthesis is that the patient does not generally need anticoagulation therapy. The disadvantage is the life

expectancy of the valve, which is about 10 years. Some vales degenerate sooner due to a wide range of disease processes that include cusp thickening (causing stenosis), torn cusps, calcific deposits, thrombi formation and infective endocarditis. Although the sewing ring creates acoustic shadowing posteriorly, it is normally possible to visualise the leaflets.

Mechanical valves have a longer life expectancy (up to or exceeding 20 years) than bioprostheses, but require that the patient be anticoagulated for the rest of his or her life. There are a number of different mechanical prostheses *in situ* in patients, including the older ball and cage type (Starr-Edwards), or the single or bileaflet tilting disc types, the former most commonly being of the Bjorck-Shiley type and the latter being from a variety of manufacturers (e.g. St Jude and Medtronic). Mechanical valves are available in a variety of sizes, depending on the size of the orifice into which it is to be stitched. A mechanical valve causes so much reflection of the ultrasound beam from its surface, with associated reverberation artefact posteriorly, that all definition of the prosthesis is lost. Any structures posterior to the prosthesis (in relation to the incident beam) are not only obliterated by the reverberation artefact but are also acoustically shadowed. This causes problems when assessing regurgitation through mitral or tricuspid prostheses.

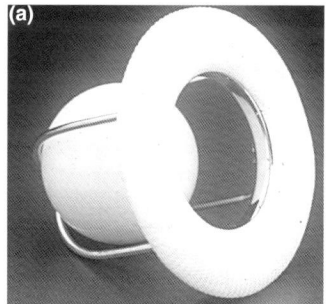
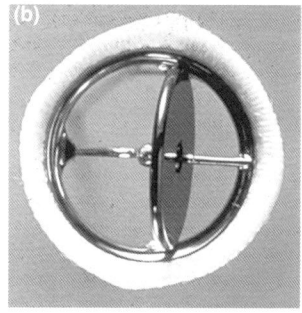
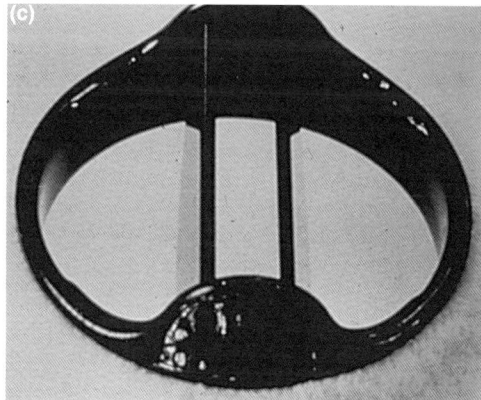
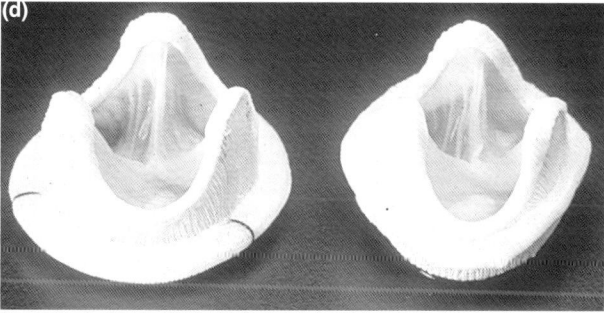

Figure 5.27 – Types of prosthetic valve: (a) ball and cage (Starr–Edwards); (b) single tilting disc (Bjorck–Shiley); (c) bileaflet tilting disc (St Jude); (d) porcine. *(Reproduced courtesy of Baxter and Medtronic).*

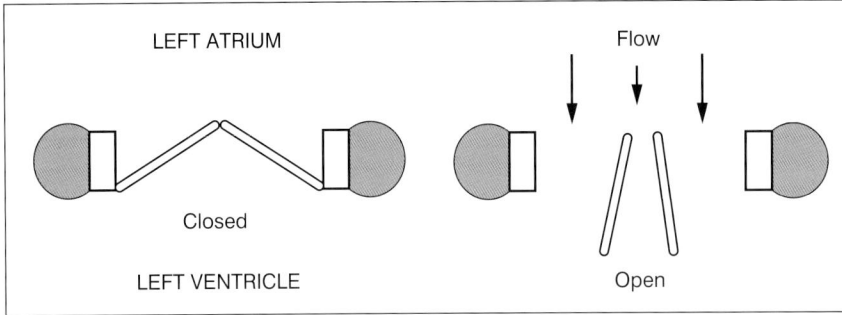

LEFT ATRIUM

Flow

Closed

Open

LEFT VENTRICLE

Figure 5.28 – Cross sectional view of the mechanism of movement of a bileaflet mechanical valve.

By their nature, all prosthetic valves are more obstructive than a normal native valve. This means that forward velocities across prosthetic valves will be higher than those across native valves. Because of the large range of normal velocities (aortic valve replacements) and pressure half times (mitral and tricuspid valve replacements) that have been quoted for each size of each type of prosthesis, it is extremely difficult to interpret individual measurements. Besides, the echocardiographer is not always informed of the type and size of the prosthesis. A patient's worsening symptoms can be due to factors other than deteriorating prosthetic function (e.g. left ventricular dysfunction). For these reasons it is suggested that a baseline study is performed on every patient undergoing a valve replacement before they leave hospital or at their first postoperative outpatient appointment. This baseline measurement should not be too early in the postoperative period, and should reflect the patient's normal outpatient medication. This will establish the 'individual normal' measurement for each patient. When follow-up scans are then performed, they can be compared with this baseline scan rather than a very wide ranging list of published normal measurements.

All mechanical prostheses give rise to a small amount of regurgitation as part of their normal function. These small regurgitant jets, often called 'washing jets', occur around the edges of the closed leaflets, inside the mechanical ring of the valve. They are usually small and are quite different to paraprosthetic jets which lie outside the sewing ring and are invariably abnormal.

ROCKING OF A PROSTHESIS

A rocking movement of a mitral prosthesis may be normal if the prosthesis is sewn to an original valve cusp rather than the valve annulus, but this attachment is unusual. Rocking movement should be recorded on the baseline scan. More usually, rocking of the mitral valve

is due to dehiscence, and it should be possible to visualise the area where the detachment has occurred. A significant amount of regurgitation will be present.

An aortic prosthesis should not present any rocking motion. If this can be visualised, it indicates dehiscence of the prosthesis, and regurgitation will be present.

PARAPROSTHETIC LEAK

This is regurgitation of blood around the outside of the prosthetic valve, through the sewing line. It may be due to an incorrectly positioned prosthesis, to some sutures having pulled through necrotic tissue, or to infective endocarditis. Paraprosthetic regurgitation and its differentiation from transprosthetic regurgitation is described in the section on each valve type, below.

When assessing flow through prostheses, Doppler filters should be increased to reduce the noise due to movement from the spectral trace. Increasing compression and rejection (if possible) will also give a clearer trace.

Mitral valve replacements

Mitral bioprostheses can be examined without too much difficulty. The leaflets can be viewed from all standard views, and M-mode traces can be obtained. The stents on which many bioprostheses are mounted can be seen clearly on the apical four chamber view. To assess forward flow, the pulsed wave sample volume should be placed at the leaflet tips, as for a native mitral valve. This will be similar to the level of the tips of the stents. Colour flow examination can help with placement of the sample volume if the forward flow is eccentric. There is one large central jet in bioprostheses. Although most studies have shown that mitral bioprosthetic flow is similar to that of native mitral valve flow, the Hatle formula[10] for converting a pressure half time measurement to an orifice area does not necessarily apply accurately, and should not be used.

The pressure half time is a valid measurement and can be compared on subsequent scans. An increase in the pressure half time indicates increasing obstruction of the prosthesis. Because most patients are in atrial fibrillation, at least three waveforms should be measured and a range of pressure half times quoted. The peak and mean forward velocities should also be recorded. In the absence of significant mitral regurgitation, a forward velocity of over 2.5 m/s indicates obstruction. A pressure half time above 200 ms also indicates obstruction. With a bioprosthesis a small amount of acoustic shadowing is present posterior to the sewing ring. The amount of shadowing will not inhibit the colour flow display, and mitral regurgitation can be assessed in the usual way.

Mechanical prostheses pose more of a problem than bioprostheses, because of the reduced visibility of the valve itself and the left atrium. Forward flow through a mechanical valve may consist of one, two or three separate jets, depending on the type of valve. In the older Starr-Edwards type valve (ball and cage) the flow is peripheral, passing around each side of the central ball (Figure 5.29). In the case of single or bileaflet valves the flow will be more central but will be divided into two streams (single leaflet valve, e.g. Bjorck-Shiley) or three streams (bileaflet valve, e.g. St Jude or Medtronic). Colour flow imaging should be used to place the pulsed wave sample volume in the largest of the jets in the most aliased part of the flow, just on the ventricular side of the prosthesis. Most forward jets are eccentric and directed towards the interventricular septum. The peak and mean

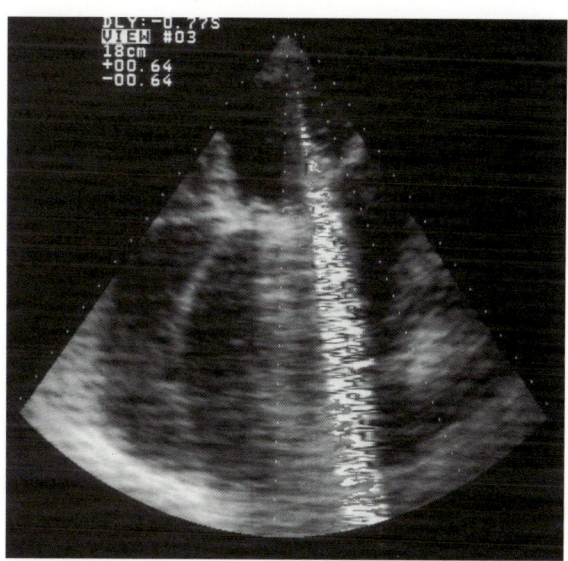

Figure 5.30 – Apical four chamber view showing colour flow 'flash' artefact superimposed on the left atrium. The artefact is caused by a prosthetic mitral valve.

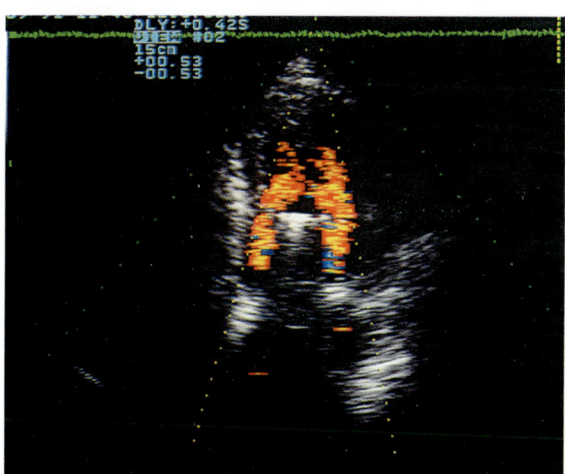

Figure 5.29 – Apical four chamber colour flow image showing two steams of forward flow through a Starr–Edwards (ball and cage) prosthetic valve.

forward velocities and a range of pressure half times should be recorded. The valve area cannot be calculated from the pressure half time measurement.

Due to acoustic shadowing posterior to a mechanical mitral valve replacement, mitral regurgitation is only detected in about 60% of cases in which it is present.[11] For this reason much care needs to be taken when checking for the presence of mitral regurgitation. Apart from a low-velocity closing volume and trivial washing jets, mechanical valves do not typically exhibit transprosthetic regurgitation. Flashes of colour are often seen within the left atrium, but do not last throughout systole and are artefactual (Figure 5.30). Important transprosthetic regurgitation will occur in mechanical valves if they are unable to close completely. This may be due to thrombus formation, growth of tissue into the orifice or infective endocarditis. If a significant amount of regurgitation is detected through a bioprosthesis, it is most probably due to degeneration of the leaflets. Significant regurgitation from a mechanical valve is most commonly paraprosthetic.

Continuous wave Doppler interrogation can be used to detect regurgitation. By slowly moving the continuous wave beam through the entirety of the left atrium, it should be possible to determine whether there is any regurgitation present and, if so, whether it is transprosthetic or paraprosthetic. Although continuous wave

Doppler traces will show the presence of regurgitation, it is not possible to quantify it from the spectral trace. If mitral prosthetic regurgitation is detected by continuous wave Doppler, it is often necessary for a transoesophageal echocardiogram to be recorded to quantify it.

'Flow convergence' is the term used to describe the phenomenon of flow acceleration on the left ventricular side of the mitral valve (Figure 5.31), which can help to draw attention to the presence and site of regurgitation. Easily detectable flow convergence seen on the apical four chamber view usually indicates at least moderate mitral regurgitation. If there is a significant amount of regurgitation the left ventricle will demonstrate volume overload and the forward velocity through the mitral prosthesis will be raised, while pressure half time will remain within the normal range.

Aortic valve replacements

Aortic bioprostheses tend to be slightly less obstructive than mechanical valves and have forward velocities slightly raised above native valve levels. Normal forward flow through a mechanical aortic valve can be quite high, particularly through the smaller sized valves (e.g. 19 and 21 mm). Velocities can vary widely and depend on volume flow (e.g. significant aortic regurgitation will result in an increased forward velocity, mimicking obstruction). It is therefore important to note the

function of the left ventricle and to grade any regurgitation when assessing forward aortic flow. As a general rule, if there is good left ventricular function and no or mild aortic regurgitation, velocities of over 4 m/s indicate obstruction. The mean velocity should also be measured. A normal mean velocity is roughly half the peak velocity. If the mean is much greater than half the peak and or above 3 m/s, this also indicates obstruction.

A more accurate way to assess aortic valvular flow is by use of the continuity equation (provided an accurate diameter of the left ventricular outflow tract can be measured). A valve orifice area of less than 1 cm² indicates obstruction. Another method for assessing prosthetic function is to note the shape of the curve of the continuous wave spectral trace. In an obstructed valve the acceleration time will be increased and the peak velocity will be attained later in systole (Figure 5.32)[12]

Regurgitation through an aortic valve prosthesis can be assessed, as for that through a native aortic valve, on the apical four chamber view, as there is no artefact anterior to the valve. Most mechanical valves exhibit a small amount of regurgitation which is considered normal. Single leaflet or bileaflet mechanical valves will show small 'washing jets' of regurgitation (Figure 5.33). Paravalvular regurgitation can be difficult to differentiate from transvalvular regurgitation due to the close proximity of the sewing ring to the walls of the aorta. Colour flow imaging in the parasternal short axis view can help to clarify the situation.

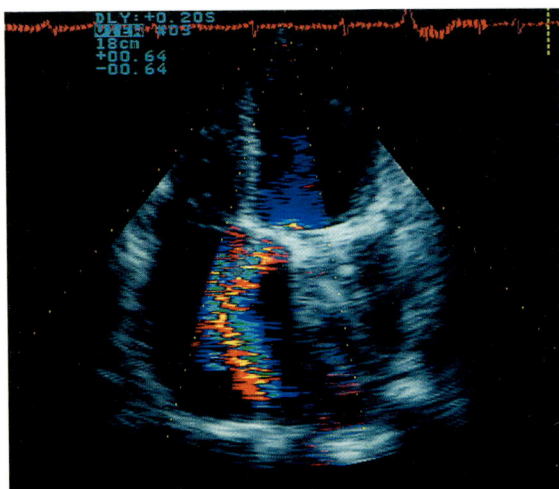

Figure 5.31 – Paraprosthetic leak around a mechanical mitral valve. The colour in the left atrium (which is unusual) is due to the large size of the left atrium in this patient and a highly eccentric jet. Note the convergence of flow in the left ventricle at the site of the defect.

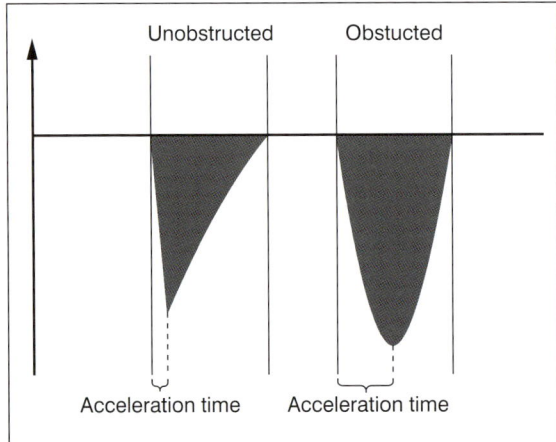

Figure 5.32 – Spectral trace recorded through an unobstructed (short acceleration time) and obstructed (longer acceleration time) aortic valve prosthesis. The valve clicks are much more pronounced than those seen for a native aortic valve.

Other observations can be used to help grade the regurgitation, such as left ventricular volume overload and reversal of flow in the descending aorta.

Tricuspid valve replacements

The evaluation of tricuspid prostheses is similar to that of mitral prostheses. Forward flow is assessed by pulsed wave Doppler. These forward velocities tend to be lower than for mitral prostheses, but the pressure half times are longer. A range of pressure half times and the peak and mean velocities should be quoted. Obstruction is indicated if the pressure half time is longer than 200 ms and the forward velocity (in the absence of significant regurgitation) is greater than 1.6 m/s.[13]

Regurgitation needs to be assessed by continuous wave and colour flow Doppler, using flow convergence in the right ventricle as an indication of regurgitation. The right ventricle should be assessed for signs of volume overload seen as a dilated, hyperdynamic ventricle.

Pulmonary valve replacements

These are extremely unusual in acquired heart disease and will be encountered in patients with congenital heart disease. They are most often used in the reconstruction of the outflow tract to the right ventricle in patients with pulmonary atresia. They are also used in the Ross procedure, in which the patient's own pulmonary valve is transferred to the aortic position (in cases of congenital aortic stenosis) and the pulmonary valve is replaced by a homograft prosthesis. Pulmonary valve replacements are usually of the biological type due to their lower incidence of thrombus formation.

Further reading

Chambers J, Fraser A, Lawford P, Nihoyannopoulos P, Simpson I. Echocardiographic assessment of artificial heart valves: British Society of Echocardiography position paper. *Br Heart J* 1994; **71**(Suppl): 6–14.

References

1. Utsunomiya T, Patel D, Doshi R, Quan M, Gardin JM. Can signal intensity of the continuous wave Doppler regurgitant jet estimate severity of mitral regurgitation? *Am Heart J* 1992; **123**: 166–171.

2. Chambers JB. *Clinical Echocardiography*. British Medical Journal Publications; London, 1995.

3. Jawad IA. *A Practical Guide to* Echocardiography and Cardiac Doppler Ultrasound. Little, Brown; Boston, 1990.

4. Samstad SO, Hengrenaes L, Skjaerpe T, Hatle L. Half time of the diastolic aortoventricular pressure difference by continuous wave Doppler ultrasound: a measure of the severity of aortic regurgitation? *Br Heart J* 1989; **61**: 336–343.

5. Jobic Y, Siama M, Tribouilloy C *et al.* Doppler echocardiographic evaluation of valve regurgitation in healthy volunteers. *Br Heart J* 1993; **2**: 109–113.

6. Berger M, Haimowitz A, van Tosh A, Berdoff RL, Goldberg E. Quantitative assessment of pulmonary hypertension in patients with tricuspid regurgitation using continuous wave Doppler ultrasound. *J Am Coll Cardiol* 1985; **6**: 359–365.

7. Simpson IA, de Belder MA, Kenny A, Martin M, Nihoyannopoulos P, on behalf of the British Society of Echocardiography. How to quantitate valve regurgitation by echo Doppler techniques. *Br Heart J* 1995; **73**(Suppl 2): 1–9.

8. Groves PH, Ikram S, Ingold U, Hal RJ. Tricuspid regurgitation following mitral valve replacement: an echocardiographic study. *J Heart Valve Disease* 1993; **2**(3): 273–278.

9. Andy JJ, Sheikh MU, Ali N *et al.* Echocardiographic observations in opiate addicts with active infective endocarditis. Frequency of involvement of the various valves and comparison of echocardiographic features of right- and left-sided cardiac valve endocarditis. *Am J Cardiol* 1977; **40**: 17–23.

10. Hatle L, Angelsen B. *Doppler Ultrasound in Cardiology*, Lea & Febiger, Philadelphia; 1982.

11. Bargiggia GS, Tronconi L, Raisaro A *et al.* Colour Doppler diagnosis of mechanical mitral regurgitation: usefulness of the flow convergence region proximal to the regurgitant orifice. *Am Heart J* 1990; **120**: 1137–1142.

12. Wranne B, Baumgartner H, Flachskampf F, Hasenkam M, Pinto F. Stenotic lesions. *Heart* 1996; **73**(Suppl 2): 36–42.

13. Pye M, Weerasana N, Bain WH, Hutton I, Cobbe SM. Doppler echocardiographic characteristics of normal and dysfunctioning prosthetic valves in the tricuspid and mitral position. *Br Heart J* 1990; **63**: 41–44.

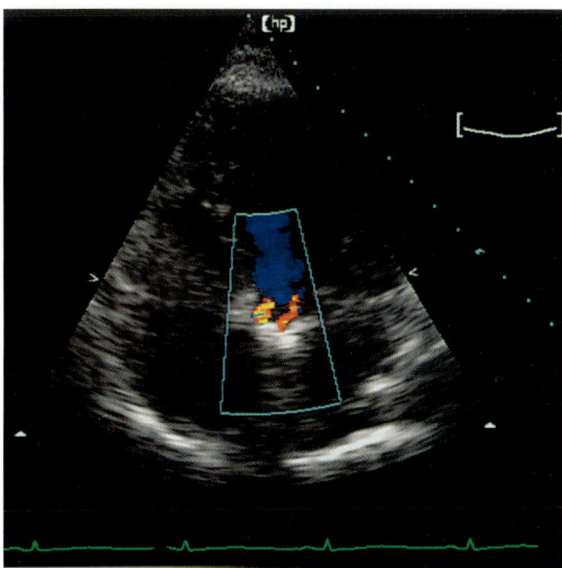

Figure 5.33 – Apical four chamber view demonstrating normal washing jets through an aortic valve prosthesis

6

HEART-MUSCLE DISEASE, PERICARDIAL DISEASE AND OTHER ACQUIRED CONDITIONS

Cardiomyopathies
Ischaemic heart disease
Myocardial infarction
Left ventricular hypertrophy
Right ventricular hypertrophy
Left ventricular dilation
Left ventricular volume overload
Right ventricular dilation
Pericardial disease
Aortic disease
Thrombus
Tumours
Implants
Interatrial aneurysm

Cardiomyopathies

Cardiomyopathy is primary disease of the heart muscle, often with no identifiable cause. It is divided into three main categories:

- dilated cardiomyopathy
- hypertrophic cardiomyopathy
- restrictive cardiomyopathy.

Dilated cardiomyopathy

Dilated cardiomyopathy is characterised by severe dilatation and diffuse severe impairment of the left ventricle (Figures 6.1 and 6.2). There are many causes such as postviral infection, alcoholic damage, diffuse ischaemic heart disease, genetic abnormalities, rare toxins and infections. The commonest group is one with no known cause, idiopathic cardiomyopathy. The walls of the ventricle may be thinned and will demonstrate poor systolic thickening. The left atrium will also be dilated. The mitral annular ring becomes stretched, causing functional mitral regurgitation which can sometimes be moderately severe. The cardiomyopathy may also affect the right side of the heart, in which case the right ventricle will be dilated and impaired, with associated tricuspid regurgitation.

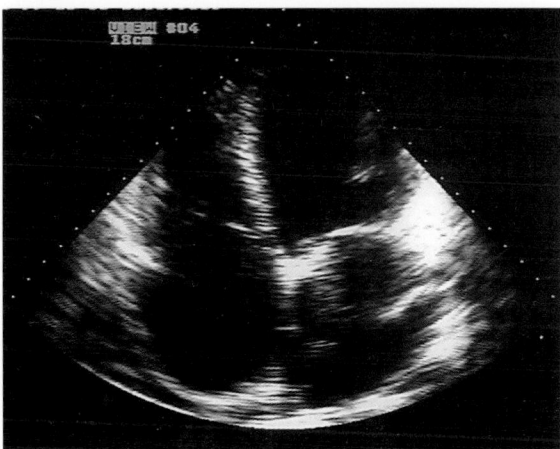

Figure 6.1 – Apical four chamber image of a dilated heart. Although all the chambers look normal in size relative to one another, the centimetre markings down the side of the sector give an indication of their actual size. Real-time scanning would show poorly contracting ventricles.

SIGNS OF DILATED CARDIOMYOPATHY
Dilated left ventricle and atrium (possible right-sided involvement)
Poorly contractile left ventricle
Thinned myocardium

Due to stasis of blood in a poorly contractile ventricle, dilated cardiomyopathy ventricles are particularly at risk of the formation of thrombus. The left ventricle and, if involved, the right ventricle should be scanned in all planes to assess for thrombus.

PITFALLS

Long-standing significant valve disease, such as aortic stenosis or regurgitation or mitral regurgitation, can produce the same effect on the left ventricle. It is therefore important that valves are carefully assessed. (Remember that low cardiac output from a poor left ventricle will underestimate the degree of aortic stenosis, if present.) Coronary artery disease with myocardial infarction can also leave the left ventricle impaired. In such cases, however, it is likely that regional differences in contractility can be detected. Occasionally, dilated cardiomyopathy can present with some regional wall-function differences. Left ventricular dilatation and dysfunction caused by known factors, e.g. viral or alcohol, will produce similar echocardiographic appearances,[1] but still tend to be termed a cardiomyopathy. The cause of dilated cardiomyopathy cannot be diagnosed from the echocardiogram alone and results from a variety of other examinations are needed.

Hypertrophic cardiomyopathy (HCM)

Hypertrophic cardiomyopathy is an inherited disease where there is unexplained hypertrophy of the ventricular myocardium. There are characteristic derangements at the cellular level and there are genetic markers. The condition sometimes presents with chest pain or syncope and often is detected following a routine examination where a murmur or abnormal electrocardiograph (ECG) is discovered. Occasionally, and tragically, it may first present with sudden death.

The condition most commonly affects the interventricular septum (55% of cases) (Figure 6.3), but may be concentric (31%) or apical (14%).[2] The right ventricle is also affected in 44% of cases[3] and so the wall thickness of the right ventricle should be measured in all cases.

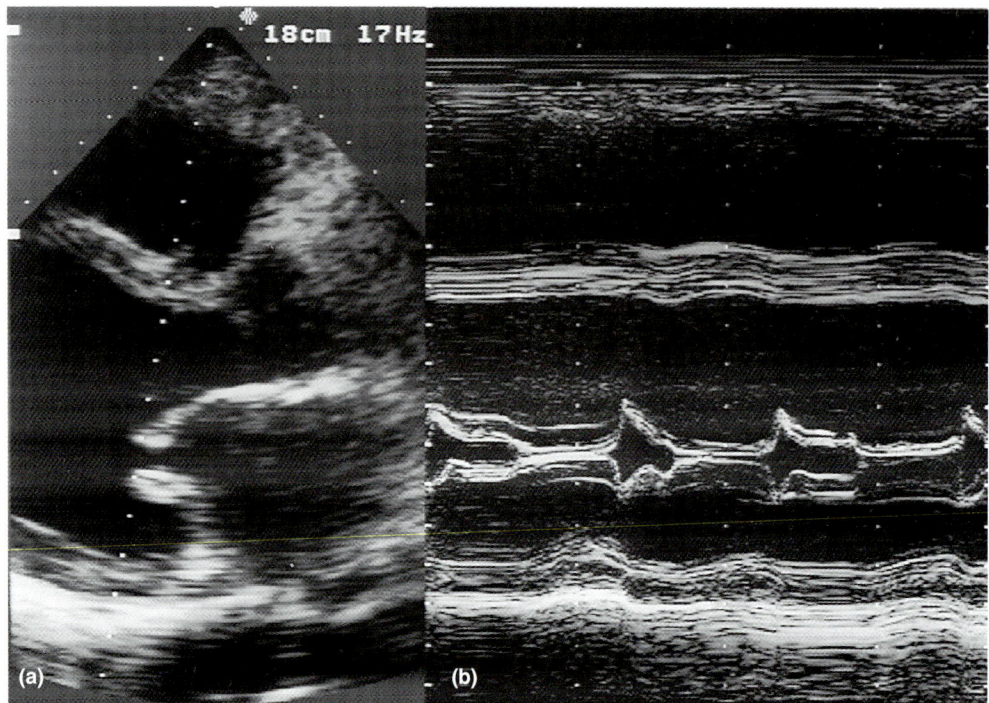

Figure 6.2 – Parasternal long axis view in a patient with dilated cardiomyopathy. (a) Two-dimensional image showing a very dilated left ventricle. The M-mode cursor lies across the base of this ventricle, including the lips of the mitral valve. (b) M-mode trace from (a), showing a very poorly contracting ventricle (end diastolic diameter 6.6 cm, end systolic diameter 6.1 cm). The mitral valve lies far from the interventricular septum due to dilatation of the left ventricle.

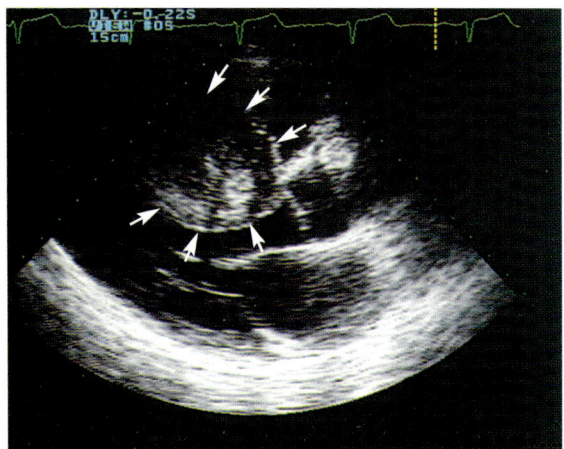

Figure 6.3 – Parasternal long-axis view demonstrating an asymmetrically hypertrophied septum. The hypertrophy is extreme (septal thickness 5 cm); the arrows indicate the edges of the septum.

The condition is frequently referred to as HOCM (pronounced 'hocum'), or hypertrophic obstructive cardiomyopathy, but this is a misleading term, as not all patients have an obstructive element to the condition. The term hypertrophic cardiomyopathy, or HCM, is generally preferred.

There is a collection of signs, some or all of which may be present (see box). It is necessary to determine how much of the left ventricle is hypertrophied. To do this successfully the left ventricle must be imaged in all planes. Difficulties arise in the diagnosis if the hypertrophy is concentric. One typical sign that can help differentiate HCM from other forms of hypertrophy is that the diastolic filling of the left ventricle will be impaired in cases of HCM. Of course, it should be noted that hypertrophy is a natural response to pressure loading over a period of time and HCM is difficult or impossible to diagnose in the presence of aortic stenosis, hypertension or other pressure-loading pathologies.

SIGNS OF HCM
Asymmetrical hypertrophy of the septum, a septum/free wall ratio of at least 1.3:1
Systolic anterior motion (SAM) of the mitral leaflets, causing left ventricular outflow tract (LVOT) gradient
Midsystolic (early) closure of the aortic valve
Hypokinesia of hypertrophied myocardium
A small cavity left ventricle, almost obliterated during systole, a with midcavity gradient
High ejection fraction

If systolic anterior motion of the mitral valve is present, it is usually accompanied by mitral regurgitation which has a similar characteristic spectral Doppler trace to that of the left ventricular outflow tract gradient trace. This phenomenon is detectable on both two-dimensional and M-mode imaging, and involves the tips of the mitral leaflets angling up towards the septum in systole and sometimes causing significant outflow tract obstruction (Figures 6.4 and 6.5). The mechanism is obscure, but is probably related to both altered geometry of the hypertrophied ventricle and altered haemodynamics in the outflow tract. Many abnormalities in this condition are dynamic and may not be present at rest (e.g. during the examination) but might be present during significant exercise. The echocardiographer and the referring physician must both be aware of this.

If a gradient is detected on a continuous wave Doppler image, it will not be possible to determine whether it is an intracavity gradient or a left ventricular outflow tract gradient. The left ventricular cavity needs to be 'mapped' using pulsed wave or colour flow Doppler in order to determine the site of increased velocity (Figure 6.6). Both midcavity and outflow tract obstruction may be present in the same patient.

PITFALLS
Other causes of hypertrophy:

- Isolated right ventricular hypertrophy will cause apparent asymmetry of the septum.

- The basal septum in the elderly often becomes thickened as the angle between the aorta and the left ventricle becomes more acute. The area of hypertrophy is highly localised and usually does not cause obstruction.

- Oblique angulation of the ultrasound beam through the myocardium will cause apparent hypertrophy of the septum. Ensure the beam is perpendicular to the axis of left ventricle when performing measurements.

- Athletes tend to have hypertrophied left ventricles with slightly greater hypertrophy of the septum. The cavity will be large (at the upper limits of normal).

- Systemic hypertension will cause symmetrical hypertrophy.

- There is a racial variation in the thickness of the myocardium, some African Caribbeans having

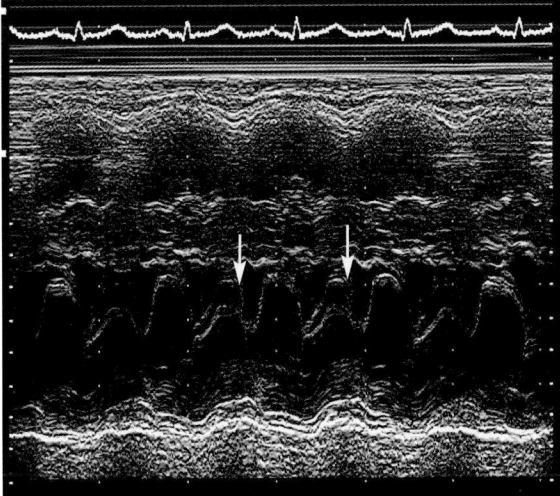

Figure 6.4 M mode trace through the mitral valve in a patient with HCM. Note the hypertrophied septum and, in particular, the marked anterior movement of the mitral leaflets during systole (arrowed).

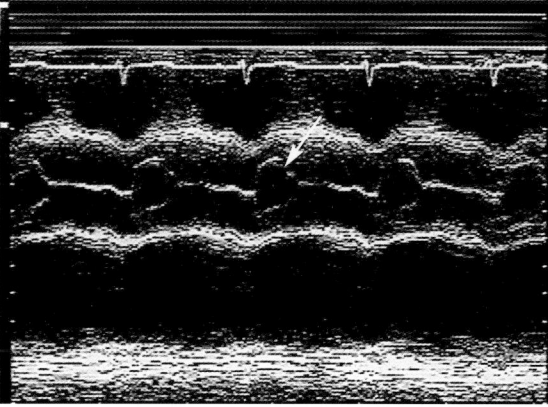

Figure 6.5 – M-mode trace through the aortic valve of a patient with HCM. Note that the aortic valve starts to close (not a square 'box') before the end of systole (early aortic valve closure) (arrowed).

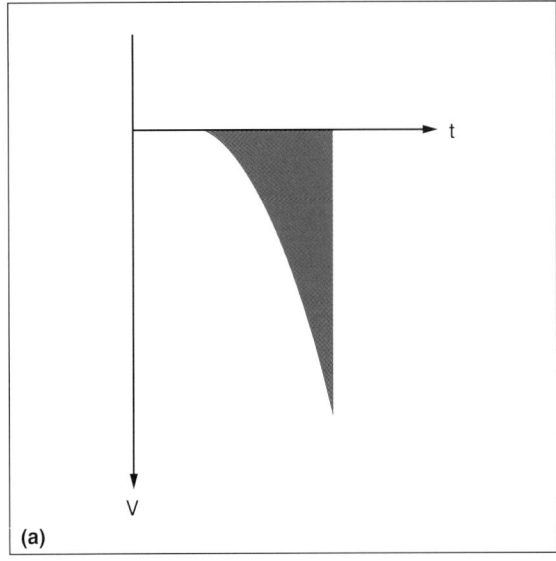
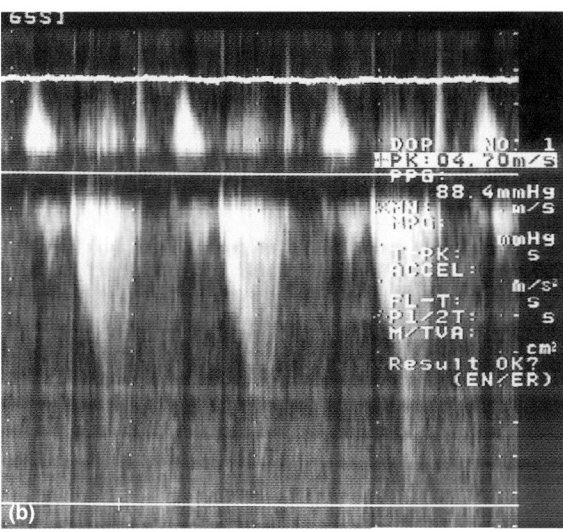

Figure 6.6 – (a) Sketch of a typical spectral trace resulting from an exponential rise in pressure, which drops off immediately at the end of systole, in a cavity or the left ventricular outflow tract. The rise in pressure is accompanied by a characteristic audio signal. (b) Apical recording of a similar trace from a patient with HCM, showing a peak velocity of 4.7 m/s.

slightly larger normal dimensions. Some of these patients also have a more florid hypertrophy response to hypertension.

- Cardiac amyloidosis can mimic HCM. The diagnosis is made clinically, but there are clues on the echo study. The condition is generally more diffuse, and the texture of the echo pattern in the myocardium is slightly more echogenic. There is generally poor contractility.

Other causes of systolic anterior motion of mitral valve:

- Hyperdynamic left ventricle.

- Redundant cusp of a prolapsing mitral valve.

Other causes of early aortic valve closure:

- Membranous subaortic stenosis.

- Severe mitral regurgitation.

Most cases of HCM are diagnosed in early adult life. However, there is a form of the disease that occurs in the elderly; it is often accompanied by calcification of the mitral annulus, which encroaches into the left ventricular outflow tract causing obstruction.

If HCM is diagnosed prior to puberty, follow-up scans should be performed every 6 months as there is rapid acceleration of the disease during puberty. If adults are newly diagnosed it may be worth screening their children in order to pick up any inheritance of the condition.

Restrictive cardiomyopathy

Restrictive cardiomyopathy is the rarest of the cardiomyopathies. The ventricles are not dilated, but both atria are markedly enlarged (Figure 6.7). There is impaired relaxation of both ventricles, which restricts the inflow of blood. Systolic function is usually noted to be normal.

> **SIGNS OF RESTRICTIVE CARDIOMYOPATHY**
> Small-cavity left ventricle
> Normal myocardial thickness
> Enlarged atria
> Impaired left ventricular filling (diastolic restriction)

Pulsed wave Doppler studies of forward mitral flow will help to determine if the left ventricle is affected by a restrictive disease, but a diagnosis of restrictive cardiomyopathy cannot be made on these findings alone.

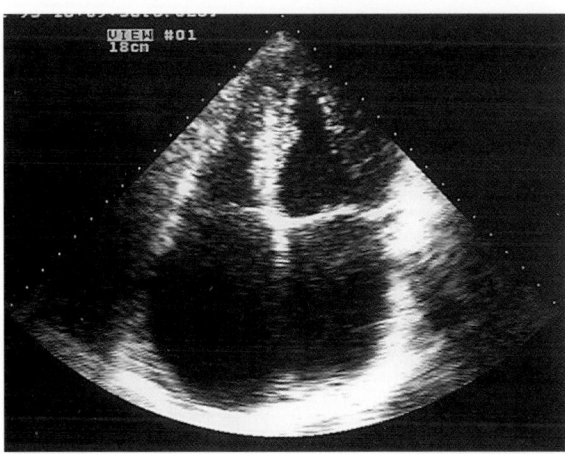

Figure 6.7 – Typical apical four chamber image of a heart showing restrictive cardiomyopathy. Note the normal or small ventricle size and enlarged atria.

If the E/A wave ratio is greater than 2.0 and/or the deceleration time of the E velocity curve is less than 150 ms then a restrictive disease is indicated.[4]

PITFALLS

Constrictive pericarditis can have a similar echocardiographic appearance to that shown by restrictive cardiomyopathy but the atria are usually small.

Ischaemic heart disease

This very common condition, usually but not always caused by coronary atheroma, is responsible for a wide variety of echocardiographic abnormalities. The coronary disease is below the resolution of the ultrasound technique, but the effects of the disease can be clearly seen.

Myocardial infarction

Infarction of the myocardial tissue occurs when there is ischaemia of the myocardium, which leads to cell death. There will be a rise in cardiac enzymes signifying tissue damage and echocardiographic changes, in addition to the classical clinical symptoms. If the infarcted area is small or subendocardial, ECG will often not be able to detect any changes. If the infarction is transendocardial (full thickness), regional wall abnormalities can be detected, the region involved corresponding to the

occluded coronary artery. In most cases the amount of muscle that appears to be affected on ECG will be greater than the actual amount infarcted. There will be reduced contraction in the affected area. *Hypokinesia* refers to contraction that is decreased but still in the same direction as normal. The myocardium will also show reduced thickening in systole. *Akinesia* is when the myocardium is static. *Dyskinesia* occurs when the most damage to myocardial tissue has occurred and the muscle moves out of synchronisation with the rest of the ventricle; often, paradoxical motion (movement in the opposite direction) will result.

In the acute period there may be no change in the appearance of the myocardium. After a few days there may be slight swelling and increased echogenicity due to tissue oedema. In early scans there may be intraventricular thrombus, but this is not easy to see as it is of low density and often disperses quickly without imparting any clinical effect.

Most studies will be on patients with healed infarction. After a few weeks the area of infarction will often have thinned myocardium (< 7 mm) and may be of increased echogenicity which is thought to be due to scar tissue.[5] Increased echogenicity will not usually be seen in the acute stages of myocardial infarction. Cardiac output will be reduced if a significant portion of the myocardium is involved. The ventricle may compensate in a number of ways to maintain output. Hyperkinesia of the surviving myocardium is a common finding where there is increased contractility and thickening of the unaffected muscle. The ventricle may also dilate to increase its output (Figure 6.8).

Although the left ventricle is by far the most usual site of infarction, the right ventricle can also be affected, and in some rare cases is the only ventricle involved. If the right ventricle is involved, it will show the same characteristics of infarction as the left ventricle (i.e. regionally impaired function and dilatation). The septum may also demonstrate paradoxical motion.

If early reperfusion of the myocardium (e.g. by thrombolytic drugs or early angioplasty) is successful, the ischaemic myocardium is referred to as 'stunned' and a follow-up echocardiogram, usually at 6 weeks, may well show normal contractility of the previously affected area.

Complications

PERICARDIAL EFFUSION

Although a small amount of pericardial fluid is typically seen following infarction, a large pericardial effusion

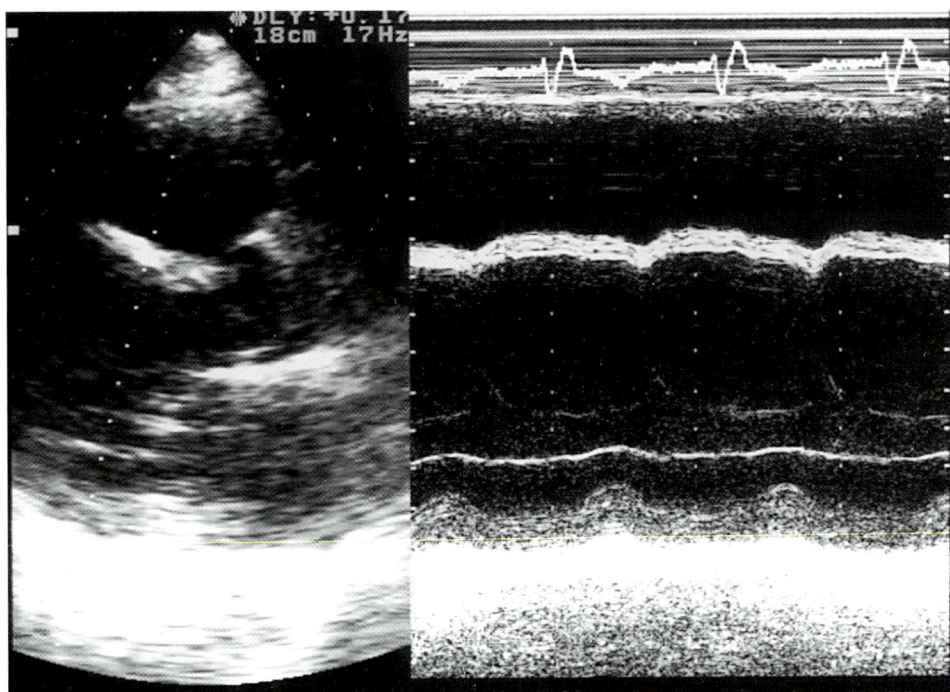

Figure 6.8 – Parasternal long axis view of the left ventricle, and the corresponding M-mode trace showing a thinned and hypokinetic septum of increased echogenicity. This appearance indicates a previous full thickness infarction. Note also the dilated left ventricular cavity.

may accumulate due to an associated pericarditis. There is also a condition called Dressler's syndrome in which a pericardial effusion develops 1 – 8 weeks after the event due to a secondary inflammatory reaction.

RUPTURED MYOCARDIUM

If ischaemia to an area of muscle is sudden and there are no collateral vessels to supply the myocardium, the risk of rupture of the affected myocardium is increased. Severe tissue ischaemia will damage the myocardium to the point where it cannot support its normal pressure stresses. If the septal region is involved, this will lead to a ventricular septal defect (VSD). The most common site for such defects is towards the anterior or apical region, but the posteroinferior area is also an important site. The defects are typically small and difficult to visualise on two-dimensional imaging, but colour flow Doppler will highlight the area and diagnosis can then be quite straightforward (Figure 6.9). The area involved will be akinetic and will often be seen to bulge towards the right ventricle. The apical four chamber view will best demonstrate apical defects, while posterior defects are often better seen from the subcostal position.

Difficulties arise if the VSD is very posterior. Continuous wave Doppler will help to pinpoint the site

of the defect. The velocity of the blood flowing from the left to right ventricle will help to determine the size of

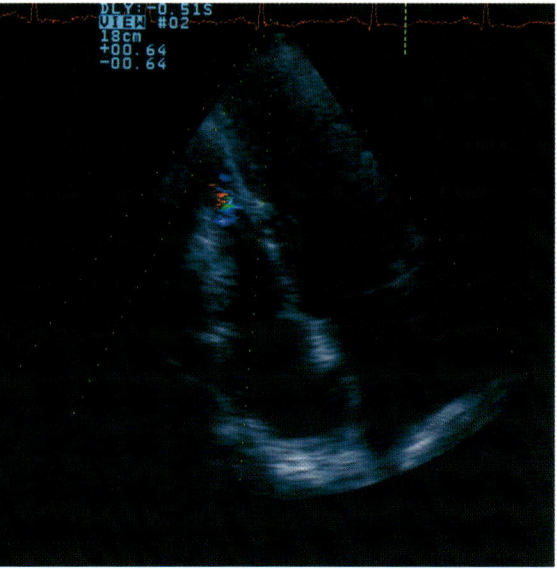

Figure 6.9 – Apical four chamber view illustrating a small apical post-infarction ventricular septal defect. (Colour flow applied to the right ventricle shows, under normal circumstances, no colour at the apex of the right ventricle.)

the VSD. A high velocity indicates a small defect. If the pressures between the ventricles equalise quickly, and the velocity is therefore low, a large defect is indicated. Remember that good alignment of the continuous wave beam and the direction of flow must be achieved or the velocity will be underestimated, falsely indicating a larger defect. If the spectral trace demonstrates flow both above and below the zero line simultaneously during systole, the beam is poorly aligned.

If the defect is large, it may be possible to image the hole and, therefore, to measure it. The larger the defect and the greater the amount of infarcted tissue surrounding it the less likely it is that successful surgery can be performed.

Ruptured myocardium may also occur in the free wall of the ventricle. The pericardium will be seen to be full of fluid (blood) and colour flow Doppler will help to determine the site of rupture. This complication is one of the causes of sudden death following myocardial infarction, but in a few patients the leak into the pericardium is contained and a false aneurysm may develop. These can become large and chronic, sometimes expanding slowly. They can often be distinguished from true aneurysms by their discontinuous margins, but in long-standing cases this may be more difficult.

RUPTURED PAPILLARY MUSCLE

If the acutely damaged and ruptured myocardium is a papillary muscle, this can cause sudden torrential mitral regurgitation. In addition to the severe regurgitation the echocardiographer may see the portion of detached papillary muscle flying back and forth across the mitral valve orifice as it remains attached to the valve by the chordae. These patients are generally very sick, but echocardiographic studies are vital in making the diagnosis and for the surgeon to decide if an operation is possible.

THROMBUS FORMATION

Thrombus is a typical late finding after a large full-thickness myocardial infarction. It will occur adjacent to sites of hypokinesia or akinesia where there is stasis of blood. The most common site is within the apex (see later in this chapter). The best way to visualise the apex is on the apical four chamber view with a high frequency transducer. This is an important diagnosis to make as there is a significant risk of systemic embolism.

ANEURYSM

An aneurysm occurs when there is stretching of scar tissue following a large full thickness myocardial infarction (Figure 6.10). Typically the myocardium will be thinned in the area of the aneurysm. The area will be akinetic, or may sometimes display paradoxical motion during systole. The most common site is at the apex. The area may calcify and hence create acoustic shadowing. Aneurysm and thrombus may co-exist in the same area.

Multiple infarcts and ischaemic cardiomyopathy

Some patients may have more than one myocardial infarction. These may involve different regions and the two areas may be distinct. In many cases patients will have had two or more infarctions, not all of which will have been definitively diagnosed either symptomatically or medically. These patients may end up with a chronically damaged ventricle with patchy impairment, thinning and scarring. Another variant is a condition where many lesions affect smaller coronary arteries and consequently produce diffuse small areas of damage and fibrosis. There is thus a spectrum of appearances between identifiable infarctions and an 'ischaemic cardiomyopathy'.

Left ventricular hypertrophy

Left ventricular hypertrophy (Figure 6.11) is most commonly a physiological response to pressure loading of

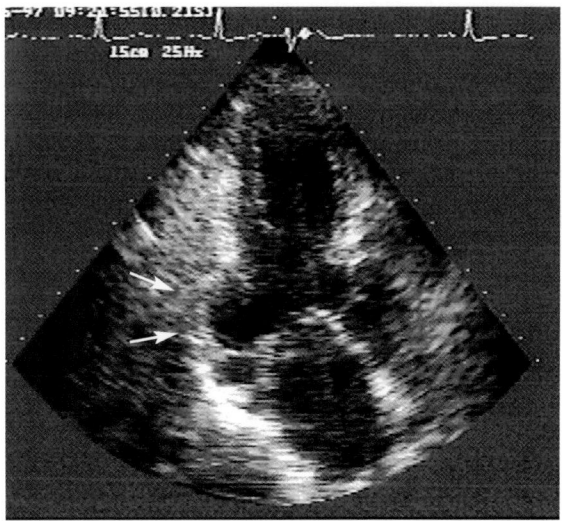

Figure 6.10 – Apical long axis view during systole, displaying normal contraction of the apex but bulging of the basal inferior region, indicating an aneurysm (arrowed).

the ventricle as occurs chronically in aortic stenosis or hypertension. It is important to quantitate the hypertrophy as this is of great significance as well as being useful for long-term patient monitoring during treatment (Table 6.1).

CAUSES OF LEFT VENTRICULAR HYPERTROPHY
Systemic hypertension
Aortic stenosis
HCM
Racial variance
Athletes

Right ventricular hypertrophy

Hypertrophy of the right ventricle is present if the wall thickness is greater than 7 mm. The right ventricle can be highly trabeculated and it is important that the measurement of wall thickness does not include trabeculations. Because axial resolution is better than lateral resolution, right ventricular wall thickness should be measured on either the parasternal short axis or the subcostal view.

CAUSES OF RIGHT VENTRICULAR HYPERTROPHY
Pulmonary hypertension
Pulmonary valve stenosis
HCM

Left ventricular dilatation

An increase in the cavity size of the left ventricle is most commonly due to impaired muscle function (commonly ischaemic heart disease or cardiomyopathy) with consequent compensatory dilatation (Table 6.2). As the effi-

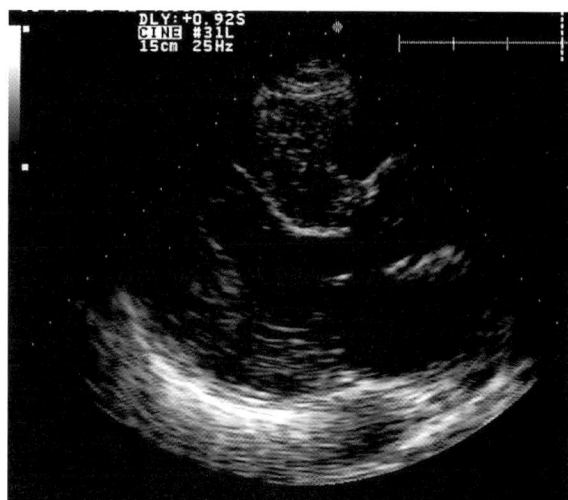

Figure 6.11 – Parasternal long axis image of symmetrical left ventricular hypertrophy.

ciency of the ventricle decreases and the ejection fraction and shortening fraction decrease, the ventricle is obliged to fill more in order to maintain an adequate cardiac output. The ventricle may also be dilated if it has to deal with an increased volume of blood to maintain the cardiac output, as occurs in valve regurgitation or VSD.

CAUSES OF LEFT VENTRICULAR DILATATION
Unknown
Myocardial infarction (long-standing ischaemia)
Volume overload (e.g. aortic or mitral regurgitation)
Chronic severe aortic stenosis with impaired left ventricle
Metabolic disease (e.g. thyrotoxicosis)

Left ventricular volume overload

Left ventricular volume overload is most easily determined from the M-mode measurements (Figure 6.12). If the end systolic diameter (ESD) is within one of the ranges given in Table 6.2 and the end diastolic diameter (EDD) is in a relatively higher range (e.g. ESD 41 mm (mildly dilated range) and EDD 65 mm (moderately dilated range)) volume overload is indicated. On two-dimensional imaging the left ventricle will appear hyperdynamic. Also take note of the stroke volume and cardiac output calculated by the system (assuming adequate quality measurements). A cardiac

Table 6.1 – Suggested guidelines for quantifying left ventricular hypertrophy in adults

Degree of hypertrophy	Wall thickness (mm)
Normal	7 – 11
Mild	12 – 13
Moderate	14 – 17
Severe	18

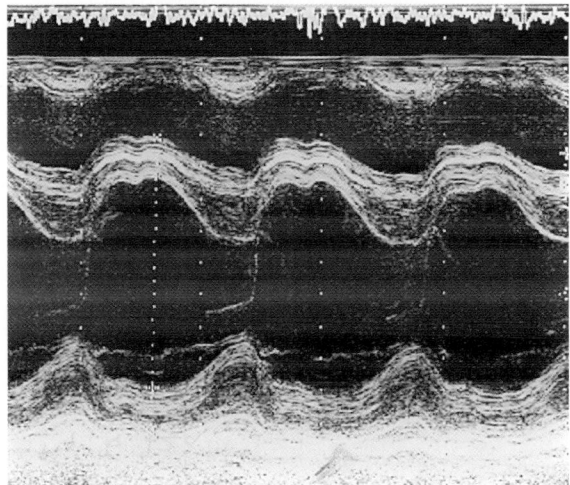

Figure 6.12 – M-mode trace showing left ventricular volume overload. Note the highly contractile myocardium (EDD 6.2 cm, ESD 3.1 cm).

output much higher than 5 l/min indicates volume overload.

Right ventricular dilatation

The right ventricle is normally assessed for size by comparing it with the left ventricle on the apical four chamber view. If the right ventricle is similar in size or larger, it is most likely to be dilated. Care must be taken in using this technique if the left ventricle is dilated. If the right ventricle looks to be in proportion with a dilated left ventricle, and so does not prompt a measurement, it is likely to also be dilated. The right ventricle is dilated if the diameter of its base (on the apical four chamber view) is greater than 30 mm.[6]

Table 6.2 – Suggested guideline measurements for quantifying left ventricular dilatation in adults

Degree of dilatation	*ESD (mm)	*EDD (mm)
Normal	23 – 36	37 – 51
Mild	37 – 45	51 – 59
Moderate	46 – 49	60 – 69
Severe	≥ 50	≥ 70

*EDD, end diastolic diameter; ESD, end systolic diameter.

> **CAUSES OF RIGHT VENTRICULAR DILATATION**
> Myocardial infarction
> Pulmonary hypertension
> Atrial and/or ventricular septal defect
> Volume overload (tricuspid or pulmonary regurgitation or left-to-right shunt)
> Dilated cardiomyopathy
> Ebstein's and other congenital abnormalities

Pericardial disease

The effects of pericardial disease that may be detected on an echocardiogram are:

- pericardial effusion
- pericardial thickening
- pericardial masses.

Pericardial effusion

A small amount of fluid in the pericardial sac is a normal finding if it is localised and measures 5 mm or less. When the depth of fluid is greater than 5 mm it is termed a pericardial effusion (Figure 6.13). The effusion may be global, surrounding the whole heart, or confined to one area. In most cases the fluid will be echo-free. Occasionally particles may be seen within the fluid, which indicates infective material (pyopericardium) or blood (haemopericardium). If there is a

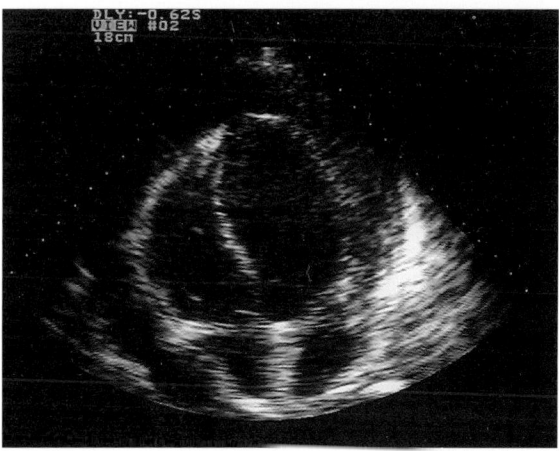

Figure 6.13 – A large pericardial effusion. Note that the fluid does not extend behind the left atrium, as there is no pericardial space in this area.

haemopericardium present the blood can clot; the resultant echo pattern is brighter and can be difficult to differentiate from the echoes normally surrounding the heart if the echo window is poor. Loculations may be present within the effusion if it is chronic and can be seen as echogenic strands attaching the epicardium to the pericardium (Figure 6.14). Chest radiograph will show an enlarged heart. It is noteworthy that there is no pericardial space directly behind the left atrium.

CAUSES OF PERICARDIAL EFFUSION
Idiopathic
Pericarditis
Congestive heart failure
Post myocardial infarction
Post cardiac surgery
Cancer of the lung or breast
Metatastic disease of the pericardium
Irradiation (e.g. therapy)
Chemotherapy
Trauma

In most cases the echocardiogram can only note the presence of a pericardial effusion and not the actual cause. One cause that can be diagnosed with certainty is rupture of the myocardium following a myocardial infarction resulting in a haemopericardium. Poorly contractile ventricles may suggest that the effusion is due to heart fail-ure, and masses within the pericardial fluid would indicate that the effusion is due to metastatic disease.

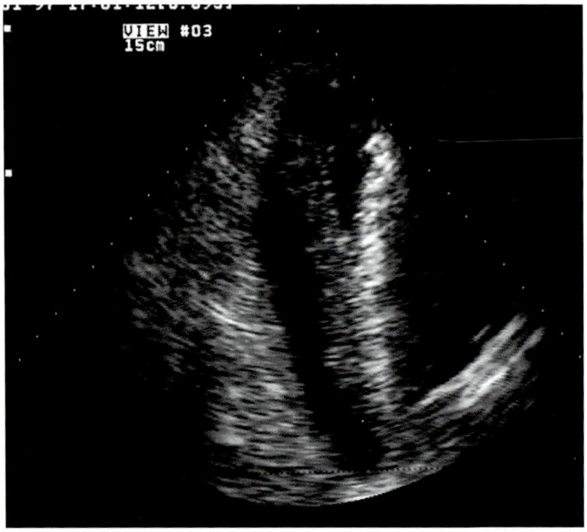

The role of the echocardiogram in pericardial effusion is to note:

- the size

- the location

- the consistency and echogenicity of the fluid

- any dysfunction (collapse) of the chambers

- any change in the subsequent follow-up scans.[7]

When scanning in the parasternal long-axis the scale of the image should always be set small enough to visualise posterior to the left ventricle in order to assess for any effusion. A left-sided pleural effusion can also be seen in this projection. An M-mode scan through the left ventricle will display an echo-free zone posterior to the left ventricle. When the M-mode beam is placed through the right ventricle on the parasternal long-axis view, mid diastolic notching can be noted, even in the smallest of pericardial effusions (Figure 6.15). This should not be confused with the more serious diastolic collapse of the right ventricle, which is described later in this section. A small right-sided pericardial effusion may be missed due to reverberations in the near field

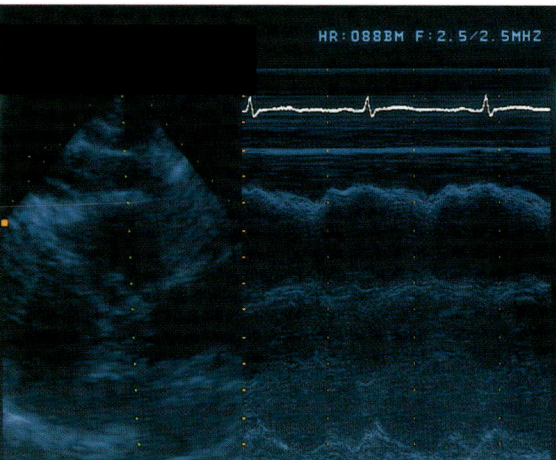

Figure 6.15 – M-mode trace through the right ventricle on the parasternal long axis view. Note the slight notch in the anterior wall of the ventricle during diastole – a characteristic finding associated with a small pericardial effusion. This notching should not be confused with collapse of the right ventricle, which will be indicated by much greater movement of the anterior wall during diastole.

Figure 6.14 – Apical long axis view of a fibrous strand within a pericardial effusion in a patient who had recently undergone complex heart surgery.

on the parasternal views. A good view of the right-sided chambers can usually be obtained by using the subcostal position. The heart can be very mobile within a large pericardial effusion, and hence assessment of ventricular and valvular function can be difficult.

Moderate or large pericardial effusions (Table 6.3) should be brought to the attention of the referring doctor, as should signs of tamponade (see below), as drainage of these effusions needs to be considered.

PITFALLS

Pericardial and epicardial fat have a low-level echo appearance similar to a haemopyopericardium and pyopericardium. However, the echoes within the area will be constant and will not change with patient position. There will be no right ventricular notching and no signs of tamponade.

A left-sided pleural effusion can have a very similar appearance to that of a pericardial effusion. Differentiation is by the location of the fluid relative to the aorta (Figure 6.16). On the parasternal long axis view a pericardial effusion will finish just anterior to the descending aorta. A pleural effusion will lie posterior to the aorta. Lung can often be demonstrated within a pleural effusion. If pericardial and pleural effusions exist side by side, the interface of the layers will be visible.

These diagnoses can be difficult and in any case of doubt the advice of someone more experienced should be sought.

Tamponade

The normal pressure within the pericardium is zero or negative. As the amount of fluid in the pericardium increases, the pressure rises. This increase in pressure does not allow complete relaxation of the ventricles during diastole, and filling is reduced. The pressure is at maximum during diastole and the ventricles may collapse. The right ventricle is typically affected, as it is usually at a lower pressure than the left ventricle (Figure 6.17). Because the right ventricle is impaired,

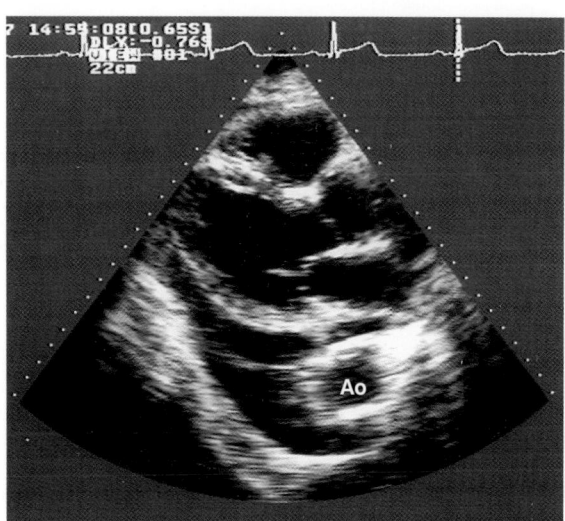

Figure 6.16 – Parasternal long axis view of pericardial and left pleural effusions co-existing in the same patient. Note that the pericardial effusion remains anterior to the aorta, while the pleural effusion extends behind it. The interface between the two effusions is indicated by an echogenic line. Ao=aorta.

there is a reduced cardiac output from the entire heart, leading to a drop in blood pressure. Characteristically the clinician will note pulsus paradoxus where the peripheral pulse will become weaker or even disappear during inspiration, which is normally a phase that improves the venous return to the heart and would tend to sustain the pulse.

If the free wall of the right ventricle is stiff or if the patient has pulmonary hypertension, the right ventricle will not demonstrate collapse. Diastolic collapse may also be observed in the right atrium (Figure 6.18) and less commonly in the left-sided chambers. This collapse can be noted on M-mode traces and seen on real-time scanning. If there is both diastolic collapse of a cardiac chamber and the blood pressure is low, this indicates that the pericardial effusion is haemodynamically significant and will require drainage. Patients will often be breathless and drainage will give immediate relief from this symptom.

Doppler studies of forward mitral flow in patients with tamponade and some with pericardial effusions will show a decrease in velocity as the patient breathes in. In the same patients, forward tricuspid flow velocity will increase at inspiration.[8] Left ventricular ejection time has been shown to be shortened on inspiration in patients with a pericardial effusion (not tamponade)[9].

Table 6.3 – Suggested guideline measurements for quantifying pericardial effusion in adults

Average depth (cm)	Size of effusion
0.5 – 1.5	Small
1.5 – 3.0	Moderate
> 3.0	Large

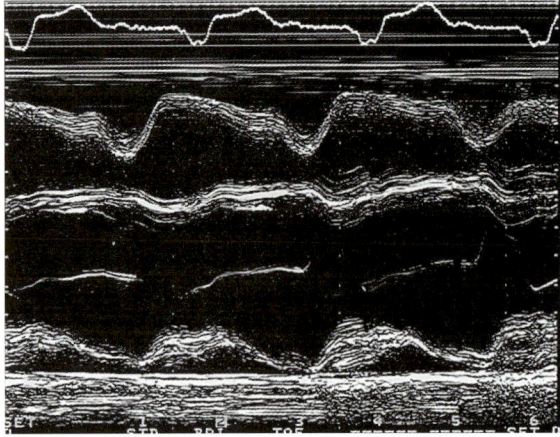

Figure 6.17 – M-mode trace in the parasternal long axis view through the right and left ventricles. Note the pericardial effusion anterior to the right ventricle and posterior to the left ventricle. During diastole (see the ECG trace) the right ventricle collapses.

Pericarditis

Many patients are referred for an echocardiogram with a history of 'any evidence of pericarditis'. Most examinations on these patients have no abnormal echocardiographic findings because pericarditis is usually an inflammation of the pericardial layers without gross change in morphology. Occasionally, a pericardial effu-

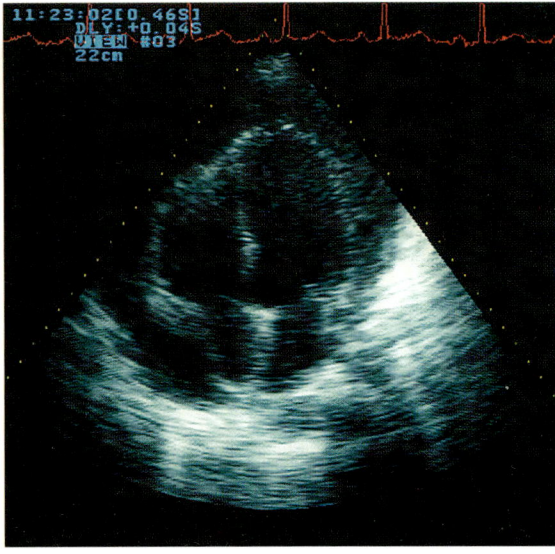

Figure 6.18 – Apical four chamber view of a large pericardial effusion with collapse of the right atrium, which is typical of tamponade.

sion may be demonstrated, but this does not necessarily imply a diagnosis of pericarditis.

Pericardiocentesis

(Pericardial tap)

INDICATIONS

1. Relief of tamponade in patients who are haemodynamically compromised
2. Large global volume (if depth $\geq$ 3 cm) if symptomatic
3. Diagnostic pericardiocentesis for aetiology of pericardial fluid, e.g. metastatic pericardial effusion
4. For instillation of therapeutic drugs, e.g. antibiotics.
5. For positioning of an indwelling catheter for continuing drainage

PATIENT PREPARATION

In an emergency no preparation is needed.

If planned   1. Informed consent
              2. Patient fasted for 6 hours prior
              3. In some instances premedication may be appropriate.

TROLLEY SET UP

Sterile pericardiocentesis kits are available commercially. If your department does not stock them the following list of items should be prepared:

- Antiseptic skin preparation
- Blade
- Sterile fenestrated drape
- 9 Fr straight catheter with side holes
- Procedure towel
- 3-way stopcock
- Gauze swabs
- 8 Fr vessel dilator
- Selection of syringes
- ECG connector wire to needle
- Selection of needles
- Silk sutures with straight cutting needle
- 1000 ml drainage collection bag
- 0. 035' (0.89 mm) × 80 cm guidewire with 3 mm J tip
- 18G procedure needle, 30 bevel, with fitted stylet.

You will also need:

- ECG electrodes
- Local anaesthetic
- Gown
- Dressing
- Gloves
- Sterile specimen containers and forms
- Skin wash

Initially, the patient is scanned to identify the optimum site of puncture. This typically is subcostally but the apical approach often allows easier access to the effusion. As long as the effusion is clearly seen from the apex, then interposed air will not be present and pneumothorax will be unlikely. In the case of the traditional subcostal approach it is often surprising to see how far the effusion is from the surface and how often the left lobe of the liver lies in the path of the needle.

Ideally the patient should be comfortably positioned (supine for the subcostal approach, rotated to the left for the apical approach) and a careful scan performed to identify (a) the exact site for puncture (b) the exact direction to orientate the needle to aim at the maximum quantity of fluid and (c) the depth of the effusion from the surface. The puncture site should be marked with a permanent marker before skin preparation.

The procedure needle is typically attached to a separate ECG lead to help identify any inadvertent contact with the myocardium. Some operators prefer to monitor the introduction of the procedure needle by ultrasound from a window at a distance from the operation site, but others prefer to use the ultrasound technique to determine the exact site and direction for puncture beforehand. The tip of the needle is characterised by a bright echo with multiple reverberations posterior to it.

A sample of fluid may be taken, the effusion may be drawn off manually or a drainage catheter may be left in situ and the patient returned to the ward. If draining the effusion completely, the pericardium should be scanned prior to withdrawal of the catheter to ensure complete removal of the fluid. This should be performed in several image planes.

POST PROCEDURE CARE

Following the procedure the patient may eat and drink normally. Bed rest for two to four hours is recommended. The puncture site should be checked half hourly for four hours. Blood pressure, pulse and respiratory rates should be checked half hourly for two hours. If there is any clinical suspicion of pneumothorax, a chest X-ray should be taken.

Constrictive pericarditis

A stiff, thickened pericardium will prevent diastolic relaxation of the ventricles and filling will be impaired. This is relatively rare and the commonest cause is old healed tuberculous pericarditis. Accurate measurement of pericardial thickness is difficult using ultrasound imaging and cannot be reliably quoted.[10] Alternative imaging modalities such as computed tomography (CT) or magnetic resonance imaging (MRI) can give accurate measurements of pericardial thickness. In some cases the pericardium can calcify, thus giving rise to very bright echoes with acoustic shadowing behind. Systolic function remains normal, but there will be diastolic dysfunction. The two-dimensional images and Doppler findings are similar to those for restrictive cardiomyopathy.

Aortic disease

The aortic root and/or ascending aorta can become dilated for a number of reasons:

- atherosclerosis
- hypertension
- severe aortic stenosis
- aneurysm/dissection
- connective tissue disorder (e.g. Marfan's syndrome)
- idiopathic cause

The diameter of the ascending aorta can be measured on the parasternal long axis view, where it should be less than 3.4 cm. Diameters greater than this indicate a dilated ascending aorta and such aortas become clearly visible on the echocardiogram. If the root of the aorta (sinus of Valsalva) is dilated, aortic regurgitation will usually be present. It is good practice also to measure the arch of the aorta and the descending aorta if the ascending aorta is seen to be dilated. If the proximal ascending aorta is dilated it overlies the right atrium on the apical four chamber view and mimics the atrium in size and shape (Figure 6.19).

Patients with Marfan's syndrome require regular follow-up scans with measurements being made (on the parasternal long-axis view) of the aortic valve annulus, the sinotubular junction, the sinus of valsalva, and the middle of the ascending aorta (Figure 6.20). In addition, if possible, the transverse arch and descending aorta should be measured using other views. The mitral valve also needs to be assessed, as these patients tend to have floppy mitral valves that prolapse.

Aortic aneurysm and dissection

The wall of the aorta may become weakened and stretched, thus forming an aneurysm. A weakened wall can lead to the intima becoming detached from the

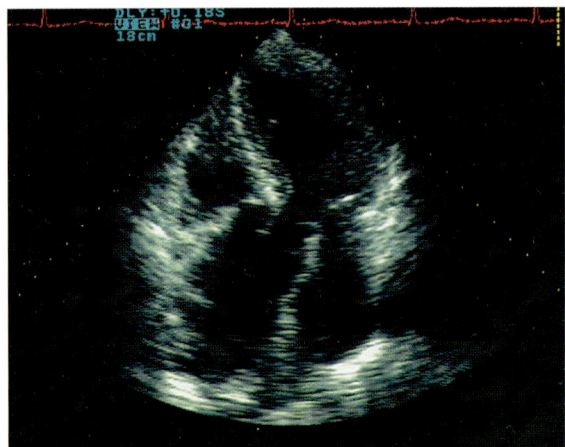

Figure 6.19 – Apical four chamber view of a dilated ascending aorta overlying the right atrium.

media layer, causing a dissection. The dissection may be localised or extend to the arch, involving the origins of the head and neck vessels. It is often possible to visualise a flap within the ascending aorta in the presence of a dissection. The flap needs to be confirmed from two separate views and should not be confused with the reverberation artefact often seen within the ascending aorta. The motion of the flap will be quite independent of the walls of the aorta. The intimal flap now separates two lumens: a true lumen and a false lumen. Colour

flow should be used to visualise the flow within the true lumen. The false lumen often has no flow within it, but if it has a connection to the true lumen, any abnormal flow will be detected in the false lumen. A dissection may extend into the aortic valve and significant aortic regurgitation can result. The origins of the coronary arteries may be occluded by the flap, causing myocardial infarction.

Aortic dissection is a very serious condition with high early mortality and it should be diagnosed rapidly. There are two main types: type A involves the ascending aorta and is the most serious type (Figure 6.21): and type B starts after the aortic arch vessels (Figure 6.22). The latter often requires medical treatment but Type A dissection usually necessitates urgent surgery.

The role of the echocardiogram in cases of dissection are:

- to note the site and extent of the flap
- to note any flow within the false lumen
- to assess any aortic regurgitation
- to assess left ventricular function/hypertrophy
- to note the presence of pericardial effusion (haemopericardium may occur if the aorta ruptures).[7]

A false aneurysm can occur after surgery on the aorta or aortic valve (Figure 6.23). This occurs when there is splitting of the wall of the aorta, usually along the

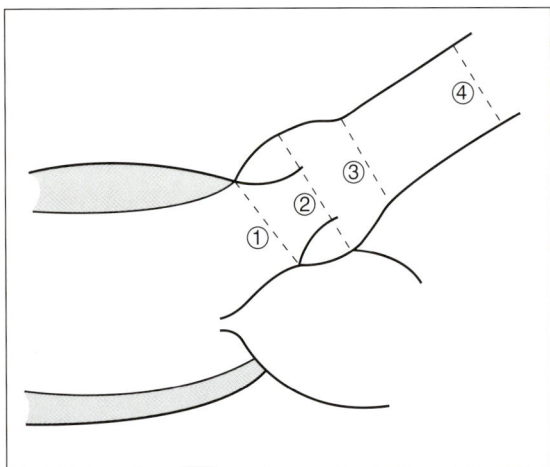

Figure 6.20 – Parasternal long axis view showing the diameters of the aorta to be measured at routine and follow-up investigations of patients with Marfan's syndrome. ① Aortic annulus diameter; ② sinus of Valsalva diameter; ③ sinotubular junction diameter; ④ diameter of the middle portion of the ascending aorta.

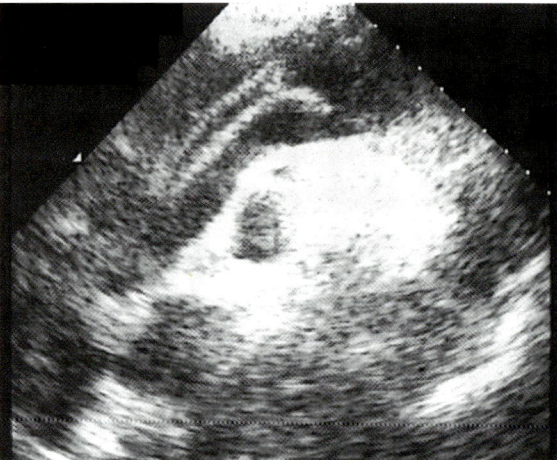

Figure 6.21 – Suprasternal image of a dissection in the ascending aorta showing a complex intimal flap, which was very mobile on the real-time scan.

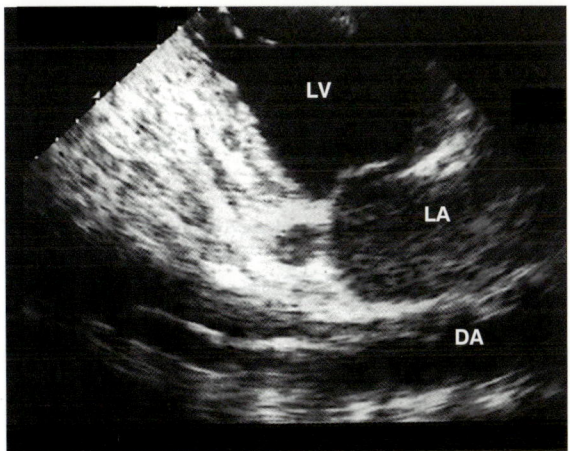

Figure 6.22 – Image from the same patient as in Figure 6.21, showing the descending aorta lying behind the heart in the apical long-axis view. The dissection flap has extended to this level. LV left ventricle, LA left atrium, DA descending aorta.

suture line (aortotomy), and a sac of blood collects anterior to the aorta. Colour flow imaging can help in identifying the connection site if it is small. If the connection between the sac and the aorta is large, both will be under the same high pressure and the velocities between the two will be small and hence not visible on the colour Doppler image.

A transoesophageal echocardiogram is often needed to visualise the aorta clearly. A CT or MRI scan shows the entire aorta, and may be the examination of choice if the patient can be moved.

Post-stenotic dilatation is due to high velocity, turbulent flow within the proximal aorta and is seen in some cases of severe aortic stenosis, especially if it is long-standing.

An aortic aneurysm (Figure 6.24) can develop without any dissection. If the ascending aorta increases beyond 5.0 cm in diameter, some authorities recommend elective aortic root replacement.

Thrombus

Often the first sign of thrombus within the cardiac chambers is an embolic event (e.g. a cerebrovascular accident (CVA)) or visual disturbances. These symptoms, of course, may be due to other intra- or extracardiac disease but if intracardiac thrombus is demonstrated on the echocardiogram immediate treatment with anticoagulants can begin and thus possible mortality may be prevented.

Echo appearances

The ultrasound appearance of thrombus is quite varied (Figure 6.25). The image of a thrombus may be quite bright and, if it is polypoid in shape, will extend into the echo-poor blood where the contrast is great. The echogenicity may be similar to that of the myocardium, in which case it can be difficult to differentiate thrombus from trabeculations or localised hypertrophy. In

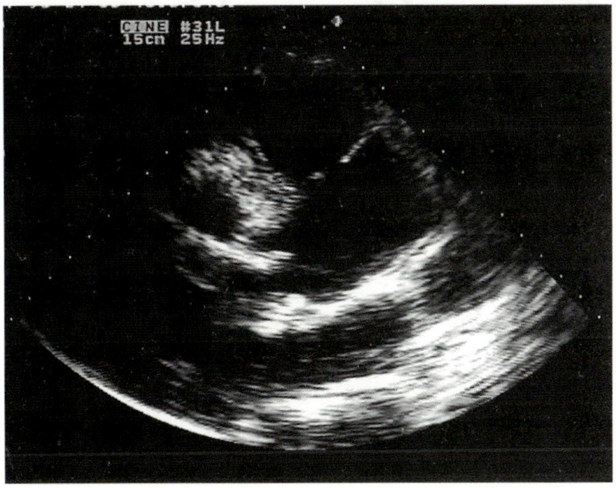

Figure 6.23 – Parasternal long axis view of a false aneurysm located anterior to the ascending aorta. The connection site can be visualised on the two-dimensional image. This patient had recently undergone replacement of the aortic valve.

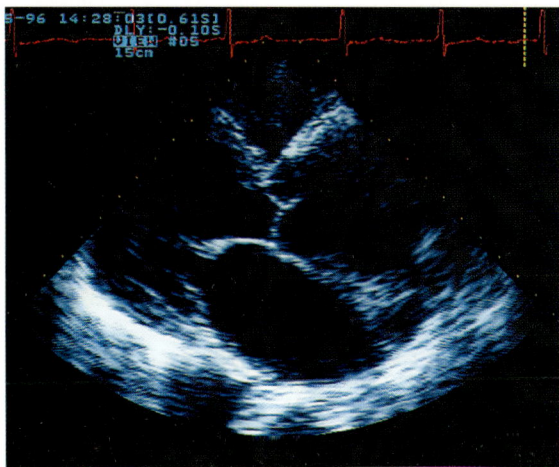

Figure 6.24 – Parasternal long axis view of an aneurysm of the ascending aorta.

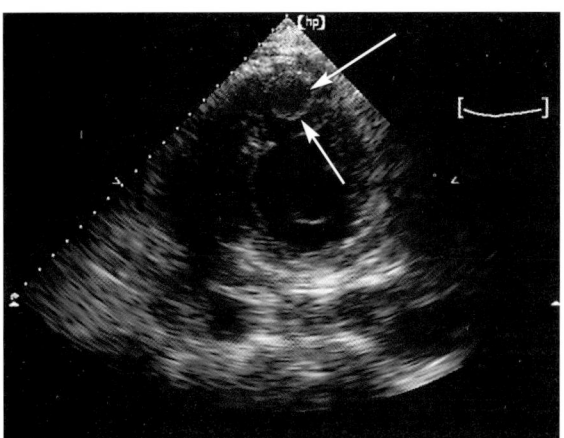

Figure 6.25 – Modified apical four chamber view demonstrating a very spherical thrombus within the apex of the left ventricle (arrowed). This patient had recently had an apical myocardial infarction.

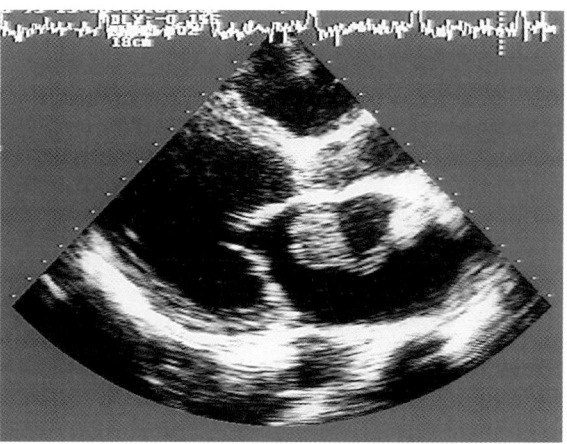

Figure 6.26 – Parasternal long-axis view showing a pedunculated (on a 'stalk') left atrial thrombus. This is a relatively unusual occurrence; more often, thrombi lie against the wall.

some instances the echogenicity will be less than the myocardium, and in these cases the thrombus is often jelly-like in its movement, which can be easily detected on real-time scanning. The thrombus may be layered along the myocardium and can be impossible to visualise. Some parts of the heart are never visualised on transthoracic echocardiography, such as the left atrial appendage, and so the presence of thrombus in the heart can never be excluded completely.

Location

Thrombus will occur at a site in the ventricles where there is impaired contractility of the underlying myocardium, allowing the movement of blood to become sluggish and then clot. By far the most common region for this to occur is in the apex, especially if there is an apical aneurysm. It can also be seen on the septum. Therefore, detailed studies for thrombus should be done in all patients with impaired ventricles (e.g. post myocardial infarction, cardiomyopathies). If a ventricle is well visualised and is seen to be contracting well with no areas of hypokinesia, thrombus can quite confidently be ruled out from the ventricles. Often the apex is not clearly visualised due to reverberation. In this case a higher frequency transducer is needed in order to look at the near field.

Atrial thrombus (Figure 6.26) is more difficult to visualise as the atria are further from the transducer. Thrombus can form in an atrium the contractility of which is impaired (e.g. atrial fibrillation) or the outflow from which is restricted (e.g. mitral or tricuspid stenosis). Patients are often referred for echocardiograms prior to cardioversion to assess the atria for thrombus. As thrombus can form during fibrillation, a shock back to sinus rhythm will cause correct contraction of the atrium and the thrombus will be dislodged and sudden death may follow. A transoesophageal echo (TOE) is needed in order to exclude completely thrombus from the atria, as small thrombi can be missed and the left atrial appendage is rarely visualised transthoracically. Right atrial thrombus may originate from veins in the extremities. When thrombus becomes dislodged from the site of origin it typically ends up in the right atrium. This thrombus will be long and thin, as it will be cast in the shape of the vein. It is difficult to differentiate such thrombus from Chiari's network (see pitfalls below).

Atrial septal defects can complicate the clinical picture of cardiac thrombus. Left-sided thrombus can then result in pulmonary emboli, and right-sided thrombus can result in systemic emboli.

Pulmonary artery thrombosis is an acute situation and can be found during pregnancy or post partum. It can also occur in chronic severe pulmonary hypertension. Occasional reports have shown the utility of echo diagnosis in the diagnosis of acute pulmonary embolism.[11]

The echo report should include the size, the site and the echogenicity of the thrombus and the contractility of the underlying myocardium, which will be useful for comparison in follow-up examinations.

PITFALLS

Artefacts can occur anywhere within the heart and mimic thrombus. The most common sites are the left ventricular apex and the left atrium. Several methods need to be used to distinguish between the two.

- If thrombus is truly present it will be possible to visualise it in at least two different planes.

- Changing to a different frequency transducer will often cause an artefact to disappear.

- Similarly, changing the depth of field will alter artefacts.

- Artefacts within the apex can be seen to pass through the myocardium rather than the thrombus, which has a definite border at the endocardium.

- Artefacts are often stationary, while thrombus will move in synchronisation with the underlying endocardium.

- The subcostal view will result in the same image as the apical four chamber view, but any artefacts will be altered due to the different angle of interrogation.

Vegetations caused by infective endocarditis have a similar appearance to thrombus and will occur in similar positions (e.g. on the tip of a pacing wire or other cardiac implant, on a valve prosthesis).

Tumours within the heart can have similar echo appearances to thrombus. Tumours may invade the underlying myocardium.

Apical HCM can also mimic thrombus within the apex. Both will show impaired contractility of the apex. It may be possible to differentiate between the two on an echocardiogram.

Papillary muscles may be confused with thrombus. After a myocardial infarction involving the papillary muscles, they can appear bright on the echo image. Papillary muscles have a characteristic shape, and careful imaging may show chordal attachment. Remember also that there are no papillary muscles at the apex or on the septum.

Left atrial thrombus cannot be excluded in the presence of a mechanical mitral prostheses due to obliteration of the left atrium by artefact (a TOE is necessary).

A mass visualised at the back of the right atrium could well be the Eustachian valve. If an image can be obtained in the subcostal view, it will help in the differentiation.

Chiari's network is present in about 3% of the normal population. It is a network of fine filaments within the right atrium. As imaging becomes better with newer machines this will become a more common echo finding. It usually originates at the inferior vena cava and floats within the atrium.

Remember that in patients with evidence of a systemic embolus, you may not find the thrombus but a predisposing cause (e.g. cardiomyopathy or valve disease) may be identified.

Follow-up

Follow-up examinations are usually requested after anticoagulation therapy has been used. If the thrombus has been present for a long period, anticoagulation may have no effect on dispersing it. A common appearance after therapy is a bright border along the endocardium where the thrombus was once present. Unfortunately, it is at this follow-up stage when an originally diagnosed thrombus may be found to be an artefact.

Tumours

Tumours of the heart are rare. About 75% of cardiac tumours are benign. The most common benign tumour of the heart is the myxoma. Primary malignant tumours are more likely to be found in the right heart chambers.

Benign tumours

MYXOMAS

Patients presenting with a myxoma often have a long history of breathlessness and embolic events. They may also present with a low-grade generalised illness, a heart murmur or an abnormal chest radiograph. The vast majority (75%) of myxomas occur in the left atrium (Figure 6.27). The echocardiogram shows a large mass of mixed echogenicity within the left atrium which pushes through the mitral valve during diastole.

Most commonly, myxomas are attached by a stalk to the interatrial septum at the site of the fossa ovalis. They are highly mobile and can be very large, obliterating the atrium during systole and obstructing the mitral valve in diastole. Less commonly they are sessile and hence are difficult to differentiate from other cardiac tumours and masses. They may also occur in the right atrium and, rarely, in the right and left ventricles. Ventricular myxomas are most commonly attached to the free wall, which will be normally contractile and so can be differentiated from thrombus, which typically forms at a hypokinetic apex or septum. Myxomas are typically solitary, but may be multiple, and so clear

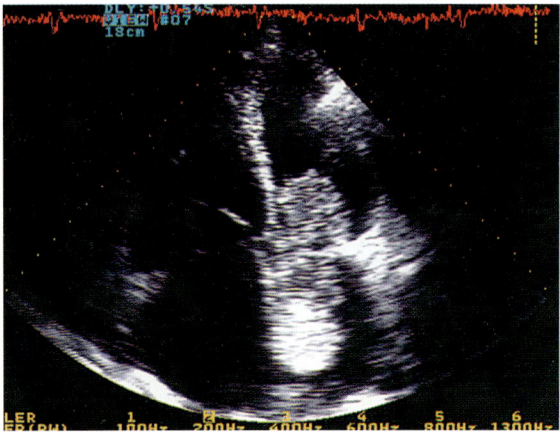

Figure 6.27 – Apical four chamber view during diastole of a large atrial myxoma pushing through the mitral valve into the left ventricle and obstructing the valve orifice.

visualisation of all cardiac chambers is necessary if one is identified. The M-mode trace often shows a characteristic appearance, with the orifice of the mitral valve being occupied by the echogenic tumour during diastole (Figure 6.28).

Immediate surgical intervention is mandatory to prevent fatal consequences from embolism. For this reason, if a myxoma is identified it should be brought to the attention of the referring doctor straight away. Follow-up of myxoma patients is necessary, as the tumours recur in 5% of cases. The role of echocardiography in the case of myxoma is to note the site of attach-

ment, the size, echo texture and mobility of the tumour, and to note any haemodynamic effect.

OTHER BENIGN TUMOURS

Other benign tumours of the heart are quite rare, and include rhabdomyoma (typically found in children), fibroma, lipoma and haemangioma. It is not possible to differentiate between benign and malignant tumours on echocardiography.

Malignant tumours

METASTASES

The most common malignant tumours of the heart are metastases. Typical malignancies that metastasise to the heart include lung, breast, leukaemia and lymphoma, malignant melanoma and renal cell carcinoma. The pericardium is the most common site for metastases (Figure 6.29), where they will often result in a pericardial effusion. A mass or masses can be identified in the presence of a pericardial effusion. If no effusion is present it may be almost impossible to visualise the small metastatic deposits. More rarely, metastases are found in the myocardium.

OTHER MALIGNANT TUMOURS

Other malignant tumours of the heart include sarcomas and direct invasion by extracardiac tumours. If a right atrial tumour is suspected, subdiaphragmatic imaging should be undertaken, especially of the IVC which provides a direct link from the abdomen to the right atrium.

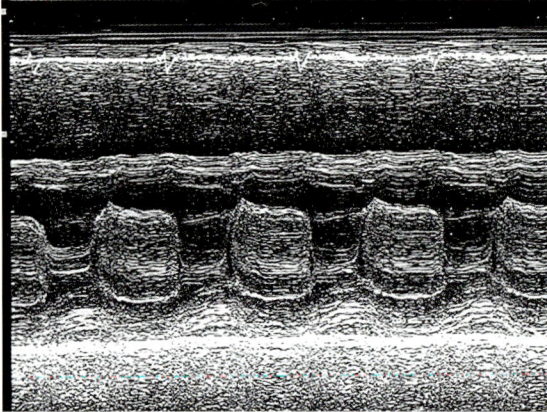

Figure 6.28 – M-mode trace through the mitral valve in the parasternal long axis view. Note that the space between the mitral leaflets, which is normally echo free, is filled with echoes during diastole. This appearance indicates the presence of myxoma.

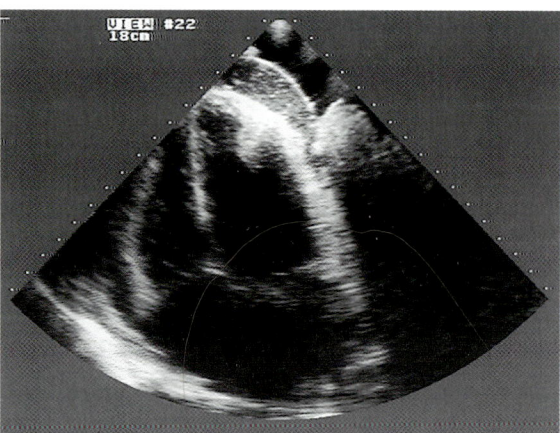

Figure 6.29 – Spherical metastasis extending through the pericardium into the pleura. There is extensive malignant pleural effusion that shows internal echoes. There is also a metastasis in the left ventricular myocardium. This patient had disseminated carcinomatosis.

Mesothelioma is a primary malignant tumour of the pericardium.

Carcinoid tumours of the liver can affect the right heart, particularly the tricuspid and pulmonary valves. They can cause thickening and restriction of the annulus and leaflets, causing both stenosis and regurgitation.

Implants

There are many man-made 'foreign bodies' that may be found within the heart. These include pacing wires, which may consist of one wire with the tip situated in the right ventricle, or two wires where one should sit in the right atrium and one in the right ventricle (Figure 6.30). Other right-sided lines include central venous lines, indwelling catheters, shunts and Swan-Ganz catheters. Although prosthetic valves may seem an obvious implant, if the operator is not informed of the presence of the prosthesis (especially a porcine aortic valve) it can take close examination to work out what is 'wrong' with the valve.

A bright, thickened area in the septum may represent a patch over a septal defect. Such areas will demonstrate reduced contractility and can be difficult to differentiate from infarcted myocardium. Suture lines will also appear as a brighter area in the myocardium. Individual stitches around valve sewing rings can appear as small mobile masses in patients when good images are obtained. Differentiation from endocarditis can be difficult.

Complications

Thrombus and infective endocarditis are typical complications of any implant. If pacing wires, catheters, etc, are affected the most common site of attachment of vegetations or thrombus is at the tip. The infection or thrombus may layer along the length of the catheter, in which case it will be impossible to visualise.

If a line passes through the tricuspid valve it may irritate the leaflets and cause localised thickening. A right-sided line will also prevent complete closure of the tricuspid valve, giving rise to tricuspid regurgitation.

The tip of a newly inserted pacing wire in the right ventricle can be seen to be quite mobile. With time, the tip should embed into the myocardium. Therefore, if a pacing wire that has been inserted for some time is seen

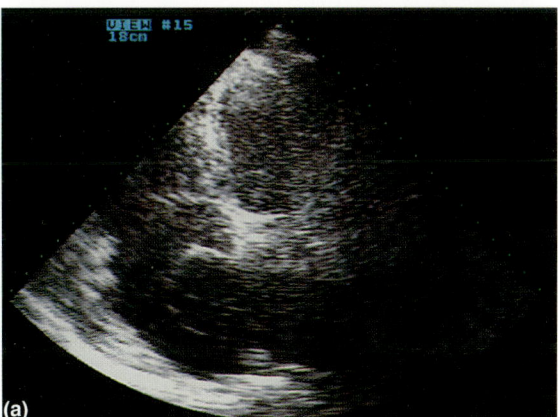

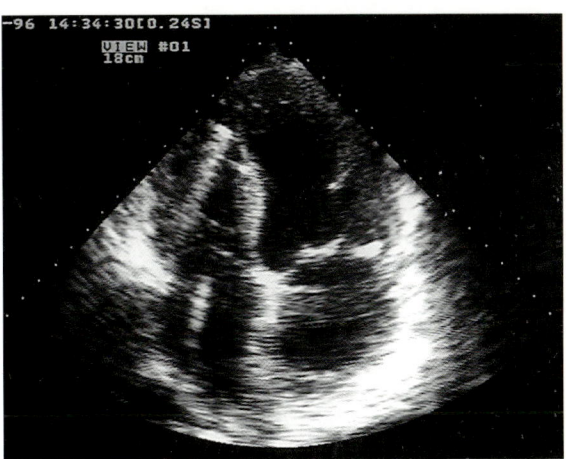

Figure 6.30 – Characteristic image of a two lead pacing system. One tip can be seen in the right atrium, and the other in the right ventricle.

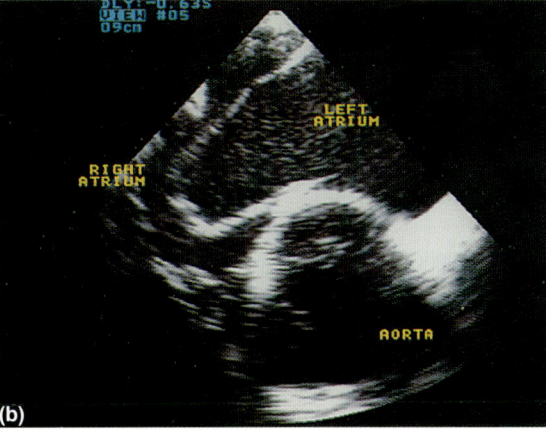

Figure 6.31 – (a) Apical four chamber view showing an interatrial aneurysm deviating into the right atrium. At this depth the image quality is limited. (b) Transoesophageal image from the same patient, showing the interatrial aneurysm much more clearly.

to move freely within the right ventricle, it should be commented on.

Interatrial aneurysm

This can be visualised in the thin membranous area between the two atria at the site of the fossa ovalis (Figure 6.31). There is redundant tissue which is very mobile and can be seen to swing from one atrium to the other during the cardiac cycle. Interatrial aneurysm can be associated with a patent foramen ovale.

References

1. Marcus ML, Schelbert HR, Skorton DJ, Wolf GL (eds). *Cardiac Imaging*. WB Saunders, Philadelphia, 1991.

2. Shapiro LM, McKenna WJ. Distribution of left ventricular hypertrophy in hypertrophic cardiomyopathy: a two-dimensional echocardiographic study. *J Am Coll Cardiol* 1983; **2**: 437–444.

3. McKenna WJ, Keleinebenne A, Nihoyannopoulos P, Foale R. Echocardiographic measurement of right ventricular wall thickness in hypertrophic cardiomyopathy: relation to clinical and prognostic features. *J Am Coll Cardiol* 1988; **11**: 351–358.

4. Yamamoto K, Redfield MM, Nishimura RA. Analysis of left ventricular diastolic function. *Heart* 1996; **77** (Suppl 2): 27–35.

5. Jawad JA. *A Practical Guide to Echocardiography and Cardiac Doppler Ultrasound*. Little and Brown, Boston, 1990.

6. Foale R, Nihoyannopoulos P, McKenna et al. Echocardiographic measurement of the normal adult right ventricle. *Br Heart J* 198; **56**: 3–44.

7. Wilde P (ed). *Cardiac Ultrasound*. Churchill Livingstone, Edinburgh, 1993.

8. Appleton CP, Hatle LK, Popp RL. Cardiac tamponade and pericardial effusion: respiratory variation in transvalvular flow studied by Doppler echocardiography. *J Am Coll Cardiol* 1988; **11**(5): 1020–100.

9. Spodick DH, Paladino D, Flessas AP. Respiratory effects on systolic time intervals during pericardial effusion. *Am J Cardiol* 198; **51**: 1033–1035.

10. Voelkel AG, Pietro DA, Folland ED, Fisher ML, Parisi AF. Echocardiographic features of constrictive pericarditis. *Circulation* 1978; **58**(5): 871–875.

11. Weston MJ, Wilde P. Echocardiographic diagnosis of massive pulmonary embolism. *Br J Radiol* 1989; **62**(740): 751–753.

7

CONGENITAL HEART DISEASE

Alison Heads

Preparing the patient
Echocardiography equipment
The echocardiographic approach
Description of the scan

Preparing the patient

By the very nature of the patient population that we deal with in echocardiography an informal and loosley structured approach is required. To settle the anxieties aroused in both patients and their relatives by the proximity of the 'high tech' equipment, a relaxed, gentle and sometimes gradual introduction to the scanning room may produce a better quality study. For example, when dealing with a child, you can introduce the echo machine as a very special computer that can magically show everyone how beautiful your heart is. Allow the child to settle and even use the keyboard, tracker ball and ultrasound gel in order to gain confidence in the situation. You may do a 'test scan' on yourself or a parent. Explain to mature children why the gel and electrocardiographic electrodes are required. Always have some bribes ready, for example sweets or congratulatory stickers and remember that every child's scan and performance are always better than those of the child who has just left! Explain to the child in terms they can understand what is on the screen. A mitral valve, for example, is a trapdoor waving up and – a lovely one, of course. A ventricle squeezes in and out. Colour mapping and Doppler patterns show the blood getting where it wants to go.

The decor of the room must also suit the patient population. Mobiles, preferably at least one musical one hung above the scan bed are of great benefit, along with wall posters, which even the babies can appreciate. A hand-held toy that spins, squeaks or tinkles is a help. The favourite in our clinic is a multi-coloured abacus and a baby mirror. If in difficulty get the parent to feed the baby. You can even a achieve good scan while a baby is being breast fed. Allow time for the infant and parent to settle themselves – a stressed and tired baby will not give a good scan. Have a pram on loan so that the baby can be walked about. Be flexible about scanning infants and children sitting or reclining upon a parent's lap, in a car seat or a buggy. Never insist a child undresses if they do not want to. If you develop a relaxed relationship with the child and their parents, will help improve on an incomplete set of data at future examinations.

If all else fails, request for the patient to be sedated. Our current practice at the Freeman Hospital is set out below. For infants older than 6 months of age and young children, sedation for echocardiography is achieved with a combination of trimeprazine 5 mg/kg and triclofos 50 mg/kg given orally. These doses are large compared with those recommended in the data sheets but have been arrived at by experience as smaller doses are often ineffective. Medication is administered by nursing staff or by the parents with nursing supervision. Satisfactory sedation is usually produced within an hour, but can sometimes take up to an hour and a half. Children often cry for some time before they fall asleep. The duration of sedation is extremely variable ranging from as little as 20 – 30 minutes up to several hours. Once asleep, children should be monitored by pulse oximetry until they awake. If a triclofos and trimeprazine combination is not effective it is reasonable to top-up the sedation using nasal Midazolam. The risk of respiratory depression increases with this combination, and close monitoring is essential. Sedation is sometimes required for infants younger than 6 months. We generally avoid the use of triclofos and trimeprazine in this age group, and use nasal midazolam instead. The Midazolam injection preparation is given as nose drops in a dose of 0.1 – 0.2 mg/kg, although up to 0.5 mg/kg is occasionally required and can be given. The injection is available in a concentration of 5 mg/ml, which limits its usefulness in older infants and children – a 10 kg infant requires a volume of 1 ml, and most infants are fairly resistant to its administration. Sedated infants should be monitored until they awake and should not be discharged until they are awake. Parents should be warned that the child's sleeping pattern may be disturbed for a day or two. The administration of sedatives should always be supervised by experienced nursing and medical staff.

Echocardiography equipment

In paediatric patients penetration is less difficult to achieve but high resolution at higher heart rates is essential. A 7.5 – 5.0 MHz transducer is thus preferable for use in infants and small children. Subcostal colour flow mapping may require better penetration, however, and a 3.5 MHz transducer may be required. In older children and adolescents a 5.0 MHz transducer should be used, with a 2.5 MHz one for some subcostal scanning. All transducers should have the capability for in-line continuous wave Doppler and duplex pulsed wave Doppler examination. Colour flow mapping is a distinct advantage and should be available wherever possible. A stand-alone continuous wave Doppler probe will allow swift and accurate velocity assessments.

The echocardiographic approach

This chapter will cover the more common congenital heart problems, to allow you to scan and describe most congenital heart defects. A logical system of interrogation must be employed in order to analyse, understand and describe the function of any heart. Therefore, a sequential, segmental analysis is the approach of choice.[1]

Much as you enter a house through the main doors, so the entrance of the veins to the atria must be located before the morphology of the atria and the septum can be studied. Moving across the atrioventricular junction (the entrance to the main rooms of the house), the atrioventricular valves and their position, morphology, chordal insertions and papillary muscles must be recognised. At this junction we must relate the atrioventricular valves to their corresponding ventricles, which are recognised by their ventricular morphology, septation and relationships one to another. The next step is to move from the first floor to the upper floor of the building, that is we cross the ventriculoarterial junction. The position of the outflow or arterial valves, their relationship to one another and their origin from the ventricles must be described. The arterial trunks themselves and their arrangement with regard to one another and the ventricles must then be recognised.

So the heart can be basically broken down into three segments: the atria, the ventricles and the arterial trunks. These three segments are connected via two junctions: the atrioventricular junction and the ventriculoarterial junction (Figure 7.1).

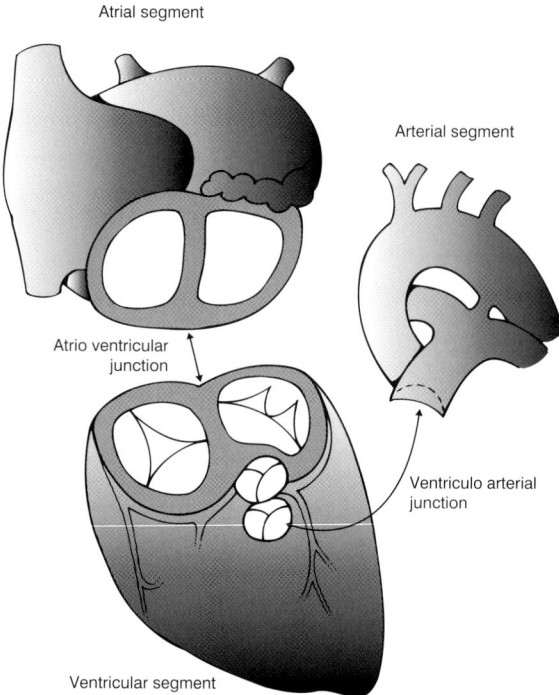

Figure 7.1 – Diagram to illustrate the major junctions of the heart, the atrioventricular junction and the ventriculoarterial junction.

Description of the scan

In this section the typical routine scan is described in the order in which the views are generally assessed. Common abnormalities and normal findings are described and illustrated, together with a description of the scanning technique used.

In this chapter, we assume that the reader has a knowledge of the standard echocardiographic views (see Chapter 4).

The subcostal approach is well tolerated by neonates and infants and provides access to all structures, except the aortic arch. Therefore, this is a commonly used point of contact and is used early in the scan. In contrast, however, in adults the subcostal approach is difficult and is thus usually performed last or not at all.

Atria and Venous Connections

The simple four chamber plane reveals the left and right atria and the interatrial septum. At this point two pulmonary veins can be seen entering the left atrium, with the inferior vena cava (IVC) and hepatic venous entry to the right atrium often also in view. Posterior (inferior) tilting of the transducer will demonstrate the coronary sinus, while anterior (superior) tilting will reveal the superior vena cava (SVC).

Views for assessing the atrial septum

There is a variety of atrial septal abnormalities and the operator must make a full inspection of the septum. From the standard subcostal four chamber view (Figure 7.2a), tilt the transducer superiorly to see the roof the atrial septum and reveal the SVC and the right upper pulmonary vein (Figure 7.2b). Now tilt the transducer inferiorly to see the posterior aspect of the atrial septum and the coronary sinus (Figure 7.2c). Rotate from the four chamber view through 90° clockwise and tilt the transducer to the right to reveal the SVC and IVC and a length of atrial septum (Figure 7.2d). Dropping down slightly leftwards from this view reveals the central atrial septum (Figure 7.2e). In the parasternal approach, long axis scans tilted inferiorly from the standard view

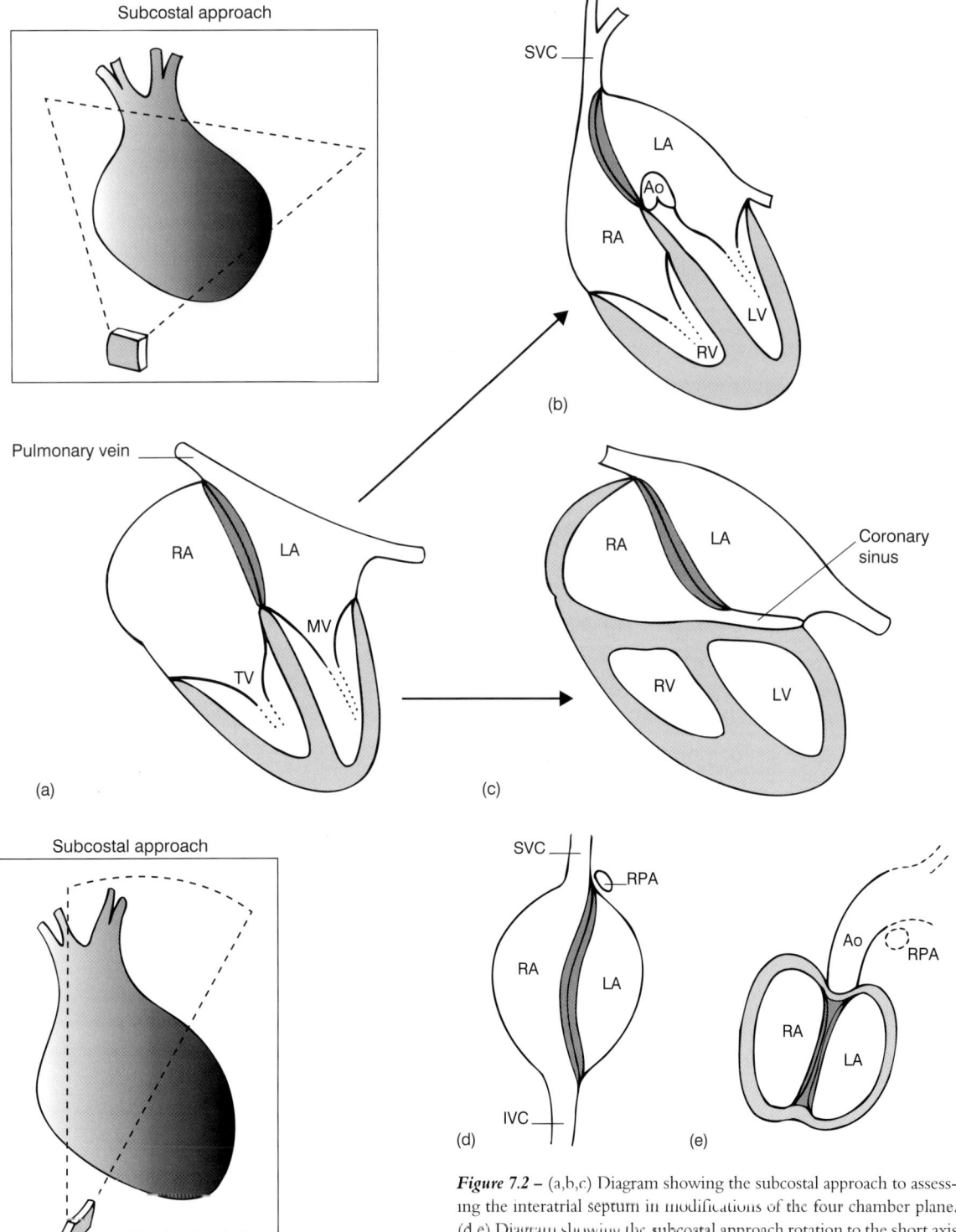

Subcostal approach

SVC

LA

Ao

RA

LV

RV

(b)

Pulmonary vein

RA

LA

MV

TV

(a)

RA

LA

Coronary sinus

RV

LV

(c)

Subcostal approach

Short axis rotation

SVC

RPA

RA

LA

IVC

(d)

Ao

RPA

RA

LA

(e)

Figure 7.2 – (a,b,c) Diagram showing the subcostal approach to assessing the interatrial septum in modifications of the four chamber plane. (d,e) Diagram showing the subcostal approach rotation to the short axis to assess the interatrial septum.

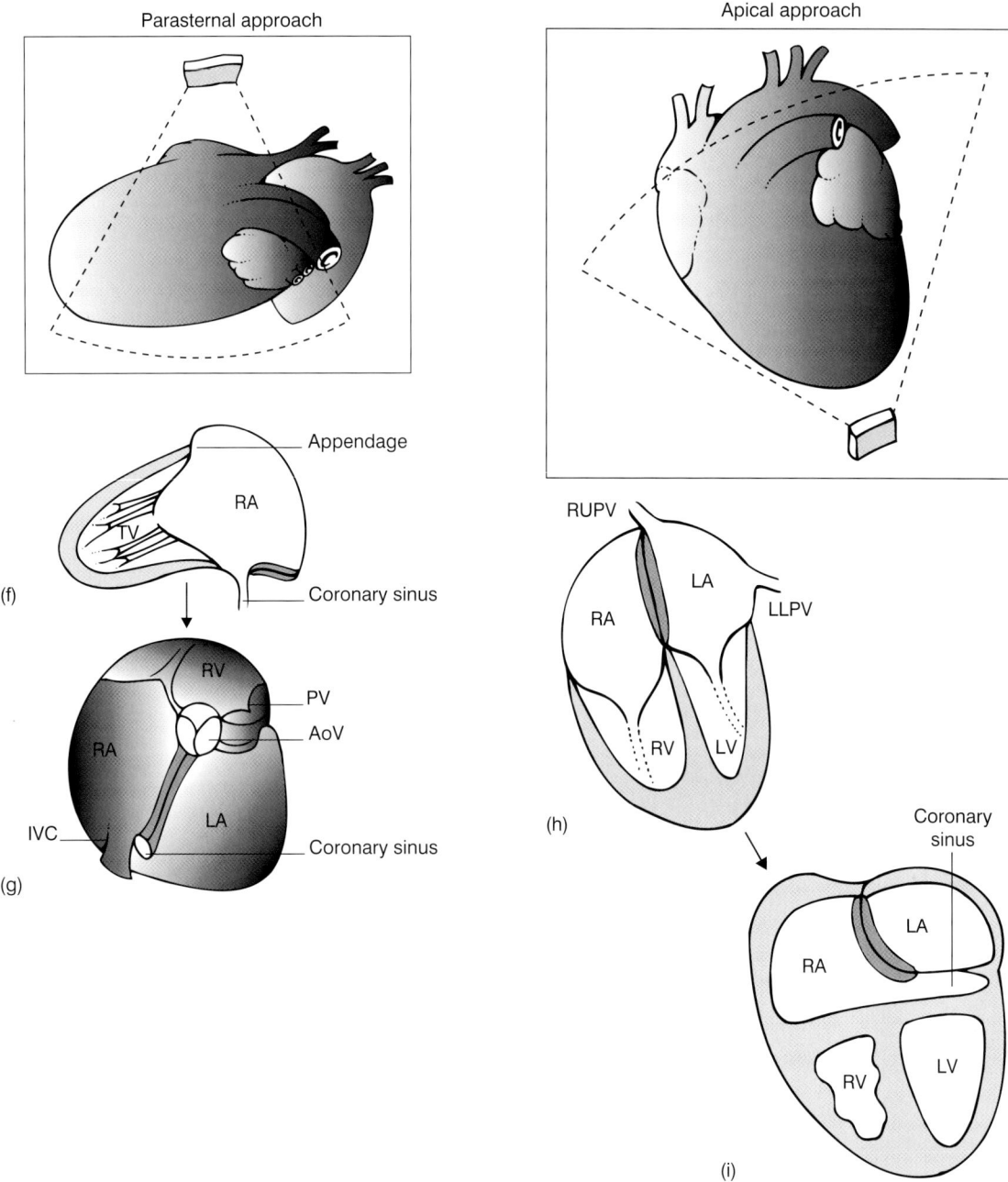

Parasternal approach

Apical approach

Figure 7.2 – (f, g) Diagram showing assessment of the interatrial septum from the parasternal view. (h, i) Diagram showing assessment of the interatrial septum from the apical four chamber view. In each illustration the atrial septum is shown in dark shading.

open up the right heart inflow area (Figure 7.2f). Rotating through 90° in the parasternal view to a superior short axis plane at the level of the atria and great vessels reveals the atrial septum (Figure 7.2g). In the apical approach the meeting of the atrial septum and the atrioventricular junction is highlighted (Figure 7.2h) and tilting posteriorly will show the coronary sinus and posterior septum (Figure 6.6i).

Abnormalities of the atrial septum and the great veins are described below.

FORAMEN OVALE AND ATRIAL SEPTAL DEFECTS

In the majority of babies, the foramen ovale, which is patent during fetal life, closes at birth. However, occasionally, it can remain open, or re-open in later life. The flap that closes the foramen ovale may be aneurysmal (Figure 7.3a). Colour mapping and pulsed wave Doppler images reveal the direction and velocity of flow (Figure 7.3b).

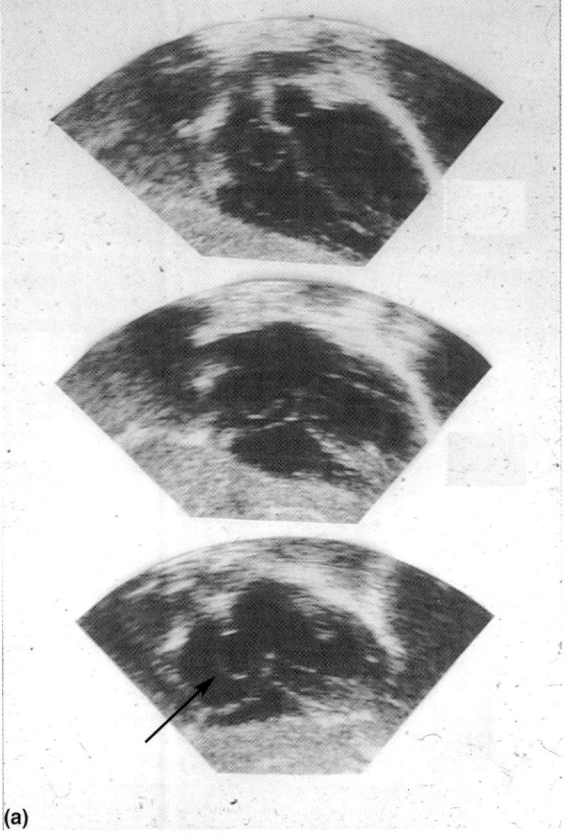

(a)

The most common type of defect of the interatrial septum is a secundum atrial septal defect. The ostium primum type defect is part of the group of the complex atrioventricular defects and is described later, but the secundum defect can be recognised and differentiated from a primum atrial septal defect by the presence of atrial septal tissue around the defect. Colour mapping and pulsed wave Doppler indicates the direction and velocity of flow (Figure 7.4a). M-mode studies of right and left ventricular wall motion in the present of large atrial shunts reveal reversed septal motion (Figure 7.4b) and a dilated right heart. Upon finding an atrial communication of any size, it is important to assess the peak tricuspid regurgitant jet velocity in order to estimate the pulmonary artery systolic pressure (Figure 7.4c).

ANOMALOUS PULMONARY VENOUS DRAINAGE

Anomalous pulmonary venous drainage (APVD) can be partial or total. In the most common type of total APVD (TAPVD) (Figure 7.5 (bottom)) the pulmonary veins form a venous confluence that ascends to meet the innominate vein draining to the heart via a distended SVC – supracardiac connection (Figure 7.5 (top)). Colour mapping almost always shows an interatrial shunt from the right to the left atrium and, more importantly, allows the operator to follow the direction and velocity of the pulmonary venous flow. Occasionally, pulmonary venous return may be obstructed, so be aware of turbulent or variant colour flow mapping.

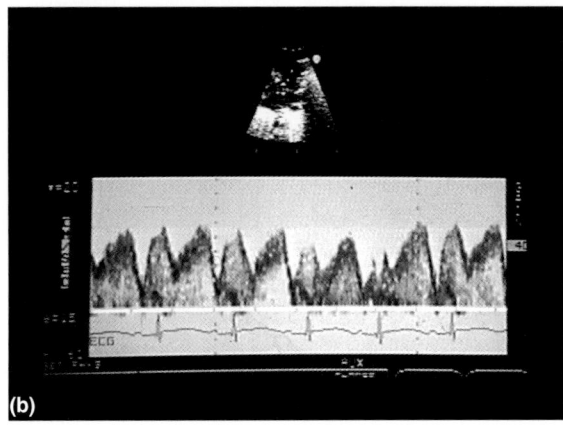

(b)

Figure 7.3 – (a) A series of three views from the subcostal four chamber view showing an aneurysm in the region of the foramen ovale (arrowed). (b) Pulsed Doppler spectral trace showing the flow pattern through a patent foramen ovale.

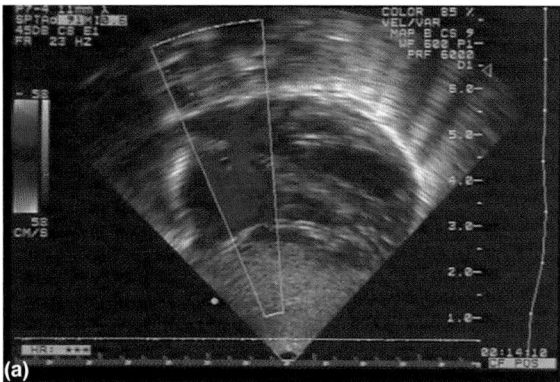

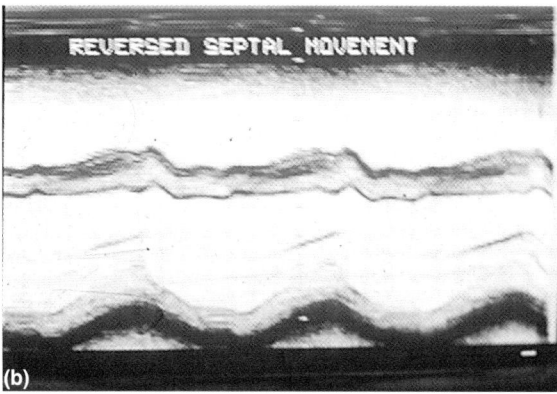

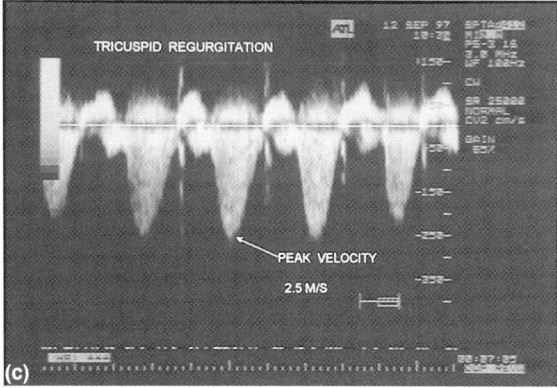

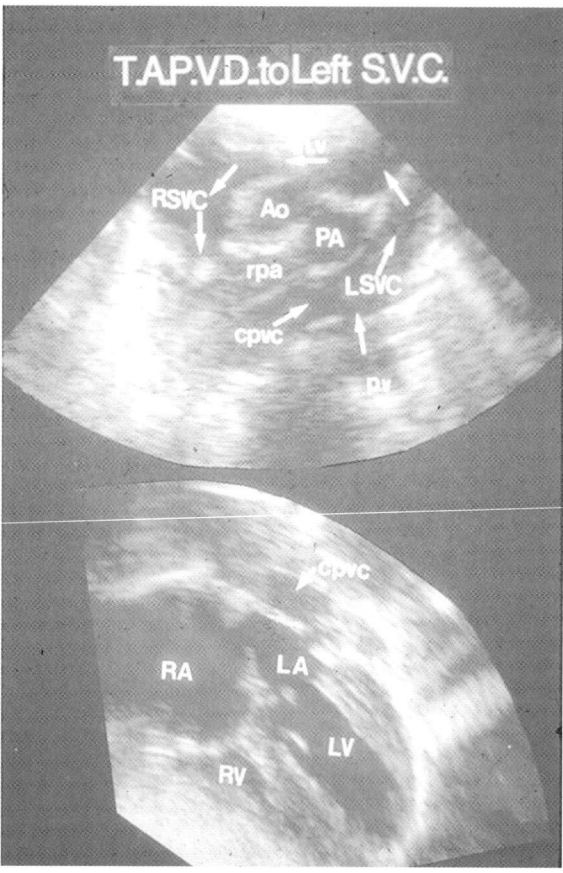

Figure 7.5 – Subcostal four chamber view showing a small left atrium and a separate pulmonary venous confluence lying behind the heart (bottom). Coronal suprasternal view showing the left-sided ascending vein and confluence with the superior vena cava (top).
RSVC – right superior vena cava
LSVC – left superior vena cava
CPVC – common pulmonary venous connection
In.v – innominate vein

Figure 7.4 – (a) Subcostal four chamber view with colour flow mapping demonstrating a broad front of flow (red) across a large atrial septal defect. (b) M-mode trace showing right ventricular volume overload and reversed septal motion in atrial septal defect (c) Continuous wave Doppler trace showing tricuspid regurgitant jet (2.5 ms⁻¹) coincidental with secundum atrial septal defect.

Anomalous pulmonary veins may also drain to other sites, such as the coronary sinus or directly into the SVC. Less commonly, drainage may be below the heart and diaphragm via the IVC and the portal vein. The latter is almost always obstructed.

If there is total lack of atrial septation a common atrium exists and a search must be made for systemic and pulmonary venous drainage.

Superior tilting from the four chamber inlet view with a minor degree of clockwise rotation will reveal the SVC running parallel to and on the right of the aorta, draining into the right atrium.

Roofing and septation of the atria can fail, in which case the right upper pulmonary vein drains directly to right atrium. This is commonly termed a sinus venosus atrial septal defect (Figure 7.6). The right heart will be

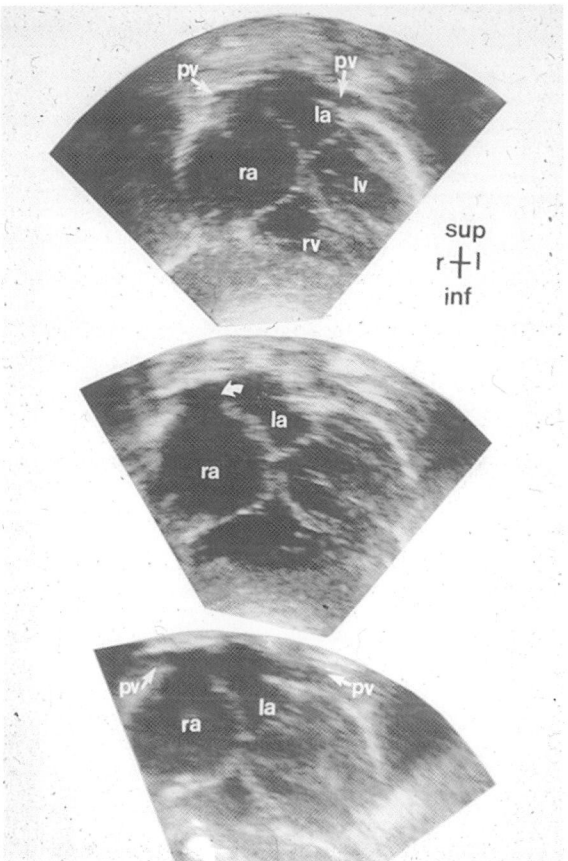

Figure 7.6 – A series of three subcostal four chamber views with increasing anterior angulation showing a high atrial septal defect of the sinus venosus type. An anomalous right upper pulmonary vein is arrowed.

enlarged and colour mapping will demonstrate the direction of flow. M-mode studies will demonstrate right ventricular volume overload with reversed septal motion.

COR TRIATRIATUM

This is a rare condition in which a membrane lies across the left atrium, separating the venous inflow from the mitral valve. The membrane usually has a small orifice through which blood flows at a high velocity. This can be seen on Doppler examination.

Atrioventricular junction

four chamber scans from the apical or subcostal approach give excellent access to the atrioventricular junction and its valves. Remember that the tricuspid valve insertion is displaced apically relative to the mitral valve (Figure 7.7). It has a single large apical papillary muscle with a number of other smaller attachments. The mitral valve inserts high on the atrioventricular septum and has paired papillary muscles attached to the lateral left ventricular wall. As in adult echocardiography, the valve structure and function must be assessed. Are the leaflets thickened? Do they prolapse? Are the chordae shortened? Is the flow through the valve normal?

PARTIAL ATRIOVENTRICULAR SEPTAL DEFECT

A partial atrioventricular septal defect (Figure 7.8) is commonly referred to as an ostium primum atrial septal defect. There is common insertion of the atrioventricular valves and interatrial communication above the valves, but the ventricular septum is intact. The defect is described as partial because there is no ventricular septal defect. Colour mapping plays an important role

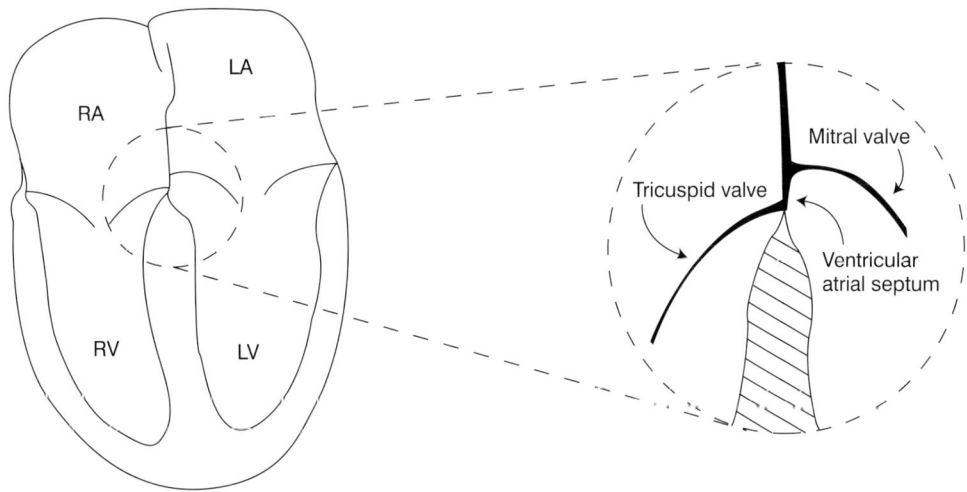

Figure 7.7 – Diagram showing the relationship of the atrioventricular valves as seen in the four chamber view.

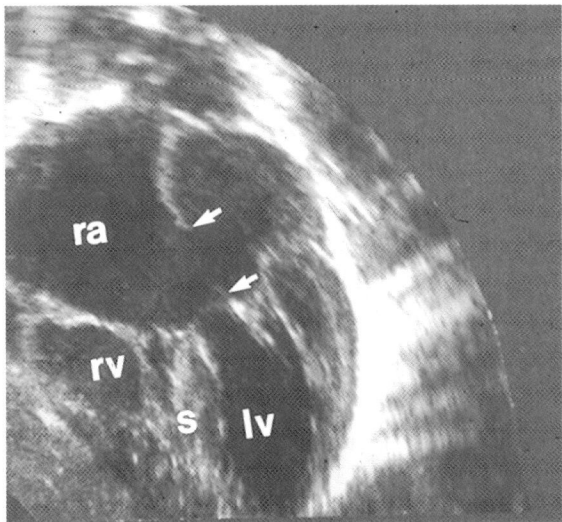

Figure 7.8 – Subcostal four chamber view showing a large atrial septal defect of the partial atrioventricular canal type (also called ostium primum ASD)

in demonstrating the function of the atrioventricular valves. Regurgitation is a common feature and often unilateral atrial enlargement is found. Regurgitation may occur from both ventricles into one atrium preferentially. Again, Doppler velocity assessment of a right ventricle to right atrium jet will aid in estimating the pulmonary artery systolic pressure. The atrioventricular junction may often be better demonstrated using apical four chamber projections.

COMPLETE ATRIOVENTRICULAR SEPTAL DEFECT

In this condition there is a complex malformation of the atrioventricular junction, involving both atrial and ventricular septal defects (Figure 7.9a). There is usually a large common atrioventricular valve with superior and inferior bridging leaflets. During systole both atrial and ventricular defects can be seen. During diastole, when the common valve is open, all chambers of the heart are in continuity. Regurgitation is common and is assessed using colour mapping and continuous wave Doppler examination. In this anomaly high pulmonary artery pressures can be expected (Figure 7.9b).

EBSTEIN'S ANOMALY

Ebstein's anomaly (Figure 7.10) is a malformation of the tricuspid valve, where the leaflets are abnormal and displaced apically, being attached to the walls of the right ventricle. There is right atrial enlargement, with atrialisation of the septal structures above the tricuspid

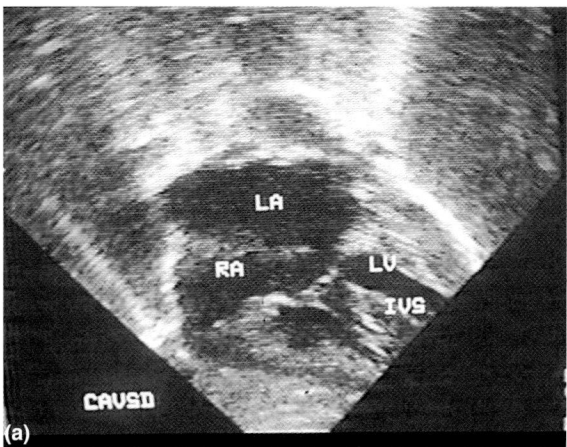

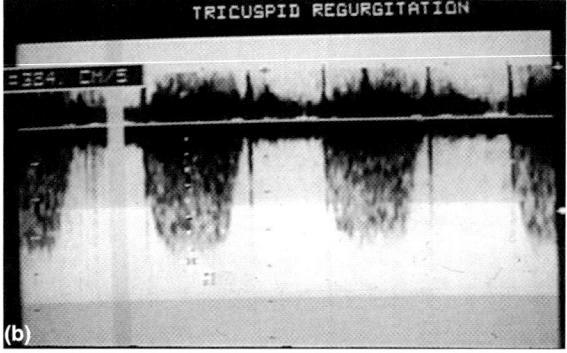

Figure 7.9 – (a) Complete atrioventricular septal defect seen in the four chamber view. The ventricular septal defect is not prominent in this example. (b) Continuous wave Doppler recording of tricuspid regurgitation showing a high jet velocity (4 m/s) which indicates severe pulmonary hypertension.

valve septal leaflet. Colour mapping reveals tricuspid regurgitation (Figure 7.10b) and continuous wave Doppler estimates of pulmonary arterial systolic pressure can be made. Secundum atrial septal defects are also common in such cases.

CLEFT MITRAL VALVE

This anomaly of the anterior leaflet (Figure 7.11) can sometimes occur as an isolated abnormality, usually with mitral regurgitation, but is more commonly associated with atrioventricular septal defects.

PARACHUTE MITRAL VALVE

Not all mitral valves will have two papillary muscles. A mitral valve with a single papillary muscle is described as a parachute mitral valve (Figure 7.12) and is commonly regurgitant and stenotic.

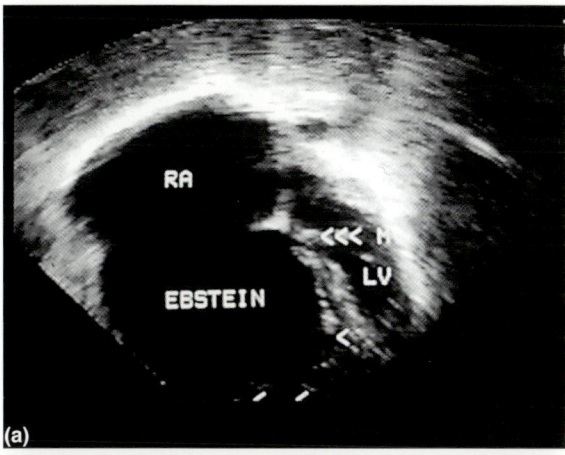

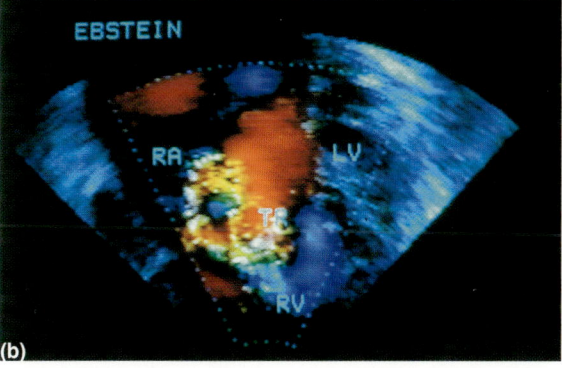

Figure 7.10 – (a) Four chamber view showing large 'atrialised' right atrium due to the abnormally positioned tricuspid valve. (b) Colour flow image of (a) showing a prominent jet of tricuspid regurgitation.

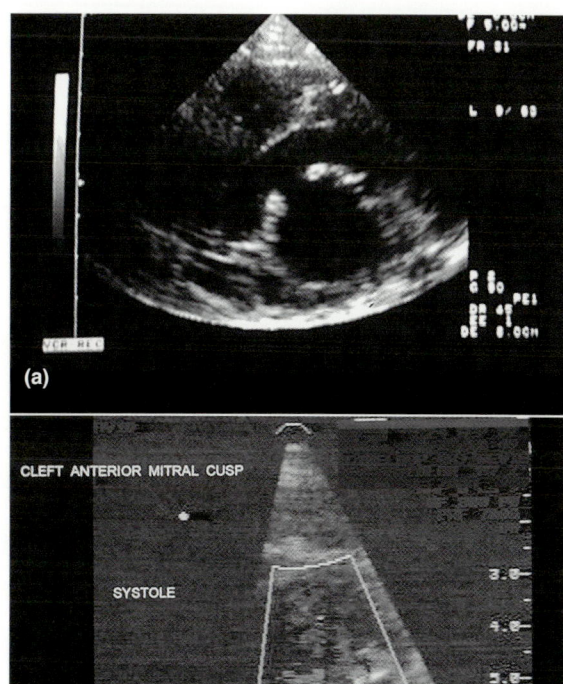

Figure 7.11 – (a) Short axis view showing a prominent cleft in the anterior leaflet of the mitral valve. (b) Short axis view of a mitral regurgitant jet through an anterior leaflet cleft.

VENTRICULAR HYPOPLASIA

Flow status during interuterine life may cause relative hypoplasia of some of the cardiac chambers. It is therefore important to assess the relative structural chamber sizes. It is equally important to assess the atrioventricular valve chordae with regard to their position and insertion, and the papillary muscles. Apical approaches often reveal more of these details and scanning 'off axis' may open up the anatomy for better assessment (Figure 7.13).

In the assessment of the atrioventricular junction the type of connection is noted. It is a general rule that ventricles follow valves. If the left atrium empties through the mitral valve into a long smooth left ventricular type ventricle, a concordant connection is made. If the left atrium connects to a tricuspid type valve leading into a coarsely trabeculated ventricle of right ventricular type, a discordant connection is pre-

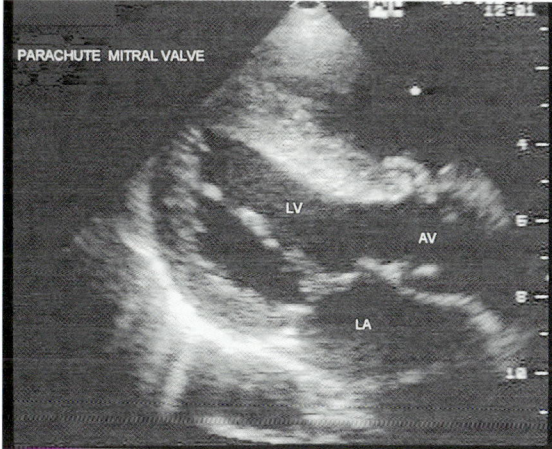

Figure 7.12 – Parasternal long axis view of a parachute mitral valve with a single papillary muscle.

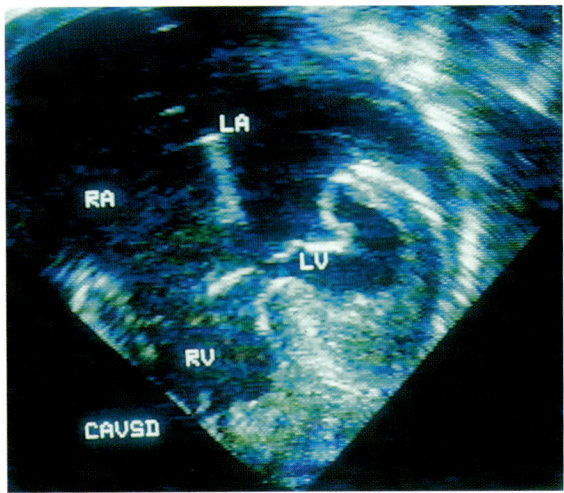

Figure 7.13 – Complete atrioventricular septal defect seen in the four chamber view, the ventricular septal defect is seen lying below the atrioventricular valves.

sent (Figure 7.14). Simply describe what you have seen in order to avoid ambiguity (e.g. 'a left atrium going through a tricuspid valve into a right ventricle with discordance'). Remember to assess ventricular function as you would in an adult scan.

DOUBLE INLET VENTRICLE

Both atrioventricular valves may direct their flow into one ventricle (usually the left ventricle). This is termed a double inlet ventricle (Figure 7.15). It is important here to search for a ventricular septal defect,

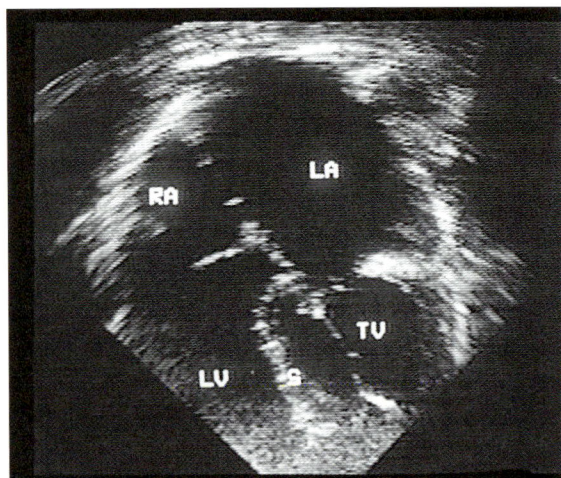

Figure 7.14 – Atrioventricular discordance. This four chamber view shows reversal of the usual mitral-tricuspid relationship.

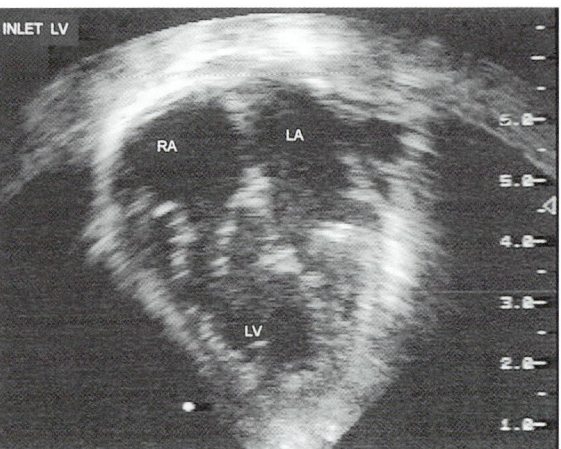

Figure 7.15 – Double inlet ventricle as seen in the apical four chamber view.

which is commonly the source of flow to a rudimentary second ventricular chamber the position of which must be identified and described, (e.g. 'superior and to the left').

ATRESIA OR ABSENCE OF AN ATRIOVENTRICULAR VALVE

There may be atresia or absence of either the tricuspid valve or the mitral valve (Figures 7.16(a), (b)). The absent valve is replaced by an echo-dense bar of sulcus tissue. Colour flow mapping will reveal an atrial communication allowing venous mixing and flow through the remaining atrioventricular valve. In both instances, a ventricular septal defect and rudimentary ventricle should be sought. Colour mapping will aid in the assessment of valve competence, and flow through an atrial or ventricular septal defect.

Views for assessing the ventricular septum

The interventricular septum is a particularly important area to study, not only because of its curved anatomy and its closely related structures, but because a ventricular septal defect is one of the commonest intracardiac defects. These defects commonly occur alone, but many other intracardiac abnormalities are associated with them.

Use standard subcostal views to assess the inlet and trabecular septum (Figure 7.17a). By tilting the transducer inferiorly the full extent of the posterior septum can be visualised (Figure 7.17b). Use colour mapping in these views to search for tiny defects. Tilting the transducer superiorly from four chamber view will reveal the subaortic septum (Figure 7.17c). Rotating clockwise

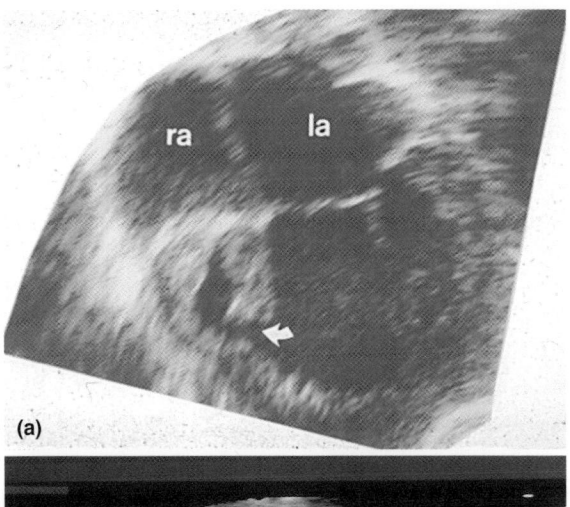

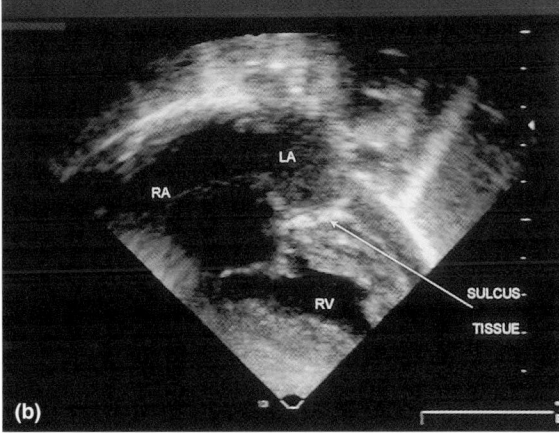

Figure 7.16 – (a) Tricuspid atresia. There is a prominent wedge of tissue in place of the normal tricuspid valve. The hypoplastic right ventricle fills from the left ventricle through a restrictive ventricular septal defect. (b) Mitral atresia as seen in an apical 4 chamber view seen with sulcus tissue in place of the mitral valve. There is severe LV hypoplasia.

from the subcostal four chamber view and tilting the transducer anteriorly opens up the right ventricular outflow tract and allows inspection of the subpulmonary septum (Figure 7.17d). Again colour mapping will reveal the origin and direction of ventricular septal defect jets; for example, a subaortic ventricular septal defect may direct its jet towards the tricuspid valve or the right ventricular outflow tract. Tilting posteriorly in this view allows an alternative view to be obtained of the trabecular septum (Figure 7.17e). Rotating anticlockwise opens a third subcostal short axis view, and again allows inspection of the subaortic and trabecular areas (Figure 7.17f).

The parasternal long axis scan gives perpendicular access to the subaortic and midtrabecular septum; therefore it is a good plane in which to study ventricular septal defect jet velocity. Very small perimembranous subaortic defects may not be visualised, except on colour mapping. While in this view look for aortic regurgitation and/or left ventricular outflow ledges, which are commonly associated with perimembranous defects and may be acquired lesions. Parasternal short axis scans superiorly from the base to the apex inferiorly demonstrate the subaortic inlet to the trabecular septum (Figures 7.17g,h,i). Use of colour flow mapping will aid in the assessment of the direction of the defect jets, their origin and velocity.

Apical four chamber scans allow inspection of the inlet and trabecular areas. Tilt the transducer anteriorly to open up the left ventricular outflow tract and image the subaortic septum, and posteriorly to demonstrate the posterior septum (Figures 7.17j,k,l).

VENTRICULAR SEPTAL DEFECTS

Ventricular septal defects (VSDs) can be grouped into three main categories (Figure 7.18)

- inlet associated with the atrioventricular junction

- outlet associated with the ventriculoarterial junction

- trabecular, in muscle away from the valves.

Their boundaries and/or margins of the inlet and outlet defects must be described. For example, a VSD under the aortic valve with only valve tissue above it is perimembranous and subaortic (i.e. there is no muscle above the defect). If there is muscle on both sides, the VSD is muscular subaortic (Figure 7.19a). Some defects, particularly perimembranous VSDs have associated redundant or aneurysmal tissue, which may partially cover the defect. Colour mapping and continuous wave Doppler examination should be used to assess the direction and velocity of the flow. However, better alignment with a subaortic VSD jet is often achieved via a parasternal long-axis approach (Figure 7.19b).

Flow velocity across a VSD reveals the pressure drop between the left and right ventricles and will therefore give an estimate of the right ventricular pressure if the patient's systemic blood pressure is also recorded. This holds true for pulmonary artery systolic pressure in the absence of any right ventricular outflow or pulmonary valve obstruction. Basically, small VSDs give rise to high velocity jets and a low pulmonary artery pressure (Figure 7.19c). Large VSDs (Figure 7.20) give low

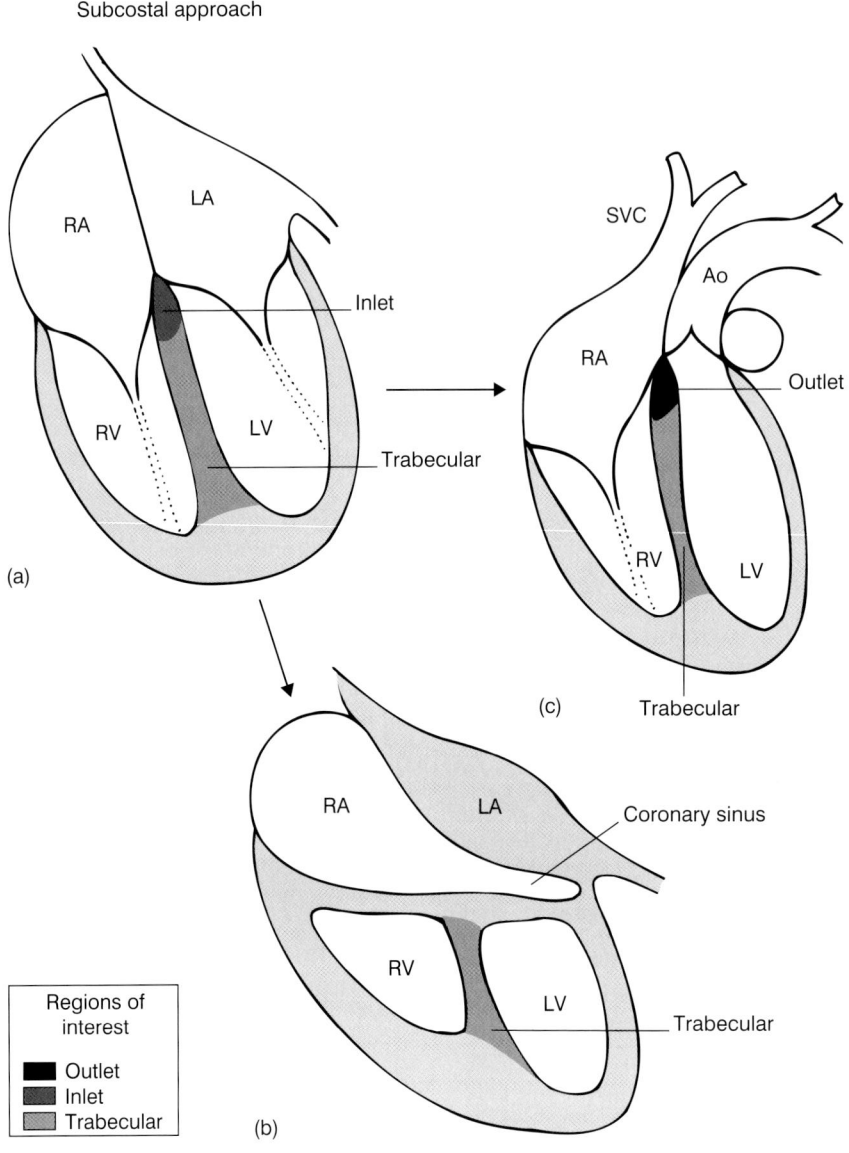

Subcostal approach

Regions of
interest

■ Outlet
■ Inlet
■ Trabecular

Figure 7.17 – (a,b,c) Diagram to show assessment of the interventricular septum from a series of subcostal four chamber views.

velocity jets and a high pulmonary artery pressure. Some VSDs shunt bidirectionally or even only right to left.

In follow-up assessment of a patient with a VSD, the size and function of the left ventricle are important measures because larger defects commonly cause left ventricular volume overload (Figure 7.21).

Remember, that more than one VSD may be present. Therefore, search over the entire ventricular septum. At the end of the examination the defect or defects should have been defined in terms of their position, size, related structures and any associated abnormality, such as redundant tissue.

Ventriculo-arterial junction

Next the operator must assess and describe the ventriculoarterial junction. A long, smooth, morphological left ventricle giving rise to the long gentle curve of the

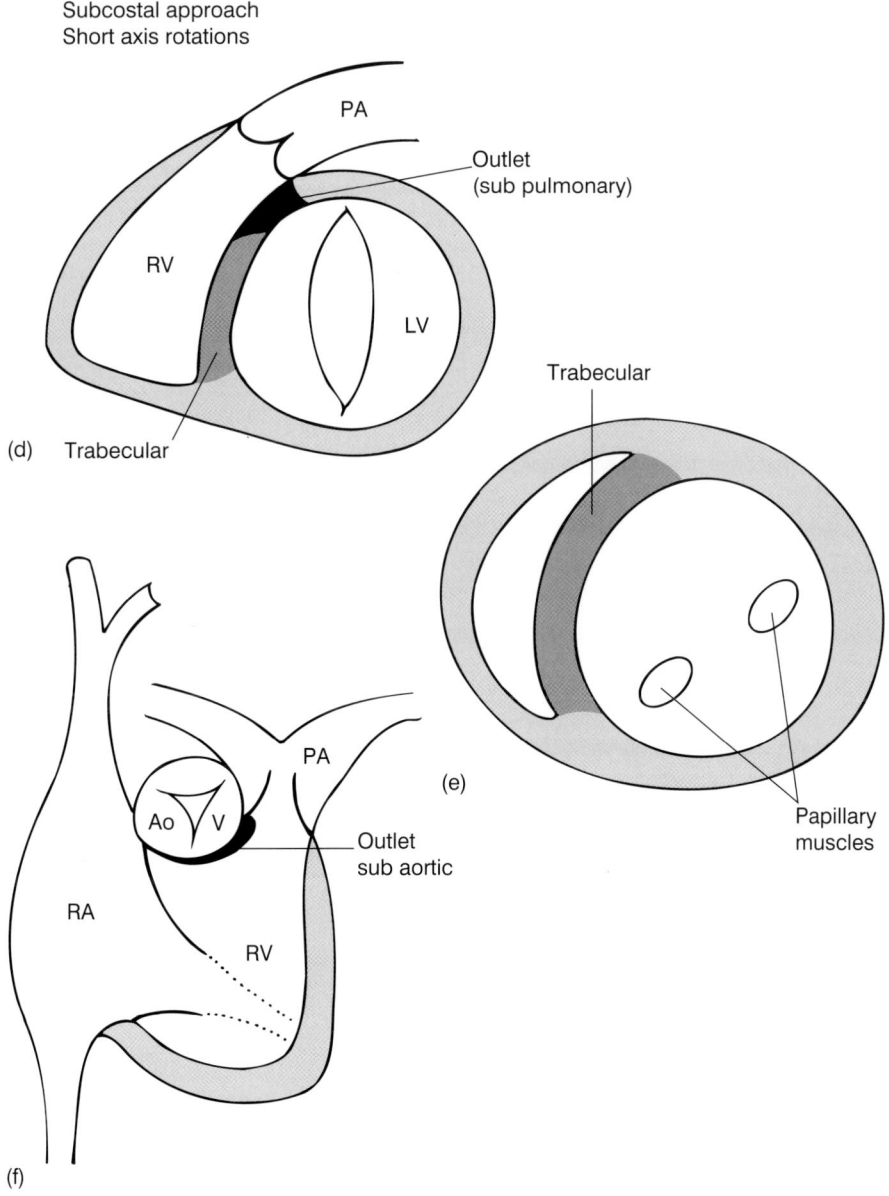

Subcostal approach
Short axis rotations

Figure 7.17 – (d,e,f) Diagram to show assessment of the interventricular septum from a series of subcostal short axis views.

aorta and a coarsely trabeculated morphological right ventricle giving rise to the short bifurcating pulmonary artery demonstrates concordant (normal) ventriculoarterial connections. In concordant connections the anterior pulmonary artery crosses over the central aorta. The ventriculoarterial valves (aortic and pulmonary) must be assessed carefully.

TRANSPOSITION OF THE GREAT ARTERIES (VENTRICULOARTERIAL DISCORDANCE)

In this condition the morphological left ventricle gives rise to the pulmonary artery and the morphological right ventricle gives rise to the aorta (Figure 7.22). Commonly, the aorta and main pulmonary artery run parallel to each other, the aorta lying anteriorly. In

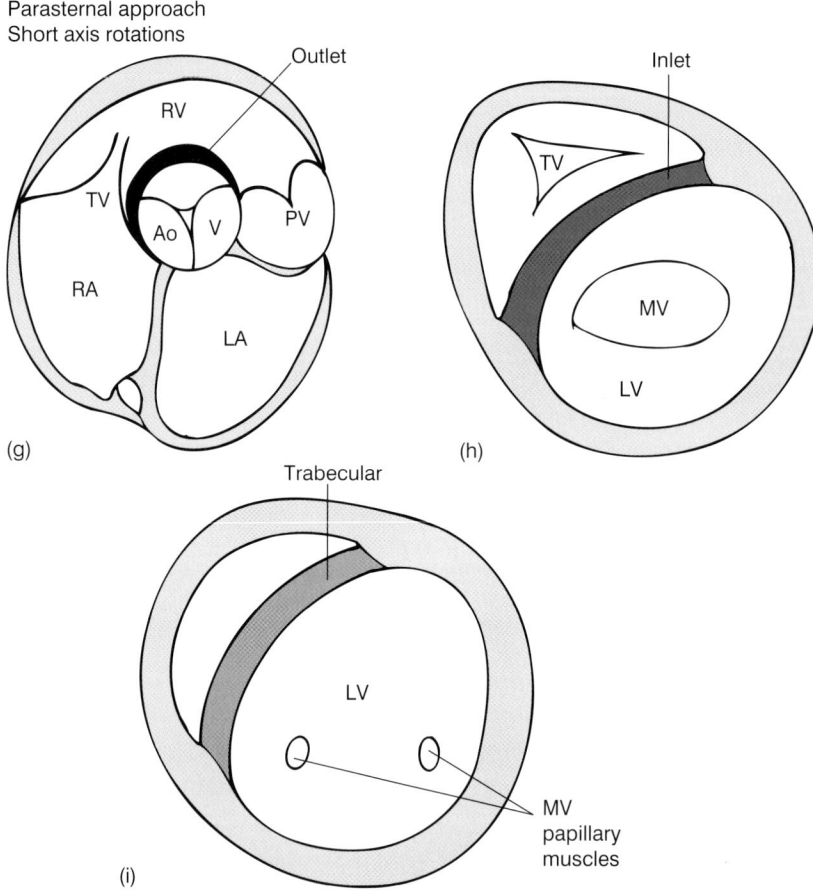

Parasternal approach
Short axis rotations

Figure 7.17 – (g,h,i) Diagram to show assessment of the interventricular septum from a series of left parasternal short axis views.

addition, the aortic valve is usually positioned more superiorly relative to the pulmonary valve, in contrast to normal position where the pulmonary valve is the more superior of the two. These relationships between the great arteries vary from patient to patient to a certain extent.

Transposition of the great arteries is one of the commoner of the cyanotic conditions presenting in infancy. Upon discovery of this condition the presence and size of an interatrial communication becomes important as this venous mixing at the atrial level will help maintain the infant until surgical repair can be made.

DOUBLE OUTLET VENTRICLE

Two great arteries may arise from one ventricle (Figure 7.23) – double outlet of either the right or left ventricles or from a single ventricle. It is necessary to describe position and laterality of the vessels one to another, (e.g. 'the pulmonary artery anterior and to the left of the

aorta'). Almost universally a subarterial VSD is present and therefore size of the defect and the flow within it must be assessed. The function and structure of the aortic and pulmonary valves must not be forgotten, and imaging and Doppler techniques are both important, as with acquired valve lesions.

There are three main conditions where there is only one great artery arising from the heart (Figure 7.24). These are distinctly different in their prognosis and treatment and therefore in all instances the aortic arch and descending aorta as well as the pulmonary artery branches should be inspected carefully to ensure correct diagnosis. The conditions are common arterial trunk or truncus arteriosus, pulmonary atresia and aortic atresia.

COMMON ARTERIAL TRUNK

In this condition a single outlet valve, the truncal valve, gives rise to a large single great artery, which immediately divides into the aorta and the pulmonary artery

Apical four chamber approach

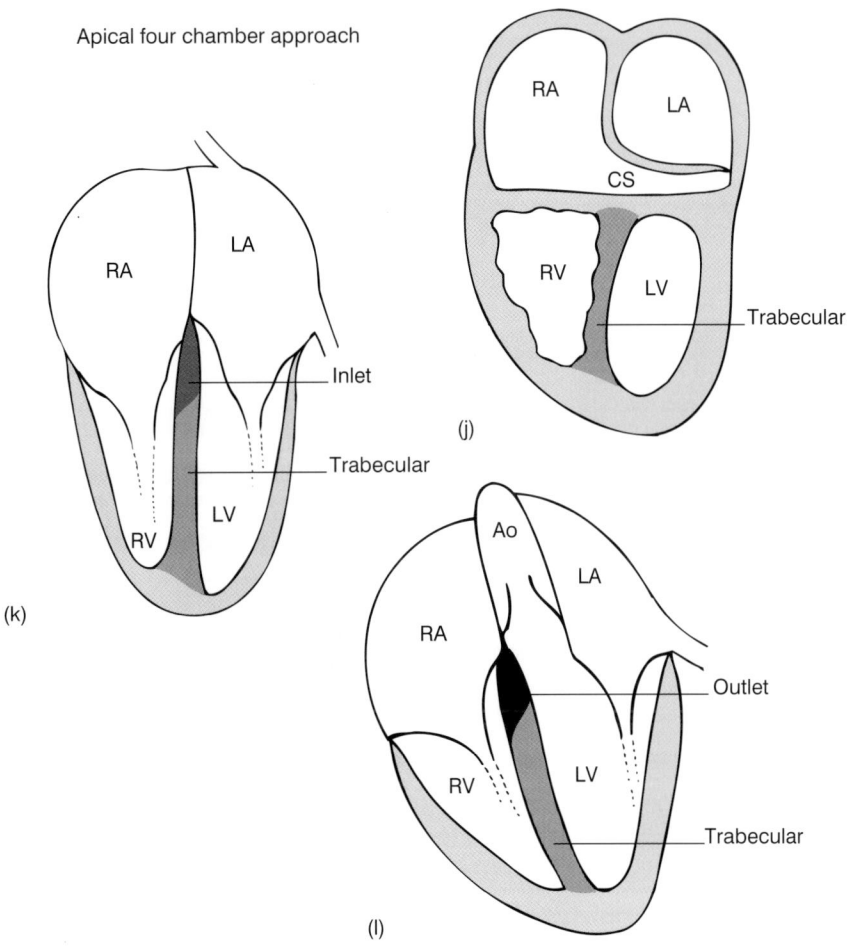

(k)

(j)

(l)

Figure 7.17 – (j,k,l) Diagram to show assessment of the interventricular septum from a series of apical four chamber views.

branches. The branching patterns vary slightly, but in all cases there is a large ventricular septal defect below the truncal valve (Fig 7.25(a,b,c)).

PULMONARY ATRESIA

Inspection of the great vessels may reveal pulmonary valve atresia with or without a coincidental defect of the ventricular septum (Figure 7.25(d)). Careful parasternal and suprasternal studies should be made to assess size of the valves and the flow in the pulmonary artery branches. In some cases of pulmonary atresia there may be no functional main pulmonary artery, but in all cases there must be some form of alternative blood supply to the pulmonary arteries; this is usually a patent arterial duct or abnormal collateral vessels.

AORTIC ATRESIA

Aortic valve atresia is commonly part of the hypoplastic left heart syndrome and goes hand in hand with atresia or severe hypoplasia of the mitral valve and left ventricle (Figure 7.26). Patent ductus arteriosus is usually present. Therefore, careful arch and parasternal studies should be made to assess the flow through the duct and the duct size. The right atrium, right ventricle and pulmonary artery in these cases are always enlarged. The left atrium will be small.

The above three causes of single great artery are relatively uncommon and the more common tetralogy of Fallot involves abnormalities of both great arteries and the heart itself.

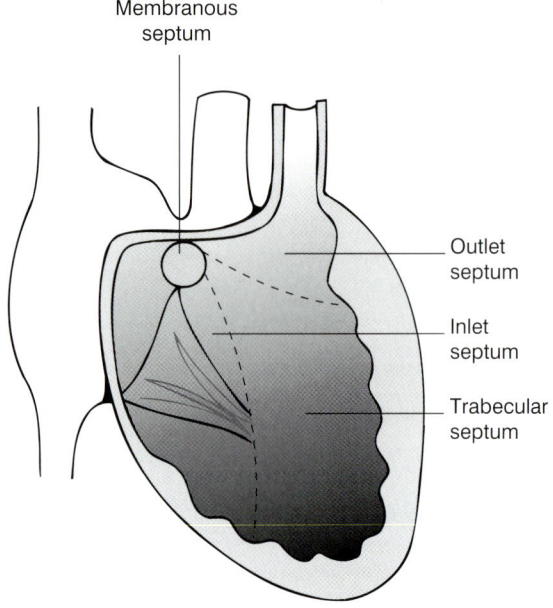

Membranous septum

Outlet septum

Inlet septum

Trabecular septum

Figure 7.18 – Diagram representing the opened right ventricle, exposing the septal surface. Typical VSD sites are shown.

FALLOT'S TETRALOGY

Inspection of the ventriculoarterial connections may reveal a combination know as Fallot's tetralogy. There are four main components (Figure 7.27(a) and (b)):

- a perimembranous subaortic ventricular septal defect

- the aortic valve overrides the crest of the ventricular septum

- infundibular (right ventricular outflow) and/or pulmonary valve stenosis

- a large muscular right ventricle.

The condition is quite variable in its expression. In some cases there is an underdeveloped main pulmonary artery and branches. In extreme cases pulmonary atresia may occur. The main pulmonary artery and branches may be seen better on the parasternal short axis view (Figure 7.27(c)).

The continuous wave Doppler wave spectral trace in the presence of infundibular and valvular pulmonary stenosis shows a characteristic double waveform. The muscular or dynamic obstruction in the infundibulum causes the velocity to increase gradually through systole, whereas the fixed or valvular stenosis causes a much sharper velocity rise at the onset of systole (Figure 7.28).

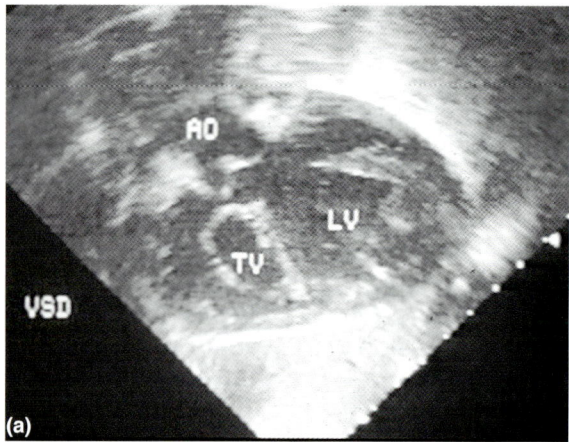

(a)

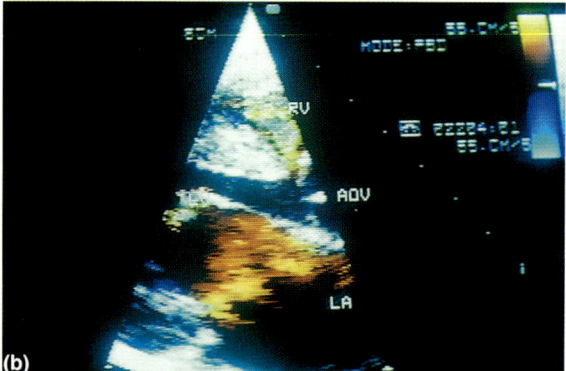

(b)

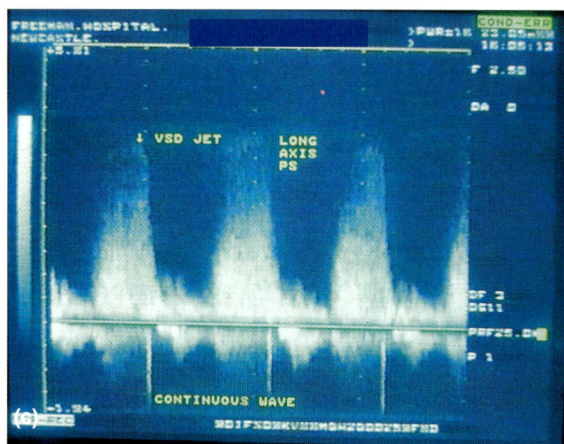

Figure 7.19 – (a) Subaortic VSD seen in the modified subcostal four chamber plane. (b) Colour flow Doppler image showing high velocity flow from the subaortic region to the right ventricle through a small VSD. (c) Continuous wave Doppler recording of a high velocity jet passing through a small VSD. The high velocity jet (5m/s) confirms low pressure in the right ventricle.

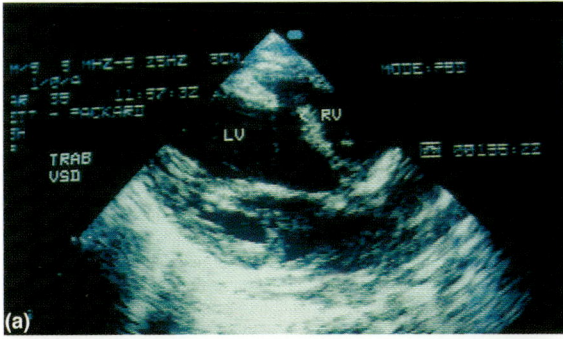

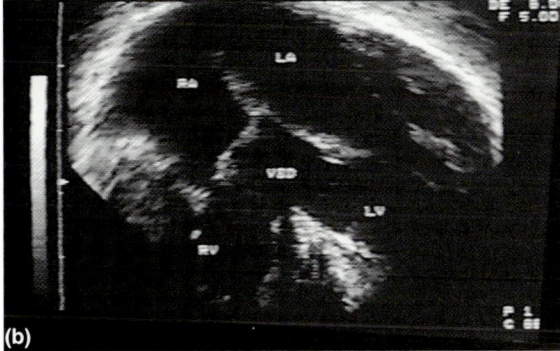

Figure 7.20 – (a) Parasternal view showing a trabecular VSD. (b) An inlet VSD, roofed by the atrioventricular valves, seen in the four chamber view.

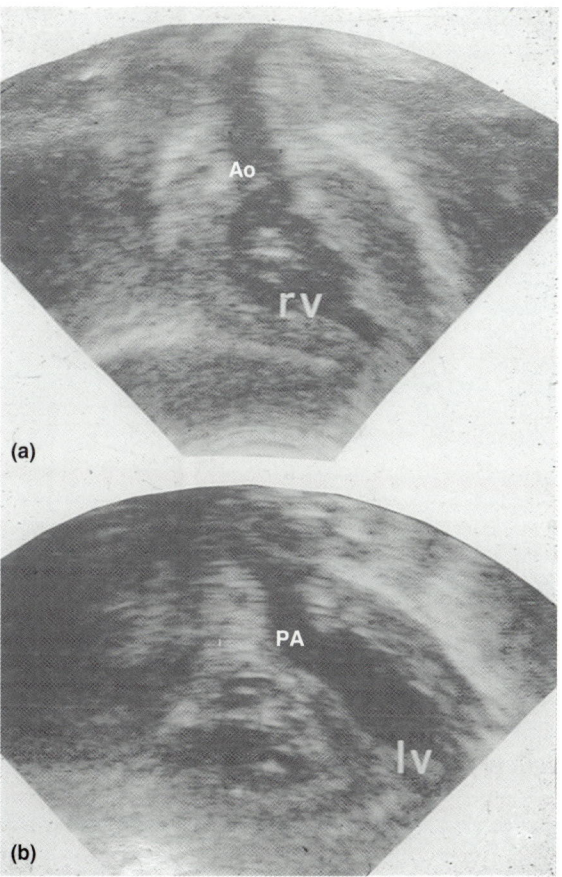

Figure 7.22 – (a) Anteriorly angled subcostal view in transposition of the great arteries showing the aorta arising from the right ventricle. (b) More posterior angulation shows the pulmonary artery arising from the left ventricle.

There are an number of other abnormalities of the outlet valves or structures near them that need to be excluded in a complete examination.

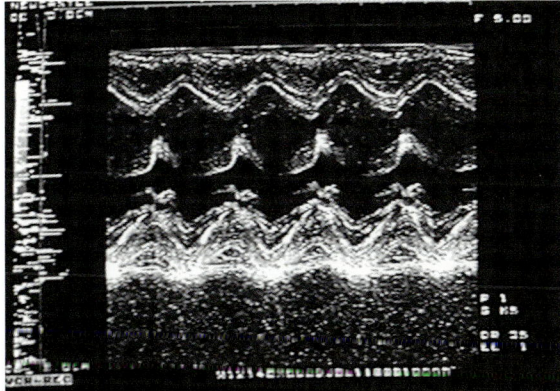

Figure 7.21 – M-mode trace showing a volume overloaded left ventricle in the case of a large VSD.

VALVE STENOSIS

This can occur with both aortic and pulmonary valves, the leaflets being congenitally fused and usually thickened with a small central orifice. The leaflets show a characteristic 'doming' appearance when open. The high velocity of the flow through the valve can be seen clearly on colour flow Doppler imaging, and careful quantitation of the velocity by means of continuous wave techniques will allow estimation the of valve 'gradients'. In some cases there is associated regurgitation through the valve, sometimes with prolapsing leaflets.

BICUSPID AORTIC VALVE

A bicuspid aortic valve (Figure 7.29) is the commonest congenital cardiac malformation and is often associated with mild restriction, which can develop into more

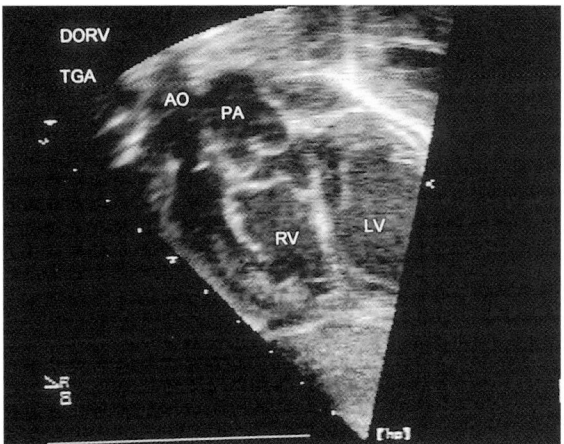

Figure 7.23 – In this rotated subcostal view the right ventricle gives rise to an anterior aorta and a centrally positioned pulmonary artery, i.e. double outlet right ventricle with transposition arrangement of the great arteries.

severe stenosis in later life. Whenever possible, the examination should include an assessment of the number of aortic valve leaflets.

SUBVALVULAR AND SUPRAVALVULAR OBSTRUCTIONS

Muscular subvalvular obstructions may be found in the left or right heart. Use of continuous wave Doppler will aid in the assessment, and colour mapping will indicate the point of acceleration and/or any regurgitant jets. It is important to describe the position and shape of the obstructing elements and any coincidental anatomical features (Figures 7.30(a) and (b)). Aortic regurgitation is commonly associated with left ventricular outflow tract obstruction. Supra-aortic stenosis is a rare abnormality. It is located just above the aortic valve and often has an hourglass shape (Figure 7.31). Stenosis of the main pulmonary artery or its branches may also be seen.

Great vessels

High parasternal views in the neonate and infant give excellent access to the main pulmonary artery and both branches. Suprasternal scans give excellent access to the arch and descending thoracic aorta.

PATENT DUCTUS ATERIOSUS

The arterial duct is a normal structure in the fetus, and usually closes shortly after birth. The duct is commonly patent in premature infants, but in a few cases it can remain patent indefinitely and causes a left-to-right shunt into the lungs. The high parasternal view is the preferred projection for viewing a patent arterial duct (Figure 7.32). Seen as a third leg, the ductal jet is towards the transducer from the descending aorta to the lateral pulmonary artery wall. The ductal velocity mirrors the pressure drop between the aorta and pulmonary artery. In neonates the pulmonary vascular resistance is still high, and the ductal flow may be of

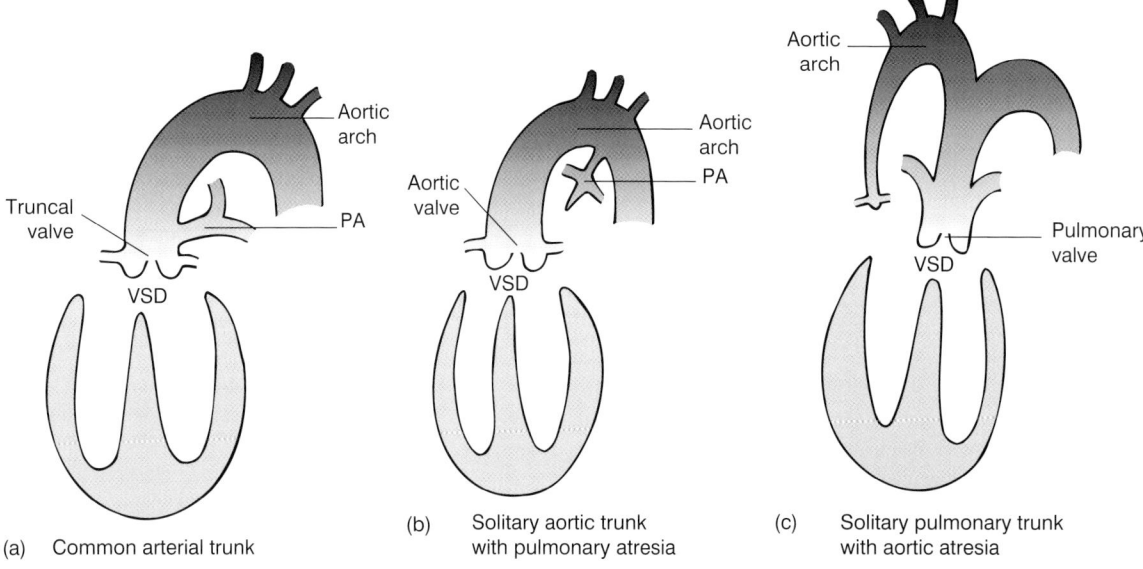

(a)   Common arterial trunk

(b)   Solitary aortic trunk with pulmonary atresia

(c)   Solitary pulmonary trunk with aortic atresia

Figure 7.24

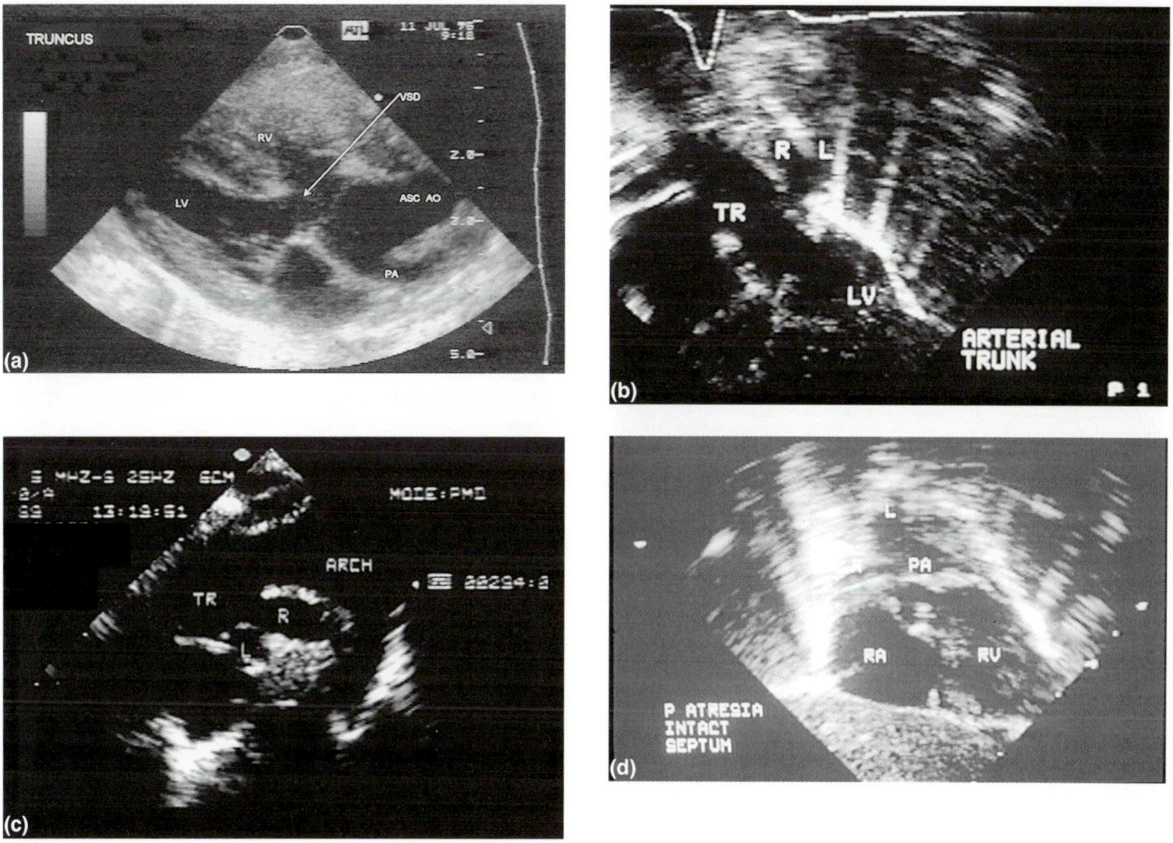

Figure 7.25 – (a) Parasternal long axis view of a common arterial trunk demonstrating the subarterial ventricular septal defect. (b) Subcostal view of a large common arterial trunk arising from the left ventricle. (c) Suprasternal view showing a common arterial trunk giving rise to posterior pulmonary artery branches. (d) Pulmonary atresia with intact ventricular septum. The right ventricle is small with no continuity to the pulmonary artery. The right atrium is large.

low velocity or bidirectional. This is, of course, the case in patients with pulmonary hypertension. Large ductal shunts will manifest themselves as left atrial and left ventricular enlargement with volume overload of the left ventricle. M-mode studies for measuring the aortic root/left atrial ratio (normal ratio about 1: 1) and left ventricular dimensions (see Chapter 4 for ranges of normal values) help in assessing therapy (Figure 7.33).

COARCTATION

In this condition there is a narrowing of the aortic arch, most commonly just distal to the left subclavian artery (Figure 7.34) The narrowing can be due to a discrete shelf, or can take the form of an hourglass type of narrowing or a long segmental narrowing (hypoplastic isthmus). Coarctation of the aorta must be described by its position and type. Continuous wave Doppler studies reveal a classical sawtooth waveform as the flow

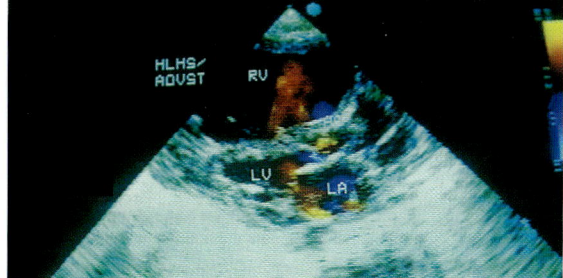

Figure 7.26 – Aortic atresia. The left ventricle is very small and the right ventricle is large. There was little or no flow detected through the aortic valve.

through the descending aorta continues through diastole (Figure 7.35). If a coarctation is found, careful left

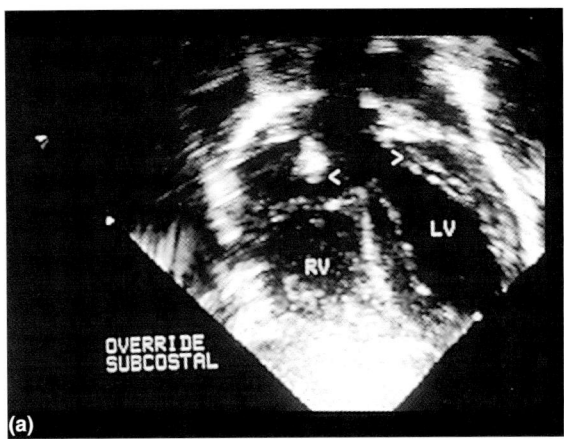

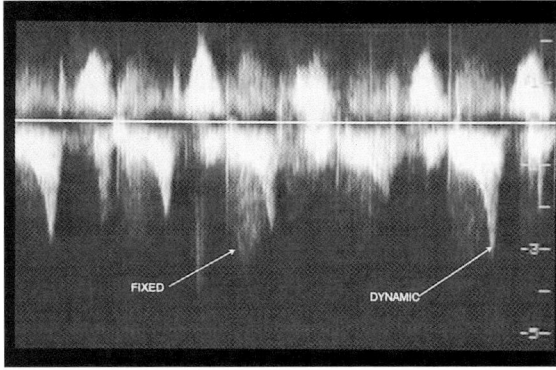

Figure 7.28 – Continuous wave Doppler study of the fixed and dynamic wave form seen in Fallot's tetralogy.

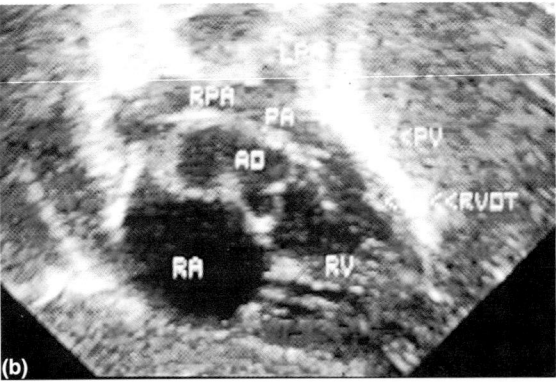

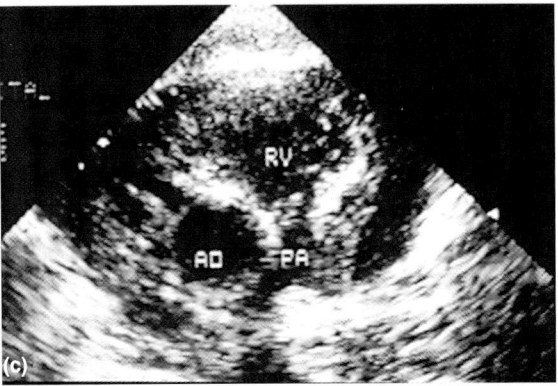

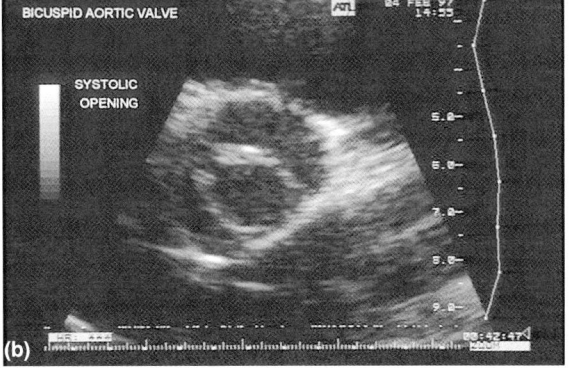

Figure 7.27 – (a) Tetralogy of Fallot showing the large perimembranous VSD. (b) Tetralogy of Fallot showing aortic override onto the right ventricle. (c) Parasternal short axis view in tetralogy of Fallot showing a thickened and stenotic pulmonary valve and a small pulmonary artery.

Figure 7.29 – Short axis view of bicuspid aortic valve in diastole (a) and systole (b).

ventricular studies should be made. Outflow obstruction will be manifested as left ventricular hypertrophy and dysfunction.

An extreme form of the condition is an interrupted aortic arch, where the descending aorta receives all its blood supply from a patent arterial duct (Figure 7.36).

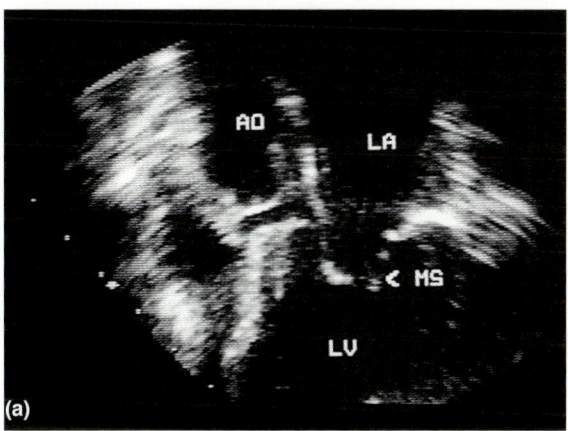

(a)

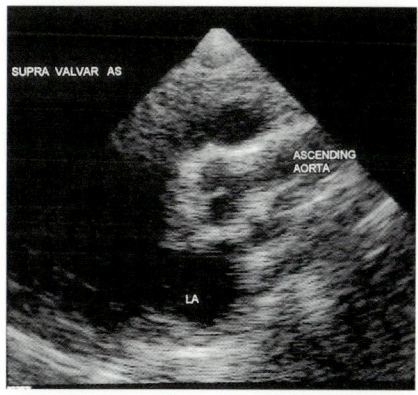

Figure 7.31 – Parasternal long axis view of an aortic root showing supravalvar aortic stenosis coincidental with William's syndrome.

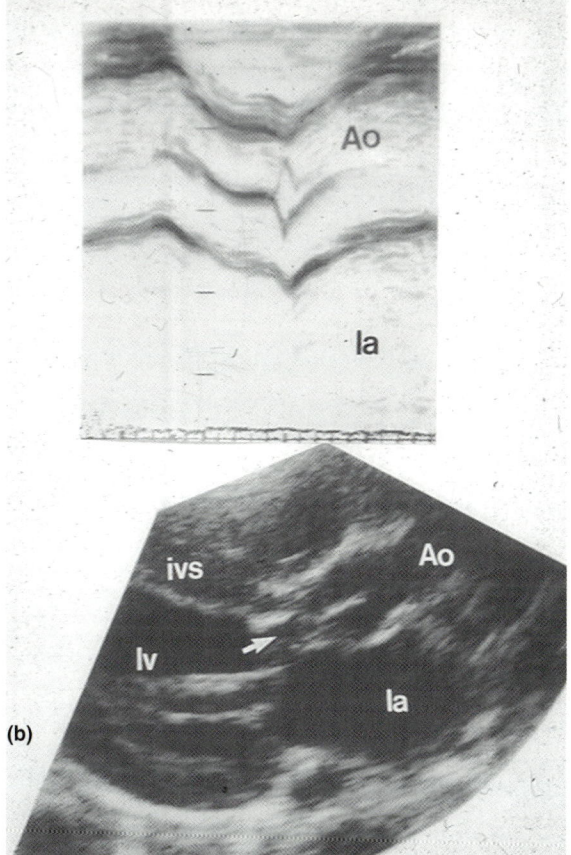

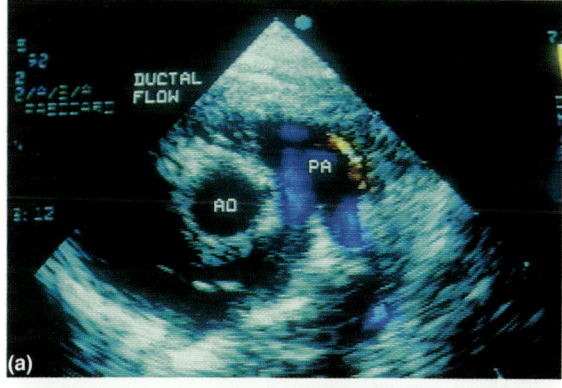

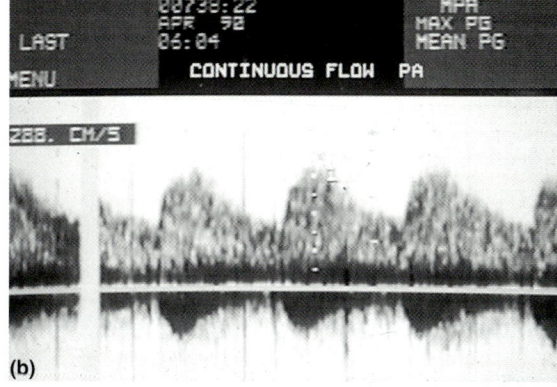

Figure 7.30 – (a) A small subaortic perimembranous VSD lies above the outlet ledge and there is coincidental mitral stenosis. (b) M-mode trace in subaortic stenosis showing early closure of the aortic wave.

Figure 7.32 – (a) Parasternal short axis view (modified) showing a colour flow jet entering the pulmonary artery from a small patent arterial duct. (b) Continuous wave recording of the typical flow pattern.

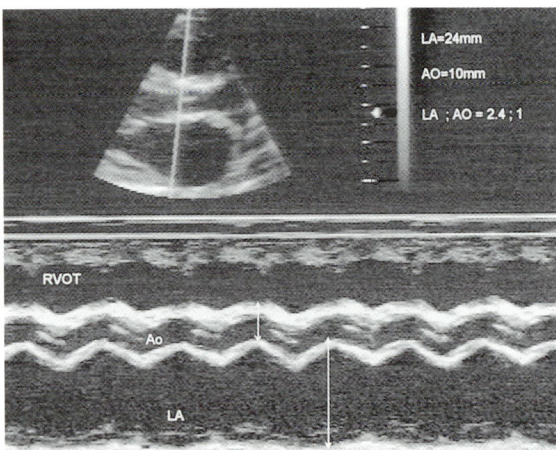

Figure 7.33 – Aortic root and left atrial M-mode trace in a patient with a significant patent ductus arteriosus shunt.

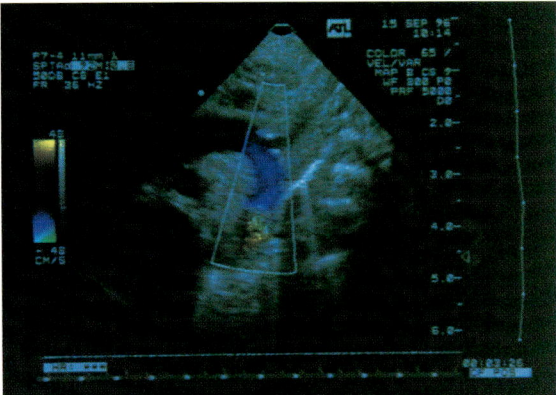

Figure 7.34 - Suprasternal view of aortic coarctation

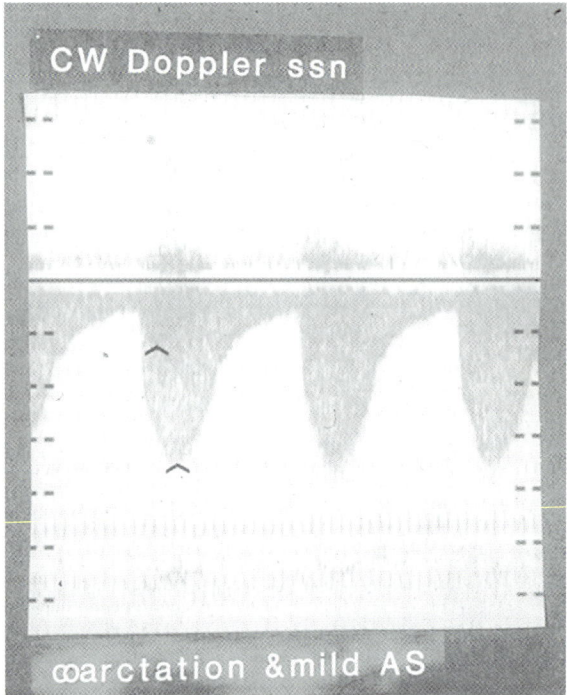

Figure 7.35 – Continuous wave pattern of typical flow in the descending aorta in coarctation.

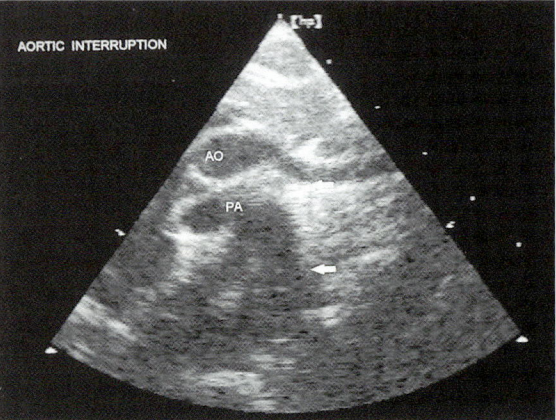

Figure 7.36 – A suprasternal view shows ductal supply to the descending aorta (arrowed) in a case of interrupted aortic arch

Summary

The above account gives an outline of the scanning technique used to assess for congenital heart disease and some of the most important conditions, but only covers the key points. Any echocardiographer scanning patients with congenital heart disease will have to study the conditions in depth from additional literature and will need a lot of supervised scanning experience before undertaking independent work.

Reference

1. Anderson RH. Simplifying the understanding of congenital malformations of the heart. *Int J of Cardio* 1991; **32**: 131–142.

Further reading

Aziz K, Tasneem H. Evaluation of pulmonary artery pressure by Doppler colour flow mapping in patients with ductus arteriosus. *Br Heart J* 1990; **63**: 295.

Bierman SZ, Williams RG. Sub-xiphoid two-dimensional imaging of the inter-atrial septum in infants and neonates with congenital heart disease.*Circulation* 1979; **60**: 80.

Cabnera A, Pastor E, Galdeano J. Cross-sectional echocardiography in the diagnosis of atrioventricular septal defects. *Int J Cardio* 1990; **28**: 19.

Capelli H, Andrade JL, Somerville J. Classification of the site of ventricular septal defect by two-dimensional echocardiography. *Am J of Cardio* 1983; **51**: 1474.

Cavalho JS, Redington AL, Shinebourne EA. Continuous wave Doppler echocardiography and coarctation of the aorta: gradients and flow patterns in the assessment of severity. *Br Heart J* 1990; **64**: 113.

Driscoll DJ, Gutgesell HP, McNamara DG. Echocardiographic features of congenital mitral stenosis. *Am J of Cardio* 1978; **42**: 259.

Gussenhoven WJ, Spitaels SEC, Bon N. Becker AE. Echocardiographic criteria for Ebstein's anomaly of the tricuspid valve. *Br Heart J* 1980; **43**: 31.

Gutgesell HP, Huhta JC, Cohen HH. Two-dimensional echocardiographic assessment of pulmonary artery and aortic arch anatomy in cyanotic infants. J Am Coll of Cardiol 1984; **4**: 1242.

Hatle L, Angelsen B. *Doppler Ultrasound in Cardiology: Physical Principles and Clinical Applications*. 2nd edn. Lea & Febiger. Philadelphia 1985.

Helmcke S, De Souza A, Nanda NC. Two-dimensional and colour Doppler assessment of ventricular septal defect of congenital origin. *Am J of Cardiol* 1989; **63**: 1112.

Houston AB, Gregory NL, Coleman NE. Echocardiographic identification of aorta and main pulmonary artery in complete transposition. *Br Heart J* 1978; **40**: 377.

Lieppe W, Scallion R, Behar VS, Kisslow JA. Two-dimensional echocardiographic findings in atrial septal defect. *Circulation* 1977; **56**: 447.

McCartney SJ, Rigby ML, Anderson RH, Stark J, Silverman NH. Double outlet right ventricle cross-sectional echocardiographic findings, their anatomical explanation and surgical relevance. *Br Heart J* 1984; **52**: 164.

Ports TA, Silverman NH, Schillar MB. Two-dimensional echocardiographic assessment of Ebstein anomaly. *Circulation* 1978; **58**: 336.

Rigby ML, Anderson RH, Gibson D, Jones DDH, Joseph MC, Shinebourne EA. Two-dimensional echocardiographic categorisation of the univentricular heart, ventricular morphology, type and mode of atrioventricular connection. *Br Heart J* 1981; **46**: 603.

Rigby ML, Gibson D, Joseph MC. Recognition of imperforate atrioventricular valve by two-dimensional echocardiography. *Br Heart J* 1982; **47**: 329.

Sahn DJ, Allen HD. Real time cross-sectional echocardiographic diagnosis of coarctation of the aorta: a prospective study of echocardiographic-angiographic correlations. *Circulation* 1978; **56**: 762.

Sahn DJ, Allen HD, Lange LW, Goldberg SJ. Cross-sectional echocardiographic diagnosis of the site of total anomalous pulmonary venous drainage. *Circulation* 1979; **60**: 1317.

Sahn DJ, Harder JR, Freedom RM. 1982.Cross-sectional echocardiographic diagnosis and subclassification of univentricular hearts. Imaging studies of atrioventricular valves, septal structures and rudimentary outflow chambers. *Circulation* 1982; **66**: 1070.

Sherman FA, Sahn DJ, Baldes-Cruz LN. Two-dimensional Dopper colour flow mapping for detecting atrial and ventricular septal defects. *Herz* 1987; **12**: 212.

Shinebourne EA, McCartney FJ, Anderson RH. Sequential chamber localisation- logical approach to diagnosis of congenital heart disease. *Br Heart J* 1976; **38**: 327.

Shub C, Dimopoulis IN, Seward JB Sensitivity of two-dimensional echocardiography in the direct visualisation of atrial septal defect utilising the subcostal approach. *J Am Coll Cardiol* 1983 **2**: 127.

Smallhorn JF, Sutherland GR, Tommasini G, Hunter S, Anderson RH, McCartney FJ. Assessment of total anomalous pulmonary venous connection by two-dimensional echocardiography. *Br Heart J* 1981 **46**: 613.

Smallhorn JF, Freedom. Post-Doppler echocardiography in the pre-operative evaluation of total anomalous pulmonary venous connection. *J Am Coll Cardiol* 1986; **8**: 1413.

Smallhorn JF, Izukawa P, Benson L, Freedom RN. Non-invasive recognition of functional pulmonary atresia by echocardiography. *Am J Cardiol* 1984; **54**: 925.

Snider AR, Silverman NH, Turley K, Ebert PA. Evaluation of infradiaphragmatic total anomalous pulmonary venous connection with two-dimensional echocardiography. *Circulation* 1982; **66**: 1129.

Sutherland GR, Godman MJ, Anderson RH, Hunter S. The spectrum of atrioventricular valve atresia – a two-dimensional echocardiographic pathological correlation. In Echocardiology. (Rijsterborgh H, ed). Martinus Nijhoff,. The Hague, 345.

Sutherland GR, Smallhorn JF, Anderson RH, Rigby MJ, Hunter S. Atrioventricular discordance. Cross-sectional echocardiographic morphological correlative study. *Br Heart J* 1983; **50**: 8.

Sutherland GR, Smyllie JH, Ogilbie BC, Keeton BR. Colour flow imaging in diagnosis of multiple ventricular septal defects. *Br Heart J* 1989; **43**: 612.

Tajik AJ, Seward JV, Hagler DM, Mair DD, Lie GT. Two-dimensional real time ultrasonic imaging of the great vessels of the heart. *Mayo Clin Proc* 1978; **53**: 271.

Tynan MJ, Becker AE, McCartney FJ, Jimenez MQ, Shinebourne EA, Anderson RH. Nomenclature and classification of congenital heart disease. *Br Heart J* 1979; **41**: 544.

8

TRANSOESOPHAGEAL ECHOCARDIOGRAPHY

Stephen Evans

Introduction

Transoesophageal echocardiography (TOE) was first introduced into clinical cardiology in the early 1980s but its usefulness was initially limited to research applications by large, cumbersome and inflexible transducers with poor image quality. Improvements in transducer technology and miniaturisation of transoesophageal probes have fuelled an explosion of interest in TOE over the past ten years with an attendant expansion of its indications. The development of the technique was initially stimulated by the diagnostic limitations of technically inadequate precordial images obtained in up to 20% of adult patients. Transoesophageal echocardiography allows the heart and great vessels to be visualised with high-frequency transducers in great detail, first, because the oesophagus lies in close proximity to the left atrium which provides a convenient echo window and, second because unlike the precordial route, there is no interposition of bone or lung between the transducer and the heart. Both bone and air transmit ultrasound poorly and limit the resolution of transthoracic images. These advantages and the development of user-friendly equipment has extended the technique far beyond limited use in patients with poor precordial windows and has allowed ultrasound imaging of the heart in ever-increasing detail.

Although TOE is now a routine investigation in many cardiovascular diseases it is not a universal panacea for imaging the heart. In common with transthoracic echocardiography (TTE) the quality of the images obtained varies between individual patients and with the structure under study. For example, in the non-dilated heart, right-sided structures, particularly the right ventricle, right ventricular outflow tract and pulmonary valve, are often not well visualised using TOE whereas in the same patient superb views of the mitral valve may be obtained. In patients with a small left atrium the available 'echo window' will be smaller than in those with a dilated left atrium. In general left sided cardiac structures are better visualised by transoesophageal echocardiography than right-sided structures. The proximal aortic arch may be obscured by the interposition of the trachea and left main bronchus and arterial branches arising from the aortic arch cannot be adequately seen by TOE. Other techniques such as magnetic resonance imaging may be preferable for examining the interrelationships between the proximal aorta, aortic arch and its branches. Transoesophageal echocardiography has proven value in the assessment of acute aortic dissection and is the investigation of choice in many centres.[1] To date, imaging of the coronary arteries is limited using TOE and the technique has no practical clinical application in quantifying coronary atherosclerosis directly. In spite of this, the coronary arteries are often well visualised (see Figure 8.16). Coronary angiography remains the gold standard for the quantification of coronary artery disease.

Transoesophageal echocardiography is a very safe procedure with few complications but it is semi-invasive and nowhere near as widely available as TTE. In addition, important information derived from transthoracic scans may not be obtainable from the transoesophageal route; for example, continuous wave Doppler estimates of aortic stenosis or planimetry of the mitral valve orifice may be much harder to achieve due to the orientation of the imaging plane. In general, with a few exceptions, such as intraoperative monitoring of left ventricular function, the results of any transoesophageal study should be integrated with those of the transthoracic examination and the clinical findings to achieve a unifying diagnosis. The aim of this chapter is to outline the basic techniques of TOE and to highlight its clinical indications, strengths and limitations.

Equipment

A modern echocardiography machine capable of providing high quality two-dimensional images, M-mode, colour flow mapping, continuous wave Doppler and pulsed wave Doppler is required. The machine must accept a TOE transducer which should be capable of

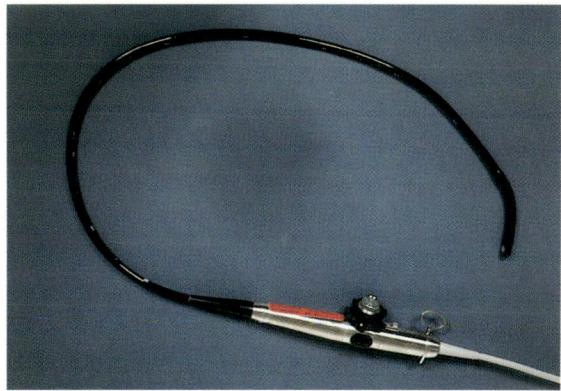

Figure 8.1 – A modern multiplane transoesophageal echocardiography endoscope. This instrument uses a phased array transducer capable of imaging the heart in many planes through an arc of 180°. Planes are selected using the handset control which rotates the transducer elements.

biplane or preferably multiplane imaging. A modern multiplane TOE endoscope is shown in Figure 8.1. The instrument is sometimes referred to as a probe or a transducer. This transducer is capable of imaging at either 5 MHz or 6.25 MHz. It contains a phased array transducer which can image planes throughout an arc of 180°, embracing within it both the transverse and longitudinal planes of the older biplane endoscopes. The transducer can be flexed or extended using controls at the handset in order to obtain optimum image positions. Controls for lateral flexion are also included but these are less frequently required on multiplane transducers which allow comprehensive manipulation of image plane. Multiplane imaging has greatly improved imaging of intracardiac structures which are often orientated obliquely and do not lend themselves to adequate imaging in two planes orientated at 90°.

The transducer should be sterilised in accordance with the manufacturer's instructions between each examination, usually with glutaraldehyde (Cidex) solution. This can be inconvenient during a busy TOE list, (unless two or three transducers are available), and an alternative is a disposable sheath which dispenses with the need for sterilisation between cases. The transducer should, however, still be sterilised frequently and between cases if there is a specific infection risk. Undoubtedly, the use of sheaths leads to some loss of image quality but this is usually acceptable for general convenience and practicality.

Indications

The recent popularity of TOE over the past few years has been accompanied by a huge increase in the number of examinations performed with an expansion of the indications for the procedure which may not be fully justified on clinical grounds. In Table 8.1 there is a list of indications for a TOE which covers the principal reasons for undertaking the examination in a typical large centre. Since TOE is a safe procedure, associated with a low risk of complications and only mild patient discomfort, it should be considered in cases where there is a good chance that it will provide additional diagnostic information. It is important to be clear what additional information is being sought before embarking on the procedure.

Complications

Complications are very rare and TOE is a safe procedure.[2] Oesophageal trauma or perforation are rare com-

Table 8.1 – Indications for TOE

Diagnostic	Intraoperative / ITU
Inadequate precordial examination	Monitoring of LV function
Assessment of prosthetic heart valves	Assessment of mitral valve repair
Investigation of infective endocarditis	Prosthetic valve function
Aortic dissection	Postoperative complications
Source of unexplained emboli	Imaging in ventilated patients
Assessment for balloon mitral valvuloplasty	
Assessment of intracardiac masses	
Congenital heart disease	

plications. There has been one reported death following TOE in a survey of 10,000 patients. This was due to oesophageal perforation during intubation of a patient with an undiagnosed invasive carcinoma. Minor throat and oral discomfort may follow the procedure in common with other forms of upper gastrointestinal endoscopy but this usually resolves rapidly. Transient arrhythmias have been reported but the overall complication rate is less than 1%. The failure rate due to inability to intubate patients is about 1–2%.

Patient Preparation

Transoesophageal echocardiography can safely be undertaken in outpatients. Patients are asked to fast for 6 hours prior to the examination. They are advised not to drive until the day after the examination and should be accompanied home as most will have been given sedative drugs. The issue of sedation seems to attract much debate. Certainly, in most patients TOE can be successfully undertaken without sedation but in general the use of sedation in small doses often makes the examination more comfortable for the patient, especially during intubation. Some patients specifically ask to avoid sedation but the majority prefer to have their anxieties about swallowing a relatively large tube alleviated by a little sedation. In some circumstances sedation is essential, for example in the investigation of acute aortic dissection where excessive stimulation and surges in blood pressure are to be avoided for fear of causing extension of the dissection. In paediatric patients or in subjects who are confused or mentally impaired sedation or even general anaesthesia is advisable. A short-acting benzodiazepine compound such as Midazolam (Hypnoval) is preferred and most adults require between 2 and 5 mg intravenously. Higher doses (above 5 or 6 mg) may lead to poor co-operation due to agitation or excessive sedation which can be counterproductive, especially during intubation when patient co-operation is essential. Midazolam rarely causes significant respiratory depression at these doses although there is considerable variation in the sedative response between individual patients. Aliquots of 1 mg at a time are generally administered over 5 minutes with careful titration against the patients' level of consciousness. There is a specific antagonist available in Flumazanil (Annexate), which should be administered if respiratory depression occurs during the procedure or if the patient is slow to recover following the examination. In practice, it is rarely necessary to reverse sedation.

Before giving sedation a final explanation of the procedure is given with particular attention to swallowing the endoscope and breathing through the nose once it is advanced into the oesophagus. Since the procedure is mildly unpleasant the sedative and amnesic properties of Midazolam are very useful especially if serial examinations are likely to be necessary. Whether sedation is used or not, the key to success is to establish a reassuring rapport with a naturally apprehensive patient. It is very important to explain in detail what will happen, how long it is likely to take and how straightforward it is going to be. All drugs should be administered under appropriate medical supervision.

It is important to ask whether the patient has ever had any problems with their stomach or oesophagus such as ulcers, bleeding, hiatus hernias or surgery. It is also important to check when they last ate or drank and whether they have any false teeth or loose crowns. The patient should sign a consent form for the procedure. Intravenous access by an indwelling cannula is essential, not only to deliver the sedation but to administer any emergency treatment. Electrodes for monitoring the electrocardiogram are applied. In most cases the transoesophageal study should be preceded by a full transthoracic examination. Once the transthoracic echocardiography is completed topical anaesthesia with Lignocaine 10% is given generously to the oropharynx, preferably about 5 minutes before the commencement of the procedure. This is especially important if sedation is not used. Pulse oximetry and blood pressure monitoring should be available throughout the procedure.

The patient is asked to turn into the left lateral position. It is preferable to have a trained nurse to assist the operator should oxygen or suction be required during the procedure. There is no reason why TOE should be limited to medical staff, provided thorough training is given, although this is often the case. However, technician operators may require medical staff to administer sedative drugs or may elect to avoid sedation altogether for convenience.

Procedure

Intubation

Before intubation, the settings on the transducer and echo machine should be checked. Patient details should be entered correctly and adequate videotape available for the whole study as it is inconvenient to have to change tapes during TOE. Presets for TOE should be selected if available on the echo machine and the transducer set in transverse imaging mode.

A bite guard is inserted to protect the patient's teeth and the expensive TOE transducer. Lignocaine jelly is used liberally to lubricate the transducer which is orientated to face anteriorly relative to the patient. The tip of the transducer is then advanced over the tongue to rest at the back of the throat, but not far enough to stimulate the gag reflex. It is essential to apply adequate flexion to the transducer so that it will pass easily into the oropharynx. At no stage should the transducer be advanced against resistance. The locks for flexion and side flexion available on some endoscopes should be disengaged. The patient is then asked to take a big swallow and the transducer gently advanced into the oesophagus. Minor gagging is almost inevitable and at this point it can be helpful to ask the patient to concentrate on breathing through their nose which takes their mind off the gagging sensation. Once the transducer is in the oesophagus a further 1 or 2 mg of Midazolam may be helpful to provide a sedative and amnesic effect for the duration of the examination which can then be undertaken calmly and thoroughly in a relaxed patient.

If difficulty is experienced in getting the patient to swallow the transducer, it is often because of excessive flexion of the transducer tip or because the transducer has not been introduced in the midline. Flexion is required to traverse the back of the tongue and oropharynx but once this has been achieved, minor extension of the transducer tip may be required to engage the oesophagus which lies posterior to the trachea. Tracheal intubation due to excessive flexion of the endoscope is uncommon but usually results in profound gagging, struggling, desaturation readings on the oximeter and very poor images. If this problem is suspected the endoscope should be withdrawn immediately and repeat intubation attempted after a recovery period with the application of minor extension of the transducer in the oropharynx.

To ensure that the transducer is introduced in the midline it may be necessary to insert a finger around the side of the bite guard to guide the tip of the transducer over the tongue using the hard palate as a marker such that the endoscope can be advanced to the oropharynx exactly in the midline. This stops the tip of the endoscope becoming lodged in the pyriform fossa. If intubation remains difficult a little further sedation may be helpful but with practice this is not usually necessary. Under no circumstances should the transducer ever be advanced against resistance, no matter how frustrated the operator might feel at not being able to pass the endoscope to the oesophagus. Causes of inability to advance the transducer to the level of the heart include tracheal intubation, oesophageal spasm or stricture or oesophageal diverticula which are relatively rare. If the endoscope is lodged in a diverticulum then excessive force may lead to oesophageal perforation.

Great caution must be exercised in the use of sedation. It is rarely necessary to use more than 5 or 6 mg of Midazolam and at all times the operator and nurse must ensure that the patient remains sufficiently conscious to understand and co-operate. If there is loss of contact or understanding with the patient, the state of full anaesthesia is present and this is not safe without the resources of an anaesthetist and their specialist equipment.

Examination

Once the transducer has negotiated the oropharynx, it should be gently advanced to between 25 and 30 cm, as marked on the shaft of the instrument. It is then flexed slightly to ensure good contact with the oesophageal wall and rotated slightly anticlockwise until the aortic valve comes into view. The minimum flexion required to produce a good image should be used since excessive flexion may cause discomfort. The endoscope should not be advanced, withdrawn or rotated in the oesophagus whilst significant flexion is applied. Transgastric views often require more flexion, and are relatively uncomfortable and for these reasons should be delayed until the end of the examination. The stimulant effects of transgastric imaging often wakes the sedated patient to some extent which is ideal prior to extubation at the end of the examination.

There is a potentially infinite number of imaging planes available during a TOE examination with a multiplane

transducer. Minor anatomical variations in the orientation of intracardiac structures, the experience of the operator and the transducer's facilities all contribute to the variation in the imaging planes available. However, Figure 8.2 shows the basic three planes which should be obtained in any transoesophageal study. In transthoracic echocardiography, established standard views are internationally recognised and provide the framework for every examination. In TOE, although some standard views are generally accepted, many variants are possible and often 'hybrid views' provide the best imaging of a particular structure. Learning the technique can be difficult initially as variant views may confuse the novice even if extensive experience of transthoracic echocardiography has been gained. The examination technique is centred around imaging a particular structure as well as possible in a variety of planes rather than simply obtaining standard views of it.

In practice it is better not to follow a rigid routine for TOE examination but rather to quickly orientate oneself and then image in detail the area of most interest in that particular case. The advantage of this flexible

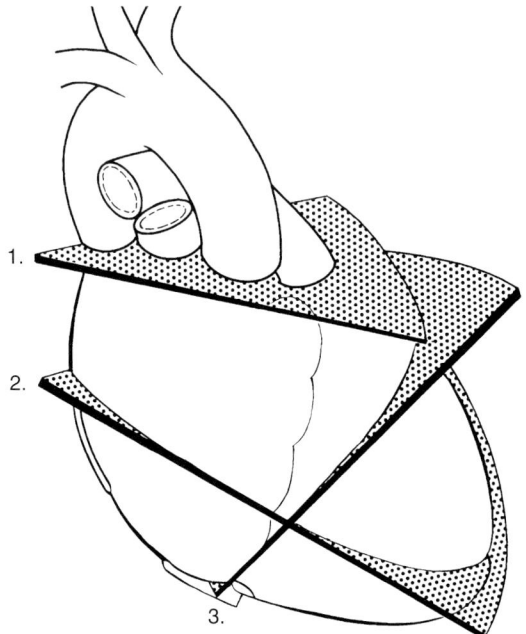

Figure 8.2 – This schematic diagram shows the three main planes obtained by transoesophageal echocardiography. These views are obtained by placing the transducer at positions 1 and 2 within the oesophagus and at 3 within the fundus of the stomach. 1. Basal short axis view. 2. Four chamber view. 3. Short axis transgastric view

approach is that if for any reason the examination has to be curtailed prematurely, at least the most important area will have been examined in detail. In the transverse plane the aortic valve serves as a useful landmark for the rest of the study. Figure 8.3 shows the aortic valve in the basal short axis view. This view is normally obtained first in order to achieve preliminary orientation. Once the main structure of interest has been thoroughly examined, it is important to perform the rest of the examination as systematically as possible. With multiplane transducers, most of the views required can be obtained successfully with a combination of three manipulations.

1. Advancement and withdrawal of the transducer within the oesophagus and stomach between 25 and 45 cm from the teeth.
2. Rotation of the transducer along its long axis in a clockwise and anticlockwise direction.
3. Rotation of the imaging plane through up to 180° by electrical manipulation of the multiplane phased array elements.

This latter manoeuvre is limited to 90° in orthogonal transverse and longitudinal planes in the case of biplane transducers. In difficult examinations it may be necessary to use side flexion in addition to obtain optimum views especially in the case of biplane or monoplane probes.

AORTIC VALVE

In the basal short axis view, the aortic valve is viewed in cross-section such that the three cusps should be seen in detail as illustrated in Figure 8.3. It is useful to adjust the position of the transducer using the manoeuvres outlined above to ensure that the valve is positioned in the centre of the screen and not imaged obliquely. For example minor withdrawal of the endoscope allows the ostia or origins of the coronary arteries to be seen just above the aortic valve and diastolic coronary flow may be confirmed on both colour flow and pulsed wave Doppler examination. When a perfect cross sectional image of the aortic valve is achieved the imaging plane is rotated through 90° to the longitudinal plane to image the valve and proximal aorta as shown in Figure 8.4. Minor adjustments in the endoscope position may be required to centre the image, especially with biplane transducers in which the two separate phased array transducers may be located a small distance apart one above the other at the end of the endoscope. Multiplane transducers allow further imaging of the valve in a variety of planes outside the orthogonal transverse and longitudinal standards.

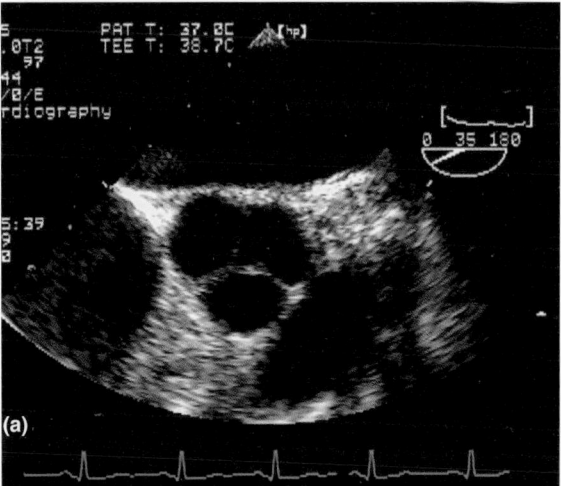

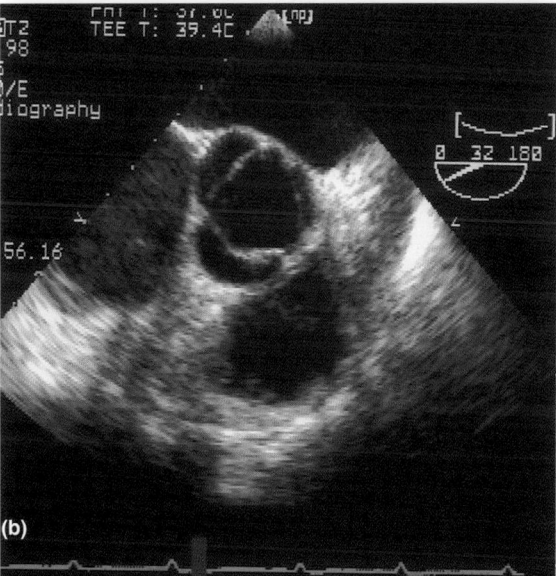

Figure 8.3 – The aortic valve in transverse plane from the basal short axis view. (a) This normal, tricuspid aortic valve is shown with leaflets closed in diastole. (b) The leaflets are open in systole.

MITRAL VALVE

The endoscope is advanced a centimetre or two from the level of the aortic valve with the imaging plane orientated transversely in order to bring into view the mitral valve. This is illustrated in Figure 8.5 which actually shows a mechanical bileaflet valve with both discs open in diastole. Once minor manipulations have centred the mitral valve, colour flow mapping and pulsed wave Doppler examination may be used to

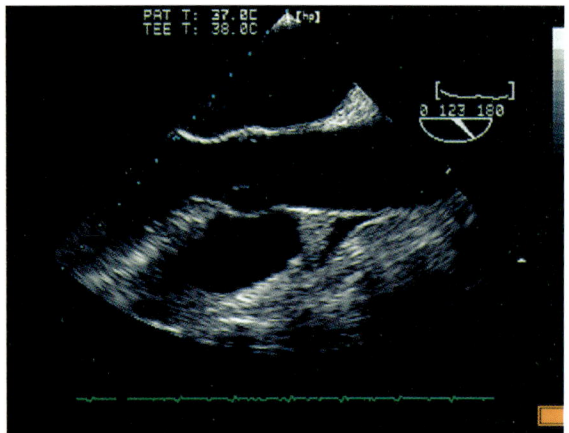

Figure 8.4 – The aortic valve in longitudinal plane from the basal short axis view. This valve is shown with the leaflets open in systole. The LVOT is to the left of the picture and the aortic root and proximal aorta to the right of the valve.

assess regurgitation and stenosis respectively. Rotation of the imaging plane allows the mitral valve to be examined in great detail in a variety of planes. The valve should be examined at least in the transverse and longitudinal planes since eccentric jets of mitral regurgitation (MR) can easily be missed, especially with prosthetic valves. Slight extension (alternatively called 'deflexion') of the endoscope allows a four chamber view in which the left atrium, left ventricle and mitral valve can be clearly seen. The right atrium, right ventricle and tricuspid valve are seen less clearly in most patients but good views are often possible in patients

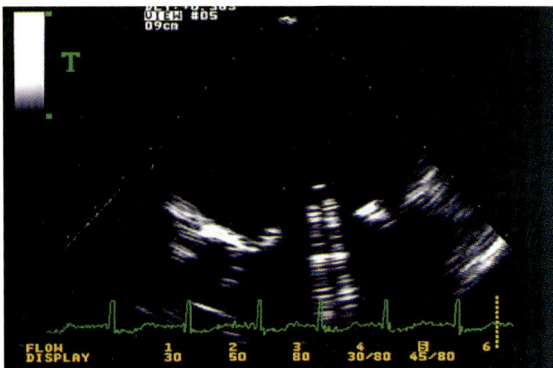

Figure 8.5 – Bileaflet mechanical mitral prosthesis shown in transverse plane from the basal short axis view. The two central discs of the valve can clearly be seen open in diastole. The left atrium is located above the valve and the left ventricle below.

with enlarged right-sided structures. Figure 8.6 shows an example of a typical four chamber view. Flexion of the transducer visualises the left ventricular outflow tract (LVOT) and aortic valve, leading to a five chamber view (Figure 8.7). This view is analogous to that obtained from the apical precordial route and is useful for the detection of aortic regurgitation since it allows an oblique view of the aortic valve and LVOT together. Extension of the transducer tends to produce a true four chamber view and optimises imaging of the mitral

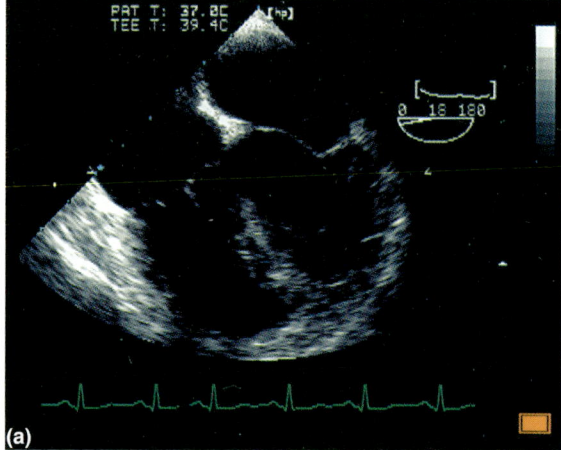

(a)

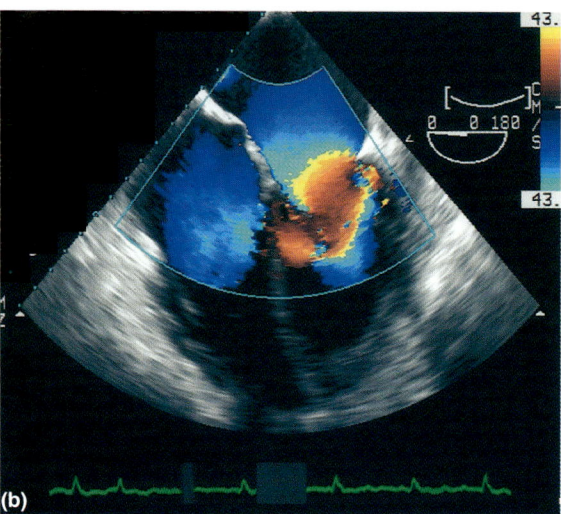

(b)

Figure 8.6 – (a) Four chamber view. This shows the left atrium at 12 o'clock with the left ventricle below it and the mitral valve between the two chambers. The right atrium at 10 o'clock is separated from the right ventricle by the tricuspid valve which is clearly seen in this example. (b) Four chamber view with colour flow Doppler mapping. Note that the normal mitral flow is slightly faster than tricuspid flow and thus causes aliasing.

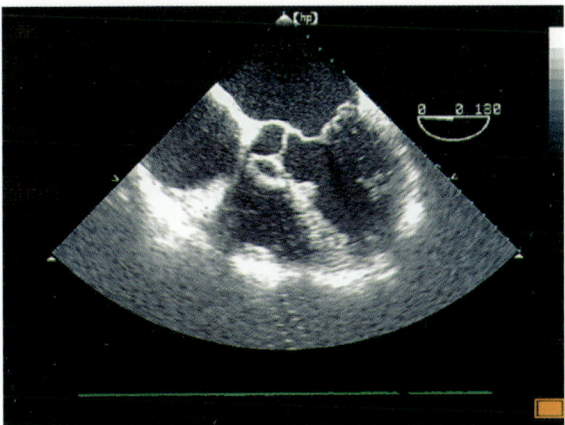

Figure 8.7 – Five chamber view. The transducer has been flexed from the four chamber view to open out the LVOT and aortic valve in the centre of the field.

valve. Anticlockwise rotation brings into view the left sided structures and clockwise rotation right-sided structures. Withdrawal of the endoscope allows imaging of the left atrium and appendage (see Figure 8.17). These structures should be carefully examined in as many planes as practical to exclude thrombus, especially if clinical suspicion is high. Identification of the pulmonary veins entering the left atrium is also possible and assessment of flow within them using pulsed wave Doppler examination may be useful in cases of MR which, if severe, may lead to reverse pulmonary venous flow during systole.

INTERATRIAL SEPTUM

Transoesophageal echocardiography is frequently used to assess the integrity of the interatrial septum in cases of unexplained pulmonary hypertension, dilated right-sided structures or paradoxical embolism. From the position of the aortic valve, clockwise rotation of the transducer allows visualisation of the septum and minor manipulations of the endoscope allow the thin part of the fossa ovalis to be seen. This is the site of the commonest atrial septal defect, the ostium secundum defect. The integrity of the atrial septum is best examined using colour flow mapping in both the transverse and longitudinal views.

Bubble contrast studies may be performed to assess the probability of paradoxical embolus by evaluating the patency of the interatrial septum. Protocols vary but a quick, simple and effective method employs 20 ml of heparinised saline mixed with 2ml of the patient's own blood which has been vigorously shaken for 5 minutes prior to intravenous injection. This is best achieved by using two 20 ml syringes connected to an intravenous line via a three way tap. The agitation of the saline is achieved by vigorously pushing an air/saline mixture between the two syringes. Visible bubbles are then left in one syringe and the other is used to inject the saline containing microbubbles. The microbubbles of air in the solution are very echo dense and provide an excellent contrast medium which is clearly seen on two-dimensional imaging. Shortly after intravenous injection, these microbubbles can be seen entering the right atrium and may cross an incompetent atrial septum, especially if the injection is combined with a Valsalva manoeuvre to raise right atrial pressure (this essentially means a straining effort against a closed glottis but this is usually hard to achieve in a sedated patient having a TOE examination). Alternatively, washout of bubble contrast may be seen on the right atrial side of the septum, indicating left to right flow across an ASD. An example of an atrial septal defect is shown in Figure 8.8. A bubble contrast study has been performed which shows mixing from right to left atrium across the defect.

Aorta

From the aortic valve in the transverse view withdrawal of the endoscope allows imaging of the aortic root and proximal ascending aorta up as far as the proximal aortic arch at which point the interposition of the left main bronchus and trachea obscures the view for a variable distance. The descending aorta can also be imaged by rotating the endoscope anticlockwise approximately 120° degrees from the aortic valve to face posteriorly. Withdrawal of the endoscope then allows imaging up the descending aorta to the distal arch. The combination of these manoeuvres enables the great majority of the thoracic aorta to be examined. The origin and extent of aortic dissections or aortic root abscesses can be accurately assessed prior to surgical intervention.

RIGHT-SIDED STRUCTURES

Variable imaging of the right ventricle is possible from the four chamber view. In general, the right atrium can usually be imaged adequately but the right ventricle is often not as well seen using TOE unless it is dilated. Right-sided structures are also better seen if the left atrium is large. Clockwise rotation and withdrawal of the transducer from the aortic valve reveals the superior vena cava, aorta and pulmonary artery. The entry of the superior vena cava and inferior vena cava into the right

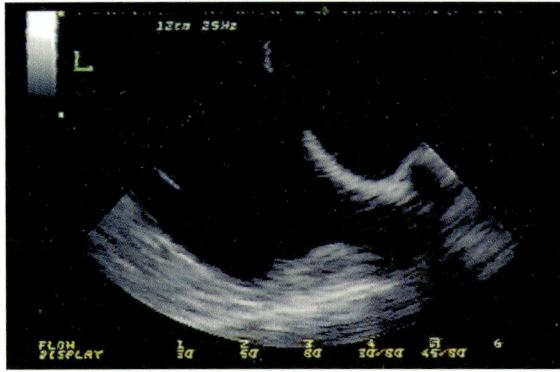

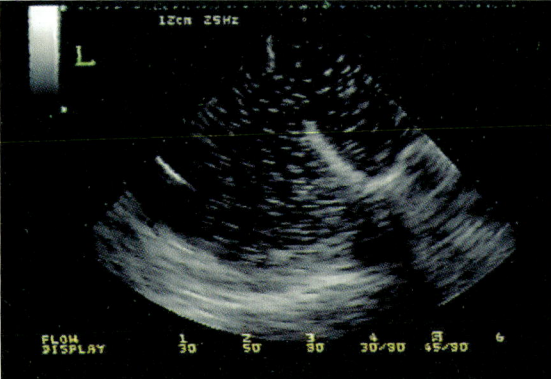

Figure 8.8 – Atrial septal defect with bubble contrast study. (a) In the longitudinal plane the right atrium is seen with the superior vena cava (SVC) entering to the right and the atrial septum above, bordering the left atrium at 2 o'clock. The interatrial septum is incompetent and a large defect is evident. (b) Bubble contrast (20 ml saline mixed with 5 ml blood shaken for 5 minutes) has been injected into the SVC via a venous catheter. The bubble contrast flows freely from the right to the left atrium confirming the presence of the ASD.

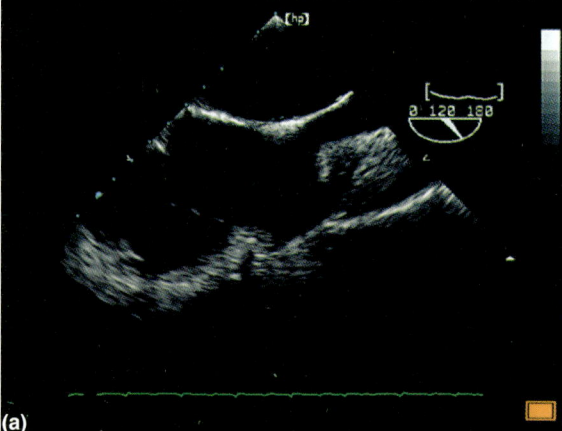

(a)

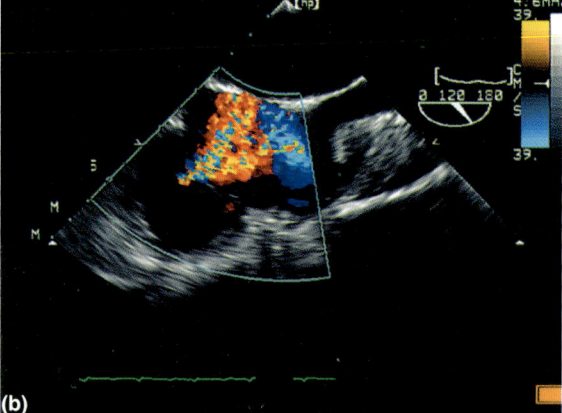

(b)

Figure 8.9 – Right-sided structures in longitudinal plane and tricuspid regurgitation. (a) The right atrium is shown in the centre of the picture with the SVC entering at 2 o'clock and the interatrial septum above bordering the left atrium. The tricuspid valve is seen with the right ventricle at 8 o'clock. (b) Colour flow mapping demonstrates a central jet of tricuspid regurgitation into a dilated right atrium.

atrium is best appreciated in the longitudinal plane. Rotation of the endoscope anticlockwise then reveals the aortic root and proximal aorta. Further anticlockwise rotation subsequently reveals the right ventricular outflow tract, the pulmonary valve (often very poorly) and the pulmonary artery which may be followed to its bifurcation. Figure 8.9 shows the right atrium, right ventricle and tricuspid valve in a patient with significant tricuspid regurgitation illustrated by colour flow Doppler imaging.

VENTRICULAR FUNCTION

Although some idea of ventricular function can be gained from the four chamber view already described,

left ventricular dimensions and function are best assessed from the transgastric route. The transducer is advanced to the fundus of the stomach, often assisted by a further swallow from the patient, and is then rotated anticlockwise and flexed until a transverse section of the left ventricle and sometimes the right ventricle is obtained. Minor adjustments of position should allow standard M-mode measurements of the left ventricle to be taken just below the mitral valve. The operator must ensure, with the use of two-dimensional imaging, that a true short axis position is achieved if M-mode measurements are to be relied upon. Care must be taken not to include the papillary muscles in these measurements as these are often prominently visualised. The ventricular short axis view is excellent for assessing left ventricular function intraoperatively and the transducer may be left in position for the duration of most surgical procedures. Care must be taken to ensure that the transducer tip does not cause thermal damage to the stomach and although most modern transducers have thermistor-driven cut-out circuits, it is sensible to disconnect the transducer when imaging is not in progress. Figure 8.10 shows the transgastric short axis view of the left ventricle.

Clinical applications

This section illustrates the use of TOE in the assessment, diagnosis and treatment of patients. It is by no means exhaustive but includes some of the common clinical circumstances in which TOE is an invaluable investigation.

Infective endocarditis

The diagnosis of endocarditis has in the past depended upon clinical criteria which assess the likelihood of endocarditis on the basis of clinical features and the isolation of a causative organism from the bloodstream.[3] These criteria allow diagnosis of endocarditis with a high degree of specificity but in practice some cases of endocarditis may be missed because they do not meet the stringent requirements for a definitive diagnosis. The criteria are more sensitive if, in addition to traditional clinical and laboratory markers of endocarditis, echocardiographic imaging criteria for vegetations and valve ring abscesses are included.[4] In modern clinical practice the technique has markedly improved the diagnosis and management of patients with proven and suspected endocarditis.[5] Echocardiography allows earlier diagnosis, identification of high-risk groups and improved clinical outcomes by guiding medical therapy and the timing of surgical intervention.[6] Transoesophageal echocardiography is valuable if TTE yields poor quality images (up to 20% of cases) and is absolutely mandatory in the assessment of suspected prosthetic valve endocarditis. It is also useful in the assessment of complications of endocarditis such as

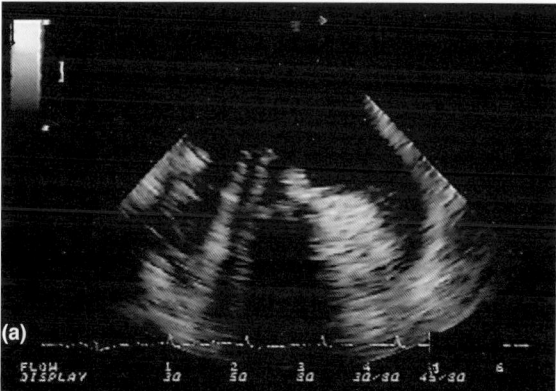

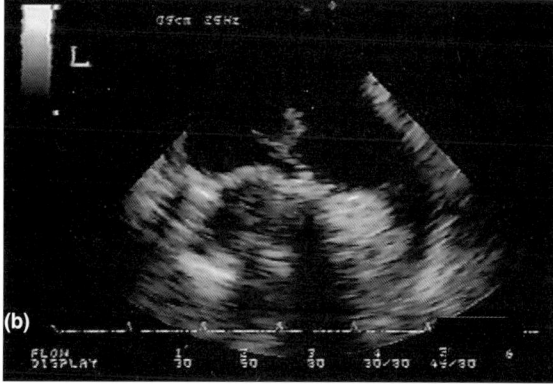

Figure 8.11 – Infective vegetation on a mechanical mitral valve. (a) The bileaflet mechanical valve is shown in diastole with both discs open. The left atrial appendage to the right of the valve has the typical 'dogs ear' appearance. (b) In systole, with the valve closed, a highly mobile vegetation can be seen arising from the atrial side of the sewing ring. This structure was not visible on transthoracic scanning, and in the absence of serological evidence of infection, proved diagnostic of prosthetic valve endocarditis.

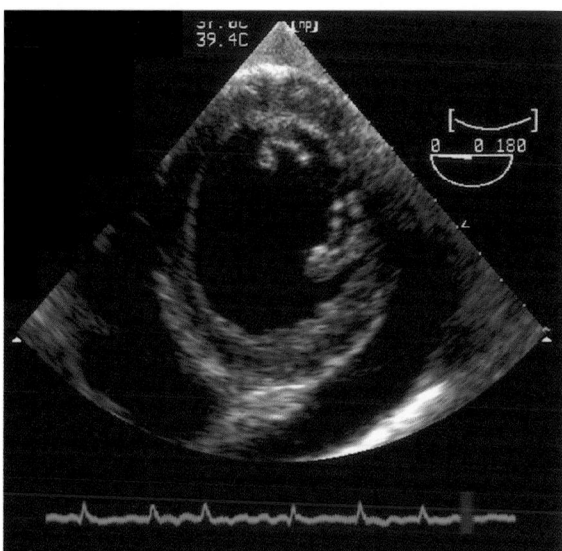

Figure 8.10 – Short axis transgastric view. The posteromedial and anterolateral papillary muscles are often well visualised and the interventricular septum is seen to the left.

valve ring or aortic root abscesses as well as mechanical valve dehiscence and regurgitation which may not be evident from the transthoracic route. Figure 8.11 shows an infective vegetation identified by TOE arising from the sewing ring of a mechanical mitral valve. In this case blood cultures were negative and no vegetation was identified by TTE.

In suspected infective endocarditis TOE should therefore be undertaken if there is doubt about the diagnosis, if TTE is inadequate, if complications are suspected and always if the patient has a prosthetic valve.

Aortic dissection

Transoesophageal echocardiography allows detailed examination of the thoracic aorta with the exception of an area of the proximal arch which is obscured by the trachea and left main bronchus. It has a proven role in the immediate diagnosis and assessment of acute aortic dissection prior to surgery[1] and provides a sensitivity and specificity in diagnosis which is superior to both angiography and computed tomography.[7] Transoesophageal echocardiography can be performed and an accurate diagnosis made within minutes of the patient's arrival in hospital. This is important as type A dissections involving the ascending aorta have a high early mortality without surgery and time is of the essence. Often, no further invasive investigation is required and higher risk angiography may be avoided prior to corrective surgery but it is essential to have good radiological advice in case angiography, CT or MRI scanning is required. Identification of the site of the intimal tear is possible in over half of cases and reliable differentiation of types A and B dissection is usual. Colour flow Doppler is useful for separating the true and false channels of the dissection.

Mitral valve repair and intraoperative monitoring

In the United States, TOE is used in over 75% of cases during valvular disease surgery. Although TOE is not as widely used in the United Kingdom, its use is increasing rapidly and it is almost mandatory for mitral valve repair surgery. Transoesophageal echocardiography is a highly specific method of identifying mitral leaflet abnormalities, annular dilatation and guiding the surgical approach to repair.[8] Transthoracic echocardiography may be sufficient for the preoperative assessment of patients with MR provided there is no mitral stenosis or previous mitral surgery and adequate images are obtained.[9] However, TOE provides enhanced imaging of the mitral valve anatomy and should be part of the routine preoperative assessment of candidates for mitral valve repair.

As experience and surgical techniques develop, fewer and fewer valves are being deemed irreparable. The complexity of mitral repair techniques is increasing and success depends upon accurate identification of the mechanism of regurgitation so that the appropriate repair technique for that particular valve can be employed. This requires the integration of data obtained from echocardiographic imaging and direct inspection of the valve by the surgeon at operation. Figure 8.12 shows an example of posterior mitral leaflet prolapse with gross mitral regurgitation. In this case, which was due to acute spontaneous chordal rupture, redundant chordal tissue can be seen attached to the posterior mitral leaflet. This chordal tissue has prolapsed into the left atrium during systole. Mitral valve repair was attempted but intraoperative TOE demonstrated significant residual MR such that mitral valve replacement was necessary. Intraoperative evaluation of mitral valve function and residual regurgitation immediately after repair allows the surgeon to decide whether the initial repair procedure has been successful or further attempts at repair are indicated.

Transoesophageal echocardiography is highly sensitive in the detection of MR. At least trivial MR is detected after the majority of mitral repairs and is usually acceptable. Mitral regurgitant jet size on colour flow Doppler evaluation decreases significantly in some patients with general anaesthesia and several factors may profoundly influence the degree of MR observed intraoperatively. These factors include systemic blood pressure, systemic vascular resistance and left ventricular volume. It is advisable to manipulate these factors to physiological levels before assessing the degree of residual MR post repair to avoid serious underestimation of regurgitation.[10] Pulmonary venous flow direction may be a better method of identifying the more severe grades of MR following mitral valve repair than colour flow mapping of jet area and length.[11] A five point scale of MR from none to severe (0 – 4) to assess post-repair MR has proved useful.[12] In patients with grades 0 – 2 results were excellent and reoperation rates low although there was a trend towards more reoperations in those with grade 2 regurgitation. Patients with more severe regurgitation (grades 3 and 4) require either further attempts at mitral valve repair or mitral valve replacement. Systolic pulmonary venous flow reversal has a high sensitivity and specificity in the prediction of grade 3 or 4

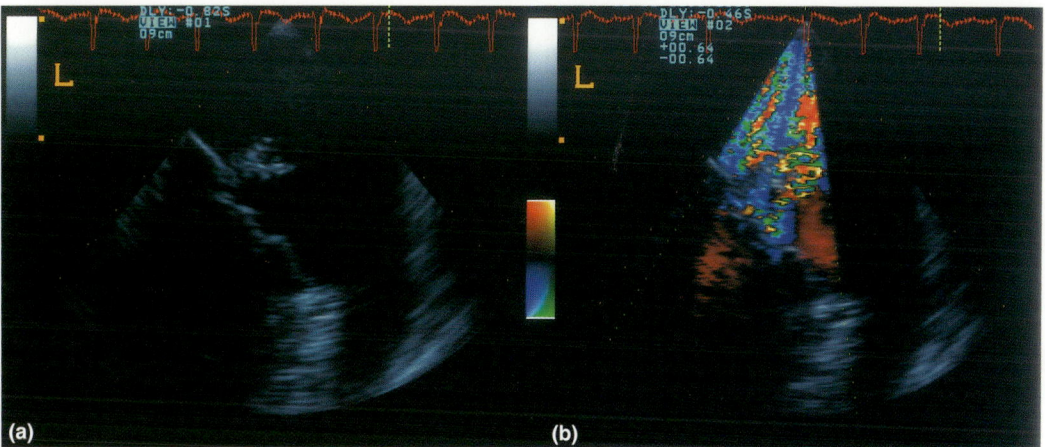

Figure 8.12 – Severe mitral regurgitation due to acute spontaneous chordal rupture. (a) In longitudinal plane gross pro-lapse of the posterior mitral leaflet (with attached redundant chordal tissue) into the left atrium is demonstrated. (b) Colour flow Doppler shows severe mitral regurgitation. This patient required emergency mitral valve replacement.

MR indicating the need for further surgery.[11] Figure 8.18 shows normal pulmonary venous flow recording.

Critical care

Transoesophageal echocardiography has an evolving role in the critical care setting. It is valuable in the diagnosis of unexplained hypotension and hypoxia and, in one study, led to a 81% improvement in survival in patients with valvular or pericardial disease and a 41% improvement in survival in patients with primary ventricular failure.[13] Transthoracic echocardiography was found to be inadequate in 64% of patients in this setting. In ventilated patients in the intensive care unit, TOE using the transgastric ventricular short axis view is invaluable for monitoring ventricular function. On the basis of this experience, there is growing interest in the technique amongst anaesthetists and intensivists. Whether or not training in TOE alone without prior training in TTE is advisable is the subject of much debate but may be acceptable for limited applications.

Prosthetic valve assessment

Acoustic shadowing limits the diagnostic resolution of TTE in the assessment of prosthetic valve dysfunction, particularly in the case of the mitral valve. Transoesophageal echocardiography, especially with colour flow mapping, is invaluable since acoustic shadowing is largely avoided through the orientation of the ultrasound to the mitral prosthesis. All prosthetic valves

'leak' to some extent in order to close and it is possible to differentiate normal 'washing' or 'closure' jets of regurgitation from pathological leaks using TOE. Paraprosthetic leaks due to incompetent sutures or infective endocarditis may also be accurately identified. Infective vegetations invisible on transthoracic scanning may appear obvious with TOE (see Figure. 8.11) and TOE is mandatory in cases of suspected prosthetic valve endocarditis. Acute prosthetic valve failure or dehiscence can be identified safely in seriously ill patients prior to emergency cardiac surgery. Prosthetic mitral valves are especially well seen with TOE but it is also invaluable in the assessment of prosthetic aortic and tricuspid valves. Figure 8.13 shows a bileaflet mechanical mitral valve with a significant paraprosthetic leak of mitral regurgitation.

In patients with both mitral and aortic prostheses acoustic shadowing may be a problem even with TOE. Acoustic masking from the mitral prosthesis often partially obscures images of the aortic prosthesis under these circumstances. The advent of multiplane probes has partially solved this problem by allowing multiple oblique views of both valves to be obtained to minimise the effects of acoustic shadowing.

Atrial septal defect

Transoesophageal echocardiography has been more slowly adopted in paediatric patients with congenital heart disease, largely because in this group excellent

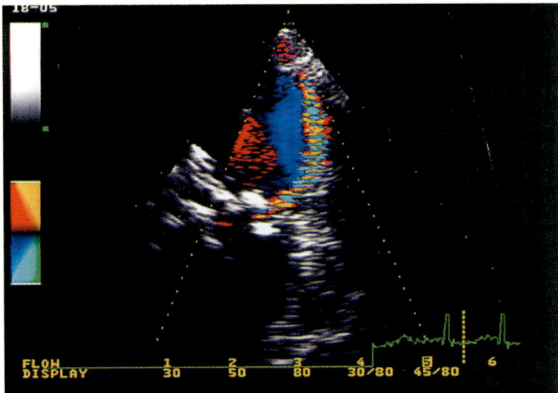

Figure 8.13 – Paraprosthetic mitral regurgitation. Colour flow Doppler illustrates this highly eccentric jet of mitral regurgitation arising from a paraprosthetic leak. It is often very difficult to quantitate prosthetic valve regurgitation by transthoracic echocardiography due to acoustic shadowing from the prosthesis. In most cases transoesophageal echocardiography should be undertaken and usually allows differentiation of prosthetic and paraprosthetic leaks.

quality images are usually obtained from the transthoracic route. Transoesophageal echocardiography is, however, useful in larger patients and in complex cases. The development of miniaturised multiplane transducers has allowed the technique to be extended into paediatric cardiology where necessary. The proximity and orientation of the transducer to the interatrial septum makes TOE an ideal method for the diagnosis and classification of atrial septal defects (ASD). It allows differentiation of ostium primum, ostium secundum and sinus venosus defects and identification of associated congenital abnormalities. Bubble contrast studies may be performed where necessary but in most cases the high resolution of two-dimensional imaging and colour flow mapping provided by modern TOE transducers is all that is required for confident diagnosis. Figure 8.8 shows an example of an ASD.

Intracardiac masses

Transoesophageal echocardiography may not make a significant contribution to the assessment of ventricular masses because the apices of both ventricles are poorly seen, being at a distance from the transducer. In many cases imaging of the ventricular cavities is suboptimal, offering no advantage over TTE. In some cases, however, TOE is still complementary to TTE in this setting especially if transthoracic images are poor. Transoesophageal echocardiography is an excellent

method of imaging atrial masses, both tumours and thrombi. The superior image resolution obtained with TOE allows precise anatomical assessment of atrial myxoma, the commonest primary intracardiac tumour. Examination prior to surgical excision guides the surgical approach and can also be used postoperatively to screen for recurrence.

Transoesophageal echocardiography is invaluable in excluding an intracardiac source of emboli in patients with unexplained neurological symptoms. Thrombus which may develop in the left atrial appendage cannot be adequately visualised using TTE but is invariably identified with TOE.[14] Patients with unexplained emboli in which clinical suspicion of an intracardiac source is high and in whom TTE has failed to identify thrombus have a high incidence of left atrial appendage thrombus visualised by TOE. Spontaneous echo contrast is a marker for thrombus formation within the left atrium and is frequently seen in patients with atrial fibrillation and mitral valve disease both of which are strong risk factors for embolic stroke.[15] Figure 8.14 shows an example of thrombus at the opening of the left atrial appendage. The presence of a patent foramen ovale can also predispose to systemic embolisation and the defect can easily be detected by colour flow mapping or microbubble contrast injection (Figure 8.15).

Since TOE is extremely effective for the detection of clot in the left atrium and appendage it has been used in some centres to exclude thrombus prior to electrical cardioversion of atrial fibrillation. However, even in patients in whom thrombus has been excluded by

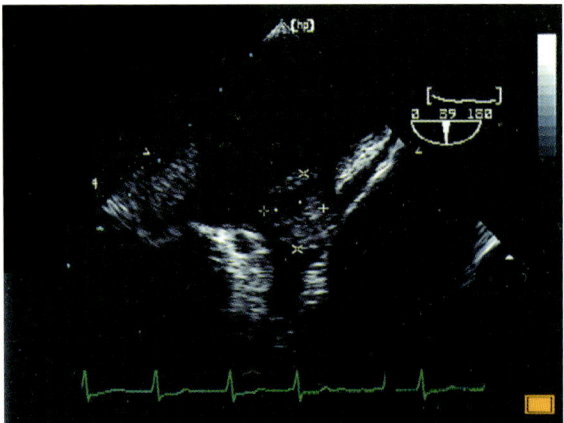

Figure 8.14 – Thrombus in the left atrial appendage. A thrombus measuring 1.6 × 1.3 cm is shown in the mouth of the left atrial appendage in a patient with atrial fibrillation. Marked spontaneous echo contrast was also evident in the body of the left atrium.

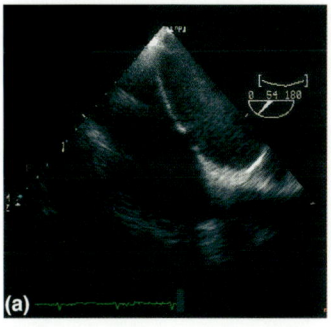
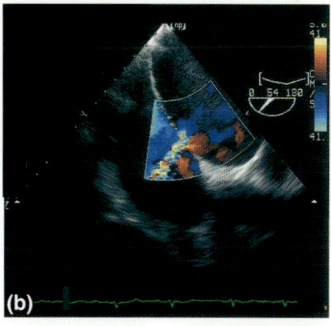
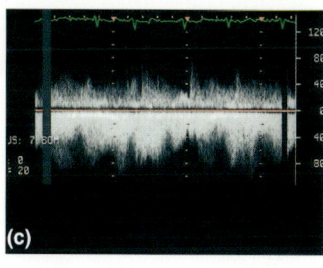

Figure 8.15 – Patent foramen ovale taken from an oblique plane. (a) the small defect in the atrial septum is seen.(b) Colour flow mapping shows a jet passing through the hole (c) Pulsed wave Doppler sample volume placed in the defect. Note that the multiplane orientation has been changed in this image.

TOE there remains a risk of thromboembolism following cardioversion unless they are anticoagulated at the time of the procedure and for a period afterwards.[16] There is an increased tendency for left atrial thrombus formation immediately after cardioversion, possibly due to atrial 'stunning' which is known to occur in this period and is associated with increased spontaneous echo contrast.[17,18] It is also possible that even with the improved resolution of modern multiplane transoesophageal transducers, some small thrombi are being missed. Despite these reservations, cardioversion of atrial fibrillation is safe following a negative TOE provided the patient is anticoagulated at the time of the procedure and for 4 weeks afterwards.[19] This approach obviates the need for anticoagulation for a period of weeks prior to cardioversion and is useful in selected patients in whom rapid restoration of sinus rhythm is desirable. However, if thrombus is identified by TOE then this approach cannot be adopted and patients should be anticoagulated for 6 weeks and a repeat TOE examination performed to ensure resolution of thrombus before cardioversion is undertaken.

Future developments

Three-dimensional image acquisition allows enhanced appreciation of the functional and spatial relationships of intracardiac structures. It is potentially of great use in the assessment of mitral valve pathology and provides detailed information on leaflet mobility, anatomy of the commissures, orifice size, and the mechanism of regurgitation.[10] Prosthetic valves are especially well seen with three-dimensional imaging. Other clinical applications

of three-dimensional TOE have yet to be firmly established, especially as the equipment required is expensive and therefore not widely available. Image acquisition and reconstruction times, although falling with technological advances, are still rather long for

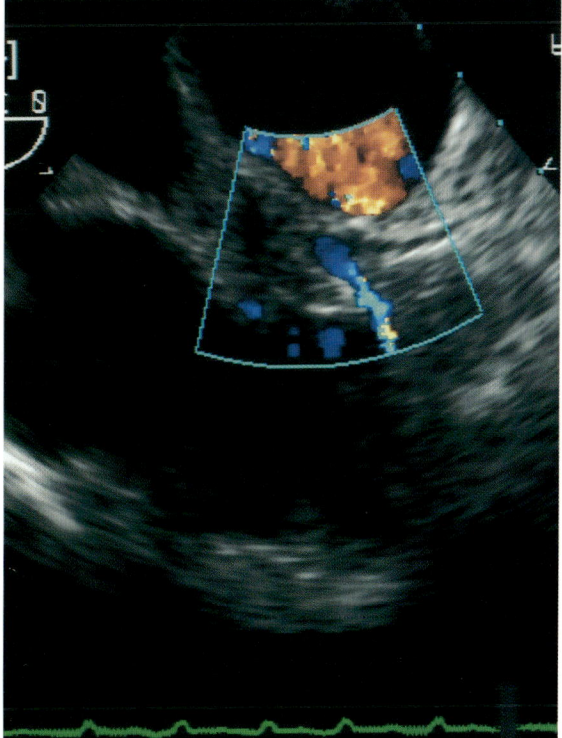

Figure 8.16 Modified multiplane view showing the proximal left coronary artery with colour flow Doppler signal in the left anterior descending vessel.

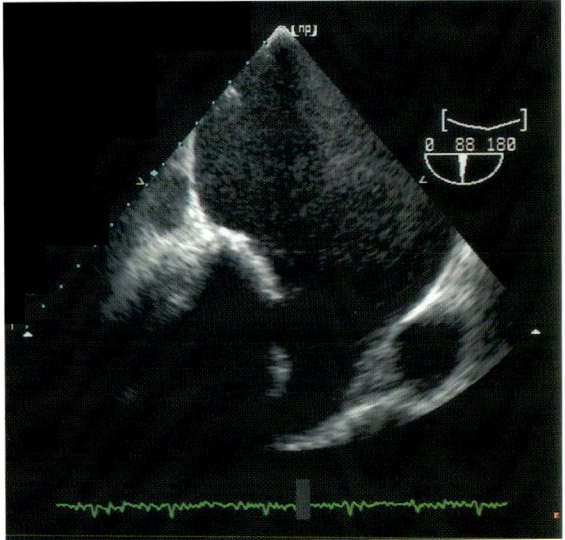

Figure 8.17 – Longitudinal view of a dilated left atrium showing the left atrial appendage.

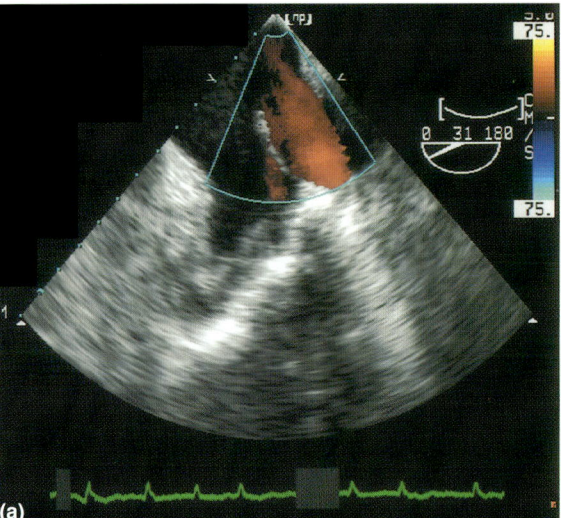

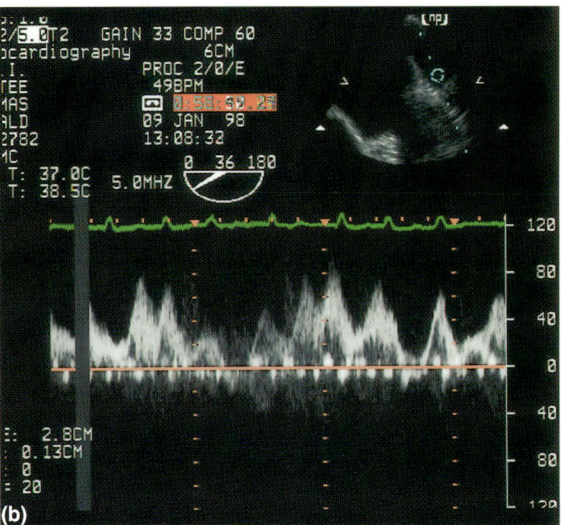

Figure 8.18 – (a) Colour image of the left upper pulmonary vein showing normal flow towards the transducer. (b) Normal pulsed Doppler signal taken from this site.

everyday clinical use. Three-dimensional assessment of atrial septal defects to facilitate the exact positioning of percutaneous closure devices and the mapping of the tricuspid annulus for the placement of electrophysiology catheters are potential future directions.

Four-dimensional echocardiography (with time as the fourth dimension) allows dynamic three-dimensional images to be displayed throughout the cardiac cycle. This evolving technique affords better understanding of direction, size and shape of regurgitant jets, and as technology advances, is likely to play an important role in the management of valvular heart disease.

Conclusion

Transoesophageal echocardiography is a powerful and safe method of imaging the heart and great vessels. It continues to develop with the advent of multiplane transducers, three-dimensional reconstruction and dynamic four-dimensional imaging. It is relatively inexpensive, semi-invasive and can be rapidly applied in emergencies. It is therefore the investigation of choice in certain circumstances and has superseded more invasive forms of investigation. Its uses are likely to expand in the future as new specialities utilise the technique. Adequate training will be important to maintain standards since, in common with other forms of ultrasound, the diagnostic power of the technique is highly dependent upon the competence of the operator.

References

1. Banning AP, Masani ND, Ikram S, Fraser AG, Hall RJ. Transoesophageal echocardiography as the sole diagnostic investigation in patients with suspected thoracic aortic dissection. *Br Heart J* 1994; **72**: 461–465.

2. Daniel WG, Erbel R, Kasper W, *et al*. Safety of transesophageal echocardiography. A multicenter survey of 10,419 examinations. *Circulation* 1991; **83**: 817–821.

3. Hogevik H, Olaison L, Andersson R, Lindberg J, Alestig K. Epidemiologic aspects of infective endocarditis in an urban population. A 5-year prospective study [Review] *Medicine* 1995; **74**: 324–339.

4. Hoen B, Selton-Suty C, Danchin N, *et al*. Evaluation of the Duke criteria versus the Beth Israel criteria for the diagnosis of infective endocarditis [see comments]. *Clin Infect Dis* 1995; **21**: 905–909.

5. Lindner JR, Case RA, Dent JM, Abbott RD, Scheld WM, Kaul S. Diagnostic value of echocardiography in suspected endocarditis. An evaluation based on the pretest probability of disease. *Circulation* 1996; **93**: 730–736.

6. Erbel R, Liu F, Ge J, Rohmann S, Kupferwasser I. Identification of high-risk subgroups in infective endocarditis and the role of echocardiography [review]. *Eur Heart J* 1995; **16**: 588–602.

7. Erbel R, Engberding R, Daniel W, Roelandt J, Visser C, Rennollet H. Echocardiography in diagnosis of aortic dissection. *Lancet* 1989; **1**: 457–461.

8. Caldarera I, van Herwerden LA, Taams MA, Bos E, Roelandt JR. Multiplane transoesophageal echocardiography and morphology of regurgitant mitral valves in surgical repair. *Eur Heart J* 1995; **16**: 999–1006.

9. Hellemans IM, Pieper EG, Ravelli AC, *et al*. Comparison of transthoracic and transesophageal echocardiography with surgical findings in mitral regurgitation. The ESMIR Research Group. *Am J Cardiol* 1996; **77**: 728–733.

10. Bach DS, Deeb GM, Bolling SF. Accuracy of intraoperative transesophageal echocardiography for estimating the severity of functional mitral regurgitation. *Am J of Cardiol* 1995; **76**: 508–512.

11. Pieper EP, Hellemans IM, Hamer HP, *et al*. Value of systolic pulmonary venous flow reversal and color Doppler jet measurements assessed with transesophageal echocardiography in recognizing severe pure mitral regurgitation. *Am J Cardiol* 1996; **78**: 444–450.

12. Fix J, Isada L, Cosgrove D, *et al*. Do patients with less than 'echo-perfect' results from mitral valve repair by intraoperative echocardiography have a different outcome? *Circulation* 1993; **88**: II39–48.

13. Heidenreich PA, Stainback RF, Redberg RF, Schiller NB, Cohen NH, Foster E. Transesophageal echocardiography predicts mortality in critically ill patients with unexplained hypotension [see comments]. *J Am Coll Cardiol* 1995; **26**: 152–158.

14. Fatkin D, Scalia G, Jacobs N, *et al*. Accuracy of biplane transesophageal echocardiography in detecting left atrial thrombus. *Am J Cardiol* 1996; **77**: 321–323.

15. Daniel WG, Nellessen U, Schroder E, *et al*. Left atrial spontaneous echo contrast in mitral valve disease: an indicator for an increased thromboembolic risk. *J Am Coll Cardiol* 1988; **11**: 1204–1211.

16. Black IW, Fatkin D, Sagar KB, *et al*. Exclusion of atrial thrombus by transesophageal echocardiography does not preclude embolism after cardioversion of atrial fibrillation. A multicenter study [see comments]. *Circulation* 1994; **89**: 2509–2513.

17. Grimm RA, Leung DY, Black IW, Stewart WJ, Thomas JD, Klein AL. Left atrial appendage 'stunning' after spontaneous conversion of atrial fibrillation demonstrated by transesophageal Doppler echocardiography [review]. *Am Heart J* 1995; **130**: 174–176.

18. Fatkin D, Kuchar DL, Thorburn CW, Feneley MP. Transesophageal echocardiography before and during direct current cardioversion of atrial fibrillation: evidence for 'atrial stunning' as a mechanism of thromboembolic complications. *J Am Coll Cardiol* 1994; **23**: 307–316.

19. Manning WJ, Silverman DI, Keighley CS, Oettgen P, Douglas PS. Transesophageal echocardiographically facilitated early cardioversion from atrial fibrillation using short-term anticoagulation: final results of a prospective 4.5-year study [see comments]. *J Am Coll Cardiol* 1995; **25**: 1354–1361.

9

STRESS ECHOCARDIOGRAPHY

Jayshree Joshi

Introduction

The diagnosis of coronary artery disease is classically based on the presence of anginal chest pain and electrocardiographic (ECG) changes. However, symptoms can be misleading and sometimes are not present (silent myocardial ischaemia) and the introduction of a stressful condition may be necessary to detect underlying or latent ischaemia.

Exercise stress testing (treadmill or less commonly using bicycle ergometer) using standard protocol has remained the commonest test for evaluating patients with coronary artery disease. It is widely available and can be performed at relatively low cost. However, as with all diagnostic procedures, there are limitations. The sensitivity and specificity may be unsatisfactory, especially in certain subgroups such as women and in patients with resting ECG abnormalities, as in post myocardial infarction, left bundle branch block, Wolff-Parkinson-White syndrome, left ventricular 'strain', digitalis and other drugs. Moreover, the ECG provides only modest localization and relatively poor quantitation of myocardial ischaemia. With the advent of therapeutic revascularization there is an increasing need for localization and quantitation of ischaemia. Such additonal information may be obtained using nuclear techniques, either by blood pool imaging or myocardial perfusion. Both techniques have proved to be useful in providing additional information of stress induced ischaemia, however they are expensive, not universally available, imply the exposure of the patients to a radio-isotope and may take longer.

Echocardiography is another technique that can be helpful in stress testing. The echocardiographic hallmark for myocardial ischaemia is the appearance of stress induced regional wall motion abnormalities. Normal myocardium will show an increase of wall thickening and movement during stress. Ischaemia is detected by a reduced systolic thickening and transient regional asynchronous contraction or asynergy. The clinical observation that wall motion abnormalities persist for several minutes allowed validation of immediate post-treadmill echocardiography for detecting exercise induced ischaemia.[1] Some of the problems that had previously limited the widespread application of the test have been solved by the development of digital recording and side by side cine loop display of two-dimensional echocardiograms. In this way respiratory artifacts, a major drawback, can be eliminated. The examination is faster, and the comparison of rest and stress images has become practical and reliable and sensitivity is improved.

Thus, during the last few years stress echocardiography has grown to become an established technique for assessing patients with proven or suspected coronary artery disease.

Myocardial Ischaemia

Myocardial ischaemia is generally associated with elimination of normal contractile performance of a localized area of myocardium resulting in asynchronous contraction. This may occur as a result of fixed atheroslerotic lesions or may be secondary to transitory reduction in blood flow caused by coronary spasm and/or platelet aggregation. Different effects of myocardial ischaemia are recognised.

After a brief period of severe ischaemia, prolonged dysfunction with gradual return of contractile activity occurs, a condition termed *myocardial stunning*.

The term *myocardial hibernation* has been given to myocardium which improves on relief of the ischaemia after being chronically depressed due to severe, chronic ischaemia.

In hibernating myocardium, perfusion is still reduced, whereas in stunned myocardium blood flow is fully or almost fully restored.[2] Both the stunned and hibernating myocardium is viable and exhibits contractile reserve, which can be evoked by an inotropic stimulus, and there may be abnormalities of systolic and/or diastolic ventricular function. Clinically, myocardial stunning occurs following successful thrombolytic therapy in patients having acute myocardial infarction and in those with severe ischaemia due to coronary vasospasm or unstable angina, or following coronary occlusion during balloon angioplasty. Hibernating myocardium results from months or years of ischaemia, and ventricular dysfunction persists until blood flow is restored.

Indications for stress testing

The rationale of stress echocardiography relies on the balance between myocardial oxygen demand and blood supply (Figure 9.1). Myocardial oxygen demand is determined by heart rate, myocardial tension and contracitility, while energy is supplied mainly by aerobic metabolism with limited anaerobic reserve. When the support of phosphates is not adequate for the request, the first cell activity to be reduced is contractility.[3] Thus, coronary artery disease detected by stress is a

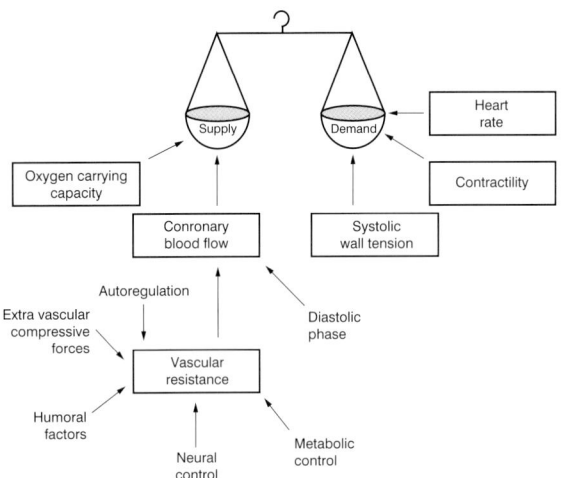

Figure 9.1 – Factors influencing myocardial oxygen supply and demand.

functional abnormality, compared to the anatomical evaluation made with coronary angiography.

Stress echocardiography is indicated for:

- prognostic value in patients referred for chest-pain complaints;

- prognostic value in patients after an acute myocardial infarction;

- prediction of functional improvement after coronary revascularization;

- preoperative cardiac risk stratification in patients scheduled for vascular surgery.

Equipment

Primarily the two-dimensional ultrasound machine requires a digital frame grabbing system, either incorporated or as a stand alone linked to it. The advantage of a stand alone system lies in the possibility of attaching this unit to any ultrasound machine. Furthermore, such a system allows review of images acquired with no interruption of the echo monitoring during the procedure and studies may be reviewed at any time leaving the ultrasound machine free for other use.

The digital frame grabbing system obtains a continuous cine-loop recording. The sequence is initiated at the peak of the R wave of the ECG and subsequent frames

are digitized at pre-set time intervals to allow the acquisition of the whole systole, and some systems even allow the display of the whole cardiac cycle. High quality data can be captured at frame rates higher than video rates by using a direct digital data link to the electronics of the ultrasound machine itself. The disadvantage is that it is only possible to capture data in real time and the interface must be compatible with the ultrasound machine.

Advantages of continuous cine-loop display are:

- elimination of respiratory artifacts, a major drawback in exercise echocardiography,

- frame by frame analysis which may improve the ability to detect subtle wall motion abnormalities,

- side by side display of different conditions, for example, base vs peak stress, or at different stages of pharmacological stress.

Other essential equipment to enable this technique to be carried out includes:

- Treadmill or an upright or supine bicycle, to exercise the patient.

- A sophisticated ECG machine designed for stress analysis.

- An infusion pump for pharmacological stress test.

- Weighing scales for pharmacological drug dosage calculation.

- Blood pressure monitoring equipment, either automated or manual.

- A couch for the patient to lie on.

- A resuscitation trolley with a defibrillator and all the necessary resuscitation drugs. Antedotes to pharmacological agents used.

- Oxygen, preferably on line.

Spatial organization of the equipment in the room is crucial to minimize the time needed for the patient to return to the couch from the treadmill (Figure 9.2)

Patient preparation

Most importantly, the patient should understand what the procedure involves and why it is being performed and if pharmacological agent/s are used, what the side

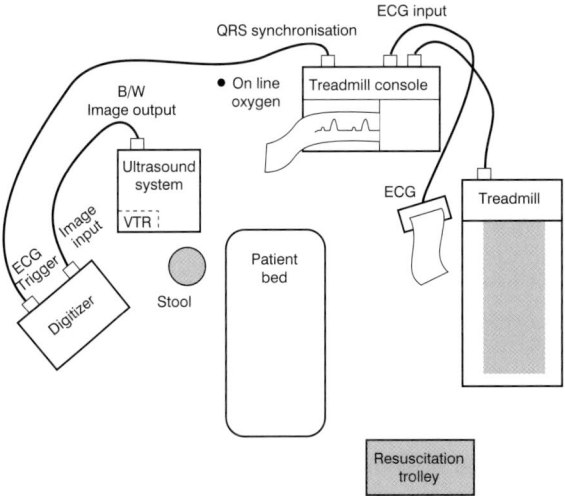

Figure 9.2 – Schematic representation of an ideal echocardiographic laboratory.

effects might be. The patient will need to be weighed for calculation of drug infusion if a pharmacological agent is used and access to a peripheral vein should be obtained for drug infusion.

It is advisable to find the echo 'windows' before applying the ECG electrodes, the positions of which can then be modified accordingly. If exercise is the mode of stress, to maintain good ECG contact during exercise, chest hair if present ought to be shaved and the skin prepared. A disposable string vest also helps to keep the ECG electrodes and cables in place. Holes may be cut in the string vest for transducer access. In our experience, before commencement of treadmill exercise test, it is helpful for the patient to practice returning from the treadmill to the same left lateral decubitus position on the couch to minimizes the lapse of time between exercise cessation and image acquisition.

Stress test modalities and protocols

The diagnostic accuracy of stress echocardiography is strongly influenced by many variables including patient selection,[4] accurate selection of the appropriate stress modality and protocol, optimal use of technology, and expertise in performing and interpreting the examinations.[5]

Exercise stress testing

Exercise is the most physiological type of stress and was the first reported mode used for stress echocardiography. Exercise increases myocardial oxygen demand by an increase in both heart rate and blood pressure. In patients with significant coronary artery disease, blood flow cannot increase sufficiently to meet demand and will lead to ischaemia. In our experience the treadmill has proved to be the preferred form of physical exercise rather than either upright or supine bicycle which invariably resulted in termination of the test due to leg fatigue before any development of cardiac symptoms. Most people are more familiar with walking than cycling and a higher level of work can therefore be performed on the treadmill.

Treadmill exercise test protocol

A two-dimensional echocardiographic study is first performed with the patient lying in the left lateral decubitus position using standard commercially available cardiac ultrasound equipment. Echocardiographic images are acquired before and immediately after treadmill exercise using parasternal long and short axis view at papillary muscle level and apical four and two chamber projections. Particular attention is paid to image all of the endocardial surface and the projections may be modified from the normal axis especially the four chamber view in order to better visualise the lateral wall. These are recorded simultaneously on high resolution videotape and in digital format using a stand alone system. Immediately after exercise, patients return to the left lateral decubitus position, and echocardiographic images are again acquired in a similar manner.

A symptom-limited treadmill exercise test is performed using the modified Bruce protocol. During exercise, 12 lead ECG is recorded every minute and blood pressure every 3 min.

In the past we employed an 11 segment model but now use the 16 segment model proposed by the American Society of Echocardiography to assess regional wall motion abnormalities (Figure 9.3).[6] Each segment is analysed individually and scored on the basis of its motion and systolic thickening. Wall motion is graded as 1(normal) to 4 (dyskinetic). Grades 2 and 3 correspond to hypokinetic and akinetic regions, respectively. A normal wall motion score is therefore 16, and any value greater than this implies myocardial ischaemia. The greater the wall motion score, the greater the amount of myocardial ischaemia. Although the normal response to exercise is to produce myocardial hyperki-

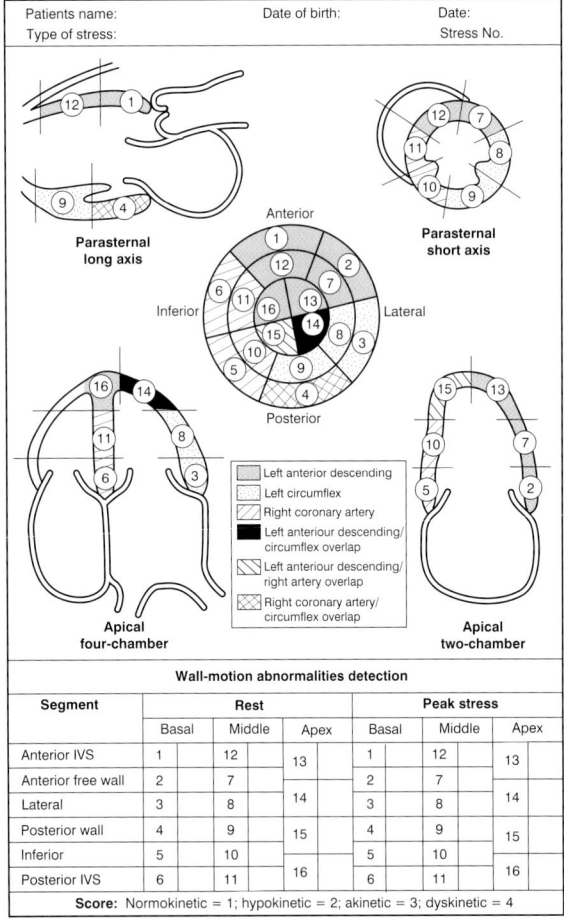

| Patients name: | Date of birth: | | Date: |
| Type of stress: | | | Stress No. |

Wall-motion abnormalities detection

Segment	Rest			Peak stress		
	Basal	Middle	Apex	Basal	Middle	Apex
Anterior IVS	1	12	13	1	12	13
Anterior free wall	2	7		2	7	
Lateral	3	8	14	3	8	14
Posterior wall	4	9	15	4	9	15
Inferior	5	10		5	10	
Posterior IVS	6	11	16	6	11	16

Score: Normokinetic = 1; hypokinetic = 2; akinetic = 3; dyskinetic = 4

Figure 9.3 – Hammersmith hospital stress echocardiography protocol with distribution of coronary perfusion using transthoracic echocardiographic images.

nesia, this is graded as normal so that total wall motion score appropriately depicts only the ischaemic segments and not the ability of normal segments to compensate.

Pharmacological stress testing

This is a useful alternative for the assessment of myocardial ischaemia in those patients who are unable to perform an adequate physical exercise, because of age and/or noncardiac diseases such as peripheral vascular disease or stroke. Two types of drugs can be used: inotropic stimulators (dobutamine, arbutamine) and vasodilators (dipyridamole, adenosine). Other types of stress have been proposed, such as rapid atrial pacing and handgrip, but they are not generally introduced in clinical practice. Pharmacological stress is also used for asssessment of hibernating/stunned myocardium.

It should be stated that in all cases of pharmacological stress testing it is essential to have full informed consent from the patient and the test should be medically supervised by a doctor familiar with the actions of the drugs being used and the clinical conditions being studied.

STRESS TESTING USING INOTROPIC AGENTS

Dobutamine is a sympathomimetic amine which stimulates β_1, β_2 and α_1 receptors. Dobutamine causes an increase in cardiac output, due to an increase in stroke volume and a decrease in systemic vascular resistance because of a secondary reflex withdrawal of sympathetic tone. Consequently systemic blood pressure usually remains unaffected during dobutamine infusion.

Low dose dobutamine has a positive inotropic effect which may improve the function of hypokinetic myocardium at rest which may return to normal movement (hibernating/stunned myocardium).

There is an increase in myocardial oxygen consumption during dobutamine infusion which closely resembles physical exercise. Besides increase in myocardial oxygen demand, dobutamine also induces coronary vasodilatation which may potentiate the ischaemic effect.

Side effects of dobutamine include chest pain, arrhythmia, headache, tremor, palpitations, and either hypertension or hypotension. If these do not revert spontaneously and quickly they can be reversed by terminating the infusion or administering an intravenous β blocking agent such as esmolol hydrochloride. Atropine is used if bradycardia and hypotension occur.

Contraindications to dobutamine include uncontrolled hypertension and uncontrolled arrhythmia. Atropine is combined with dobutamine in those patients who fail to reach test end point(target heart rate or signs or symptoms of ischaemia) with maximal dobutamine dose alone.[7] A starting dose of 0.3mg up to a maximum of 1.2mg is given intravenously.

Arbutamine is a newly developed catecholamine with β agonist activity developed specifically as a stress agent.[8] Unlike other pharmacologic stress agents, arbutamine is administered by a computerized closed-loop delivery system. The computer algorithm controls the rate of arbutamine infusion in response to the patient's heart rate, according to the rate of heart rate rise and maximal heart rate limits selected. As needed (e.g. during echo image acquisition), heart rate can be maintained using the HOLD HR feature. In addition, the system monitors blood pressure and issues visual and audible messages to identify potentially significant changes in heart rate or blood pressure. Alarm messages also stop arbutamine infusion.

Dobutamine stress protocol

As with exercise echocardiography, patients undergo a resting two-dimensional precordial echocardiographic examination and a 12 lead ECG. Graded dobutamine infusion is then administered through a peripheral vein in 3 minute stages at infusion rates of 5, 10, 20, 30, and 40μg, kg./min. In patients not achieving 85% of their age-predicted maximal heart rate (220-age) who have no symptoms or signs of ischaemia, atropine (starting with 0.3 mg increasing to 1.2 mg) is given intravenously at the end of stage 5, while dobutamine infusion is continued. Throughout the infusion the ECG is continuosly monitored, the 12 lead ECG is recorded each minute and the blood pressure is measured manually or by automatic device every 3 minutes. The two-dimensional echocardiogram is continuously monitored and recorded on a stand alone digitizer for side by side examination. The resting and stress images are also recorded on high resolution video tape during the final minute of each stage.

STRESS TESTING USING VASODILATORS

The practical difference between adenosine adminstration and dipyridamole is the duration of action, half-life time of adenosine is less than 10 seconds compared to 20 minutes of dipyridamole. The vasodilatation induces ischaemia by coronary steal. In the coronary steal phenomenon (normal vs stenosed arteries) there is increased flow to the normal vessels which can respond to the vasodilator. This has been described as the 'reversed Robin Hood' effect, they steal from the poor (myocardium at risk) and give to the rich (myocardium well nourished in resting conditions).[10]

Side effects include flushing, headache, dyspnoea, throat or chest tightness, nausea or emesis, heart block and hypotension. These are more common with adenosine but more profound and longer lasting with dipyridamole. These effects can be reversed by terminating the infusion or administering aminophylline, an adenosine receptor blocker.

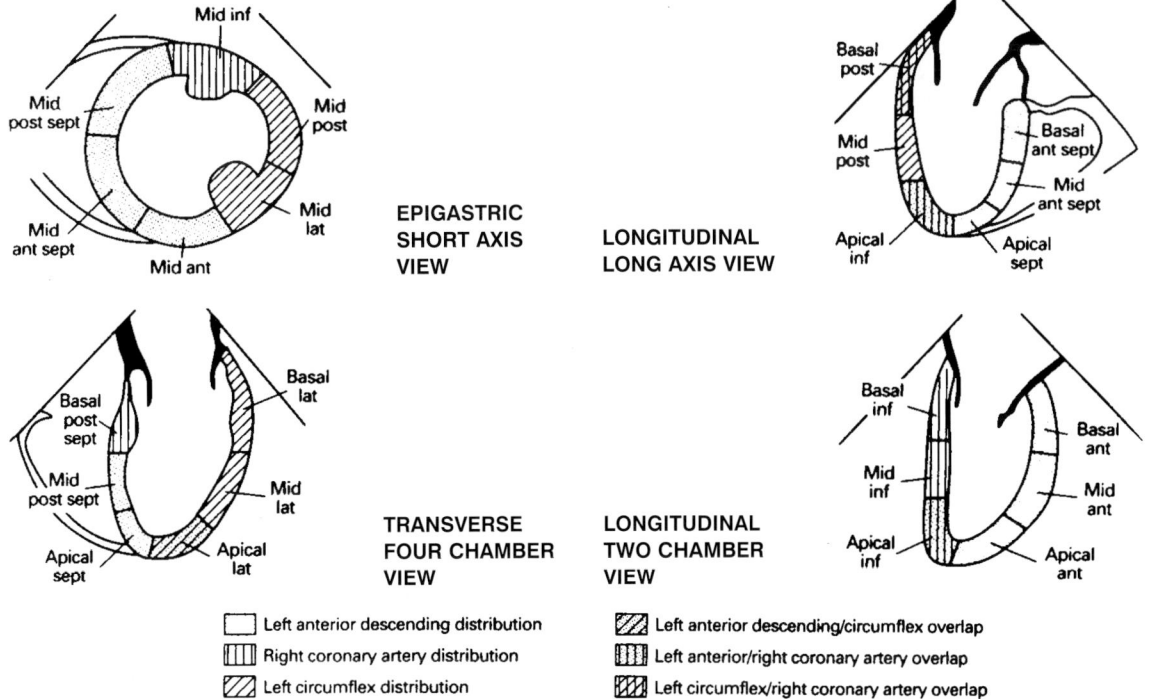

Figure 9.4 – Model of left ventricular segmentation and distribution of coronary perfusion using transoesophageal echocardiographic images.

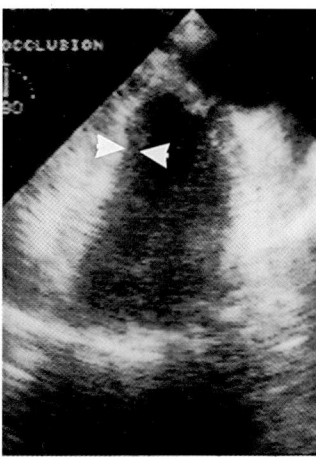

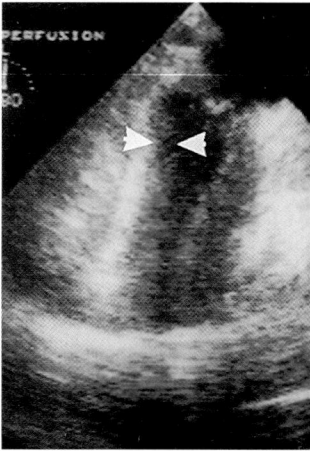

Figure 9.5 – Transoesophageal two chamber view of the left ventricle from the longitudinal plane to demonstrate akinetic inferior wall on occlusion of the right coronary artery.

Contraindications to both agents include severe obstructive lung disease (forced expiratory volume 1 second (FEV_1), less than 40% of predicted) or pronounced bronchospastic airways disease (clinical history of asthma or FEV_1 response to bronchodilator greater than 15%). Additionally, patients taking oral dipyridamole therapy should not be given adenosine, and patients who have a risk of severe complications from prolonged hypotension, such as those with clinically active carotid artery disease or aortic stenosis, should not take dipyridamole. Xanthine derivatives interfere with the effectiveness of these agents. Theophylline-containing medications and caffeine

should not be consumed preferably for 72 hours and 24 hours, respectively, before testing.

Dipyridamole stress test protocol

The procedure is carried out in the same fashion as for the dobutamine test apart from the infusion rates.

The dosage regimen is a 'high-dose dipyridamole echocardiography test': Infusion of 0.56 mg/kg for 4 minutes, then no dose for 4 minutes. If the test is still negative, an additional dose of 0.28mg/kg is infused for further 2 minutes.

Aminophylline is administered if ischaemia or side effects occur. The recovery period should last 15–20 minutes to fully offset the action of dipyridamole.

Adenosine stress test protocol

The protocol of adenosine infusion is the shortest of the pharmacological stress tests. Adenosine is infused at a dose of 0.14 mg/kg for 6 minutes. Maximum coronary blood flow is obtained 2 minutes after the start of infusion and coronary blood flow returns to the baseline less than 2 minutes after termination of the infusion (Figure 9.6).

The side effects are similar to those observed with dipyridamole but are milder and rapidly resolve after cessation of adenosine infusion.

Clinical applications

Accuracy of exercise echocardiography by experienced personnel has been shown to be excecellent with average sensitivity of 85% and specificity of 87%.[11–14](Figure 9.7)

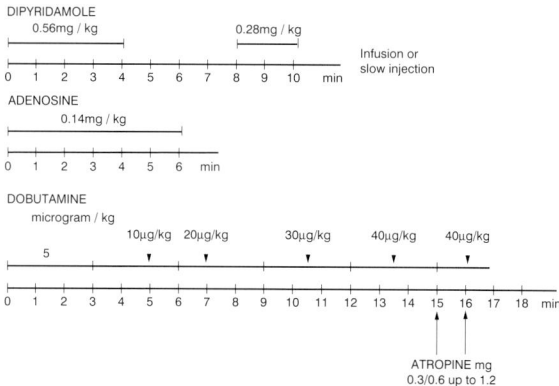

Figure 9.6 – Schematic representation of pharmacological stress echocardigraphy protocols.

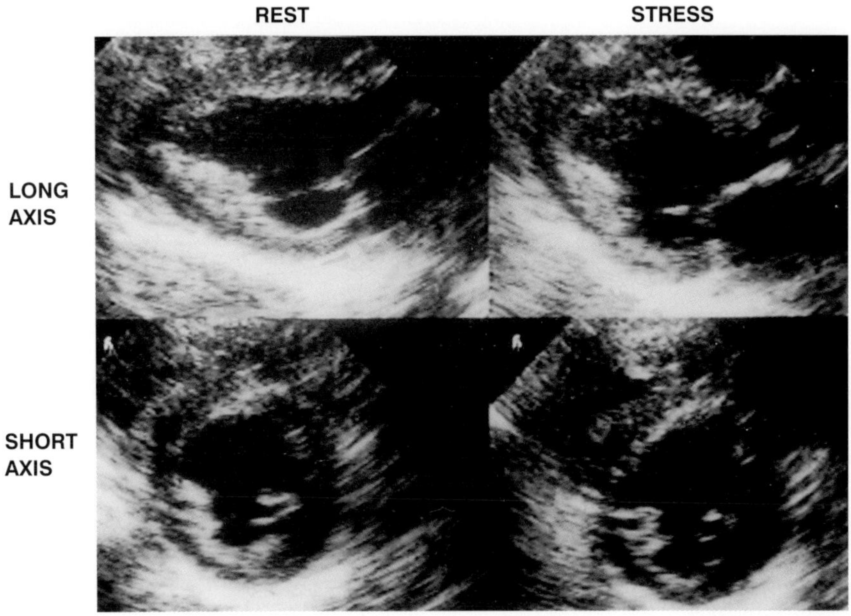

REST STRESS

LONG
AXIS

SHORT
AXIS

Figure 9.7 – Digitized side by side representation of rest and post exercise long and short axis views of the left ventricle showing the presence of anterior akinesis post exercise.

The exercise stress protocol should be the first choice for most clinical applications of stress echocardiography.

Pharmacological stressors are needed in patients unable to exercise or in whom exercise is contraindicated. Dobutamine stimulates physical exercise closely and has a great sensitivity for detecting even mild coronary artery disease.[15,16] It has been shown to be a safe and feasible diagnostic test for the noninvasive diagnosis of coronary artery disease.[17–19] Furthermore, the ischaemic threshold measured during dobutamine stress echocardiography has been shown to correlate with both the number of stenosed vessels and the left ventricular ejection fraction response to exercise.[20] It also provides invaluable information about both myocardial ischaemia and viability[21–26] in the same patient (Figures 9.8 & 9.9). It is important to recognize myocardial viability in patients with coronary artery disease and ventricular dysfunction because of the possibility of recovery after complete revascularization. Observational studies indicate that patients with nonvascularized hibernating and stunned myocardium may do worse than those with vascularized myocardium. The ability to predict myocardial recovery is therefore crucial in selecting patients with impaired left ventricular function for surgery.

	Baseline	Low dose	High dose
Normal	↑	↑↑	↑↑
Viable	–	↑	↑
Viable but jeopardised	–	↑	–
Ischaemic	↑	↑↑	–
Scar/necrotic	–	–	–

–, No contractions; ↑, contraction; ↑↑, increased contraction.

Figure 9.8 – Schematic representation of dobutamine stress echocardiographic findings in coronary artery disease. Low dose dobutamine administration improves thickening of viable myocardium. Deterioration in contractility indicates that viable myocardium is jeopardized. Ischaemia predicts significant distal vessel disease. Scar/necrotic myocardium remains akinetic.

Future developments

This chapter has concentrated on the application of stress echocardiography in the assessment of coronary artery disease. However, stress echocardiography is now also being used in the assessment of the functional consequences of valvular lesions.[27] With respect to coronary artery disease, clinical trials are already underway to assess myocardial perfusion using intravenous contrast agents.[28] Perfusion studies using ultrasonic contrast agents and 3D imaging should extend the role of echocardiography significantly in the assessment of ischaemic heart disease.

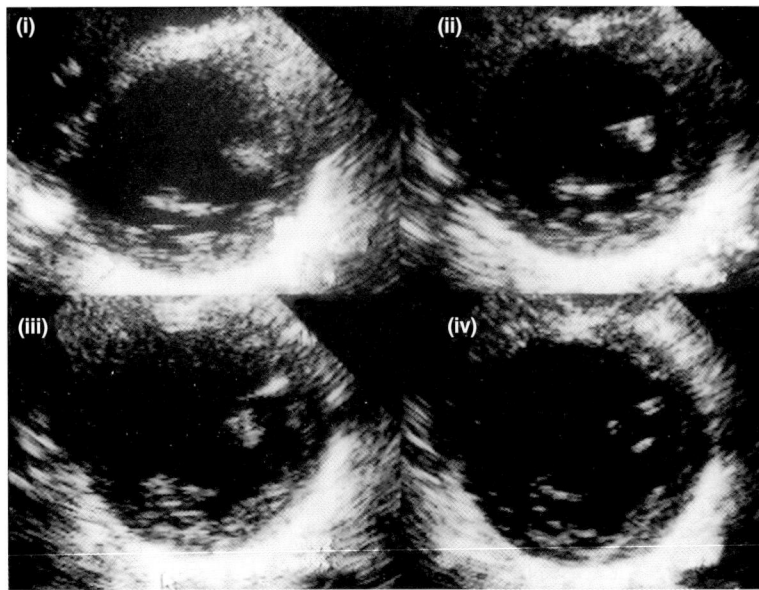

Figure 9.9 – Digitized short axis views of the left ventricle showing increase in contractility of lateral wall with low dose dobutamine (ii) comparing with rest (i). At higher dose (iii) it becomes hypokinetic again and at peak dose (iv) is akinetic suggesting the myocardium is viable but jeopardized.

References

1. Robertson WS, Feigenbaum H, Armstrong WF, Dillon JC, O'Donnell J, McHenry PW. Exercise Echocardiography: A clinically practical addition in the evaluation of coronary artery disease. *J Am Coll Cardiol* 1983; **2**; 1085–1091.

2. Sculz R, Heusch G. Characterization of hibernating and stunned myocardium. *Eur Heart J* 1995; **16**: 19–25.

3. Braunwauld E. *Heart Disease*. Saunders. Philadelphia: 1992.

4. Nihoyannopoulos P, Marsonis A, Joshi J, Athanassopoulos G, Oakley CM. Magnitude of silent ischaemia is greater in painful than in painless myocardial ischaemia: an exercise echocardiographic study. *J Am Coll Cardiol* 1995; **25**: 1507–1512.

5. Roger VL, Pellika PA, Oh JK, Miller FA, Seward JB, Tajik AJ. Stress echocardiography. Part I. Exercise echocardiography: techniques, implementation, clinical applications, and correlations. *Mayo Clin Proc* 1995; **70**: 5–15.

6. Schiller NB, Shah PM, Crawford M *et al*. Recommendations for quantitation of the left ventricle by two-dimensional echocardiography. *J Am Soc Echocardiogr* 1989; **2**: 358–367.

7. McNeill AJ, Fioretti PM, El-Said EM, Salustri A, Forster T, Roelandt JRTC. Enhanced sesitivity for detection of coronary artery disease by addtion of atropine to dobutamine stress echocardiography. *Am J Cardiol* 1992; **70**: 41–46.

8. Young M, Pan W, Wiesner J *et al*. Characterization of arbutamine: A novel catecholamine stress agent for diagnosis of coronary artery disease. *Drug Dev Res* 1994; **32**: 19–28.

9. Picano E, Lattazzi F. Dipyridamole echocardiography: A new diagnostic window on coronary artery disease. *Circulation* 1991; **83** (suppl 111): 19–26.

10. Panza JA, Laurienzo JM, Curiel RV, Quyyumi AA, Cannon III RO. Transoesophageal dobutamine stress echocardiography for evaluation of patients with coronary artery disease. *J Am Coll Cardiol* 1994; **24**: 1260–1267.

11. Limacher MC, Quinones MA, Poliner LR, Nelson JG, Winters WL, Jr, Waggoner AD. Detection of coronary artery disease with exercise two-dimensional echocardiography. *Circulation* 1983; **67**: 1211–1218.

12. Ryan T, Vasey CG, Presti CF, O'Donnell JA, Feigenbaum H, Armstrong WF. Exercise echocardiography: detection of coronary artery disease in patients with normal left ventricular wall motion at rest. *J Am Coll Cardiol* 1988; **11**: 993–999.

13. Crouse LJ, Harbrecht JJ, Vacek JL, Rosamond TL, Kramer PH. Exercise echocardiography as a screening test for coronary artery disease and correlation with coronary arteriography. *Am J Cardiol* 1991; **67**: 1213–1218.

14. Marwick TH, Nemec JJ, Pashkow FJ, Stewart WJ, Salcedo EE. Accuracy and limitations of exercise echocardiography in a routine clinical setting. *J Am Coll Cardiol* 1992; **19**: 74–81.

15. Reis G, Marcovitz PA, Leichtman AB, Merion RM, Fay WP, Werns SW, Armstrong WF. Usefulness of dobutamine stress echocardiography in detecting coronary disease in end-stage renal disease. *Am J Cardiol* 1995; **75**: 707–710.

16. Cohen JL, Ottenweller JE, George AK, Duvvuri S. Comparison of dobutamine and exercise echocardiography for detecting coronary artery disease. *Am J Cardiol* 1993; **72**: 1226–1231.

17. Salustri A, Fioretti PM, Pozzoli MMA, McNeill AJ, Roelandt JRTC. Dobutamine stress echocardiography: its role in the diagnosis of coronary artery disease. *Eur Heart J* 1992; **13**: 70–77.

18. Poldermans J, Fioretti PM, Boersma E et al. Safety of dobutamine-atropine stress echocardiography in patients with suspected or proven coronary artery disease. *Am J Cardiol* 1994; **73**: 456–459.

19. Poldermans D, Fioretti PM, Forster T *et al*. Dobutamine stress echocardiography for assessment of perioperative cardiac risk in patients undergoing major vascular surgery. *Circulation* 1993; **87**: 1506–1512.

20. Panza JA, Curiel RV, Laurienzo JM, Quyyumi AA, Dilsizian V. Relation between ischaemic threshold measured during dobutamine stress echocardiography and known indices of poor prognosis in patients with coronary artery disease. *Circulation* 1995; **92**: 2095–2101.

21. Salustri A, Elhendy A, Garyfallydis P et al. Prediction of improvement of ventricular function after first acute myocardial infarction using low-dose dobutamine stress echocardiography. *Am J Cardiol* 1994; **74**: 853–856.

22. Smart SC, Sawada S, Ryan T *et al*. Low-dose dobutamine echocardiography detects reversible dysfunction after thrombolytic therapy of acute myocardial infarction. *Circulation* 1993; **88**: 405–415.

23. Barilla F, Gheorghiade M, Alam M, Khaja F, Goldstein S. Low-dose dobutamine in patients with acute myocardial infarction identifies viable but not contractile myocardium and predicts the magnitude of improvement in wall motion abnormalities in response to coronary revascularization. *Am Heart J* 1991; **122**: 1522–1531.

24. Haque T, Furukawa T, Takahashi M, Kinoshita M. Identification of hibernating myocardium by dobutamine stress echocardiography: comparison with thallium-201 reinjection imaging. *Am Heart J* 1995; **130**: 553–563.

25. Chen C, Li L, Chen LL et al. Incremental doses of dobutamine induce a biphasic response in dysfunctional left ventricular regions subtending coronary stenoses. *Circulation* 1995; **92**: 756–766.

26. Afridi I, Main ML, Grayburn PA. Accuracy of dobutamine echocardiography for detection of myocardial viability in patients with an occluded left anterior descending coronary artery. *J Am Coll Cardiol* 1996; **28**: 455–459.

27. Tischler MD, Plehn JF. Applications of stress echocardiography: Beyond coronary disease. *J Am Soc Echocardiogr* 1995; **8**: 185–197.

28. McDicken WN, Moran CM, Hoskins PR, Monaghan MJ, Sutherland GR. New technology in echocardiography II: imaging techniques. *Heart* 1996; **75** (suppl 2): 9–16.

10

THE CARDIAC SURGERY ENVIRONMENT

Preoperative assessment

Echocardiographic assessment before cardiac surgery is becoming more common and cardiac surgeons are becoming increasingly familiar with and reliant on echocardiographic diagnosis. There are a number of ways in which echo studies can help the surgeon preoperatively.

The aim of a preoperative examination is to inform the surgeon about the current state of the ventricular contractility and valve function. It is possible that the cardiac function may have changed between the time of diagnosis and listing for operation and the time of surgery itself, particularly if waiting time has been long. Echocardiograms can also be of benefit when it is not possible at cardiac catheterisation to pass a catheter across a stenotic aortic valve to assess the left ventricular contractility or valve gradient. Another common application is where a patient with valve disease is followed for several years and regular monitoring is needed to choose the ideal time at which to intervene. Yet another example is the need to determine preoperatively, if possible, the type of surgery that might be necessary. Mitral valve repair is becoming increasingly common and it is important for the surgeon to know preoperatively if this will be an option (rather than valve replacement). The surgeon can then plan the operation appropriately and will also have an opportunity to discuss the options with the patient.

WHAT THE SURGEON NEEDS TO KNOW

- Left ventricular function – including regional abnormalities as well as overall function.

- Degree of valve disease – i.e. mild, moderate or severe stenosis and or regurgitation.

- As much detail as possible about the morphology of a diseased valve (e.g. thickened, irregular, vegetations, prolapse).

- Detail about the great arteries, particularly the aorta.

OTHER INFORMATION

- In mitral valve prolapse it is important to determine which leaflet is involved (see Chapter 5). If only the posterior leaflet is affected, repair of the valve is possible. If the anterior leaflet is involved, it is more likely that the surgeon will want to replace the valve.

- Associated dilatation of other chambers (e.g. degree of left atrial dilatation in mitral regurgitation or aortic root dilatation in severe aortic stenosis).

- Do not just look at the valve in question. It may be that, while the heart is open, other valves with less severe disease may require attention.

- Look for patent foramen ovale, which can be closed during surgery.

- Note any masses under the sternum (e.g. aortic aneurysm) that may impede the opening of the chest.

- Autografts – it is necessary to know the annular size of the aortic and pulmonary valves and to check that they match.

- The presence of abscess cavity in infective endocarditis.

Intraoperative assessment

Transoesophageal echocardiography

The use of transoesophageal echocardiography (TOE) (see Chapter 8) in the operating theatre has been a major advance in recent years (Figure 10.1). Immediate preoperative assessment of the heart followed by immediate postoperative checking of results (both while the chest is open) have proved immensely valuable. The procedure can be performed by any experi-

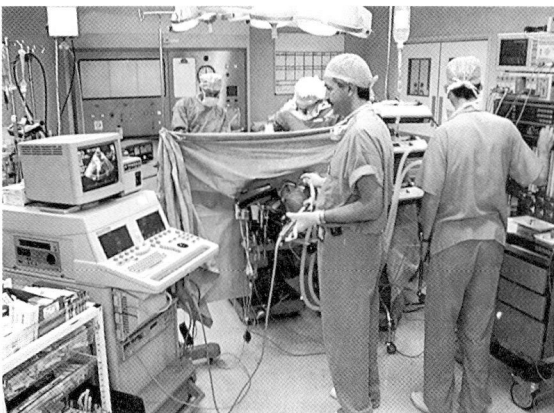

Figure 10.1 – A typical surgical environment. The anaesthetist and anaesthetic machine are seen on the right, the transoesophageal operator is seen in the centre, manipulating the endoscope.

enced TOE operator, but there has been particular interest by anaesthetists who are present throughout the operation and who are closely concerned with monitoring the haemodynamic condition of the patient. The anaesethetist is also ideally suited to the tasks of introducing and manipulating the endoscope.

It should be said, however, that the application of TOE in theatre is as complex as, if not more than, any other form of echocardiography. If mistakes and misinterpretations are to be avoided, anaesthetists should have proper training in the full scope of TOE work, including a general understanding of transthoracic echo studies and a full knowledge of the physics and interpretation of the various ultrasound modalities being used.

The technique should be carefully co-ordinated with the surgical team as it ties up equipment and operators for quite long periods of time. Some departments have dedicated resources, but this is not always the case.

Cardiac surgery us usually carried out 'on bypass', with the heart opened and excluded from the circulation. During this period TOE is of no use because the heart is not functioning and is filled with air, which prevents imaging. It is for this reason that TOE in theatre is usually done in two stages: before and after bypass. These two examinations may be separated by 1 – 2 hours.

A number of phases of the procedure can be identified: -

1   *Anaesthesia phase* — This is the time when it is most convenient to introduce the probe. Once the anaesthetist has the patient anaesthetised and ventilated, it is a relatively easy matter for them to pass the probe into the oesophagus, under direct vision if necessary. Intubation with the TOE probe at a later stage in the operating theatre is often more difficult as the patient has been draped and positioned for surgery and access can be difficult.

2   *Surgical preparation phase* — During this period the patient is being draped and prepared for surgery in the operating theatre. This is a good time to perform the initial scan as there is no disturbance of the heart or the images. A full examination should be undertaken at this stage and the surgical team must be aware that a little time (10 – 15 min) may be necessary for this. All measurements and data should be collected for postoperative comparison. If a preoperative scan has been performed, it is important to correlate the results. At this stage any indwelling catheters in the heart can be identified (Figure 10.2).

3   *Opening the chest and cannulating for cardiopulmonary bypass* — This stage involves the use of the sternal

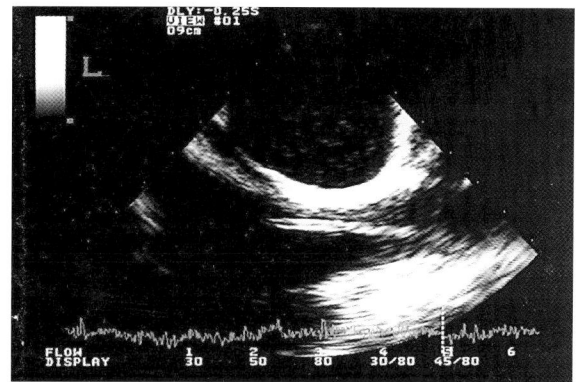

Figure 10.2 – Longitudinal projection showing a central venous line entering the right atrium via the superior vena cava.

saw, surgical diathermy to control bleeding and manual manipulation of the heart. Many technical and physiological artefacts are produced at this stage and it is not a good time for imaging.

4   *Cannulated pre-cardiopulmonary bypass* — This is the last time the heart can be imaged in a relatively normal state prior the the open heart procedure. Any last imaging must be completed during this phase.

5   *Cardiopulmonary bypass and aortic cross-clamping* — As the circulation is taken over by the 'pump' the intracardiac flows begin to slow and the blood becomes more echogenic. The rhythym of the heart may become irregular. After cross-clamping of the aorta there is no more flow and after the heart is opened, air is admitted and no more imaging is possible.

6   *Coming 'off bypass'* — At this stage the cardiac repair is completed and air should have been expelled from the heart by the surgeon. It is a good time to check for residual air but the normal action of the heart is only gradually restored as the bypass is weaned off in stages (Figure 10.3).

7   *'Off bypass'* — At this stage the heart has taken over its own action but remains cannulated for cardiopulmonary bypass. It is the most appropriate time to check all the details of the intracardiac repair. This is the time when it is least difficult to 'go back onto bypass' if the repair is unsatisfactory. At this stage the echocardiographer and the surgeon must confer over the findings and come to an agreement over the interpretation of the findings.

8   *Follow up* — No more imaging may be required if the operation is considered to be satisfactory but if the TOE probe is still available it can be left in situ to allow continued monitoring in the intensive care unit.

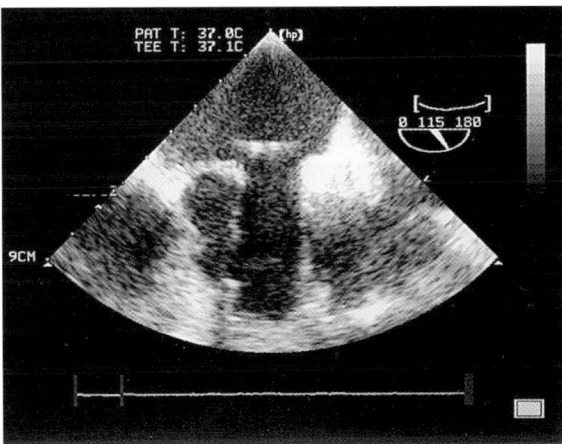

Figure 10.3 – Postoperative appearance showing a residual air bubble in the left atrium. The bubble produces a large echo signal with acoustic shadowing behind it.

There are three main indications for TOE in theatre: assessment of ventricular function; assessment of intracardiac repairs, most commonly mitral valve repair; diagnosis of uncertain problems.

LEFT VENTRICULAR FUNCTION

An evaluation of left ventricular function is of use when the surgeon is particularly concerned about a poor left ventricle. Careful assessment with recordings is needed before bypass to allow precise correlation with the images recorded after bypass.

MITRAL VALVE REPAIR

This is a specialist area and requires considerable experience and co-operation between the echocardiographer and the surgeon, both of whom need to appreciate much about the other's technique. It is often on the final 'say so' of the echocardiographer whether the course of the planned procedure is fundamentally changed.[1]

INTRAOPERATIVE DIAGNOSIS

A variety of problems may be encountered during surgery, from general considerations, such as why a heart is failing to do well after the procedure, to specific factors such as whether a prosthetic valve is working or whether a patch is intact. TOE may also be of considerable use in haemodynamic assessments such as monitoring the circulating volume or the effects of drugs. This specialist area will not be covered in more detail; full description of TOE techniques is given in Chapter 8.

Epicardial echocardiography

A small-faced, high-frequency transducer is placed directly on the heart after the chest has been opened. The transducer is placed in a sterile sheath and is usually manipulated by the surgeon, although it may be operated by a scrubbed sonographer. As the heart is moist, it may not be necessary to use coupling gel. If it is necessary, sterile gel must be used. The machine needs a separate operator. The transducer can be placed on the heart from any direction (except posteriorly) and exceptional images can be gained of a particular structure in multiple planes. For this reason, excellent knowledge of heart anatomy is needed. Some manufacturers have refined the possibilities of this technique and designed very small transducers that can be attached to the surgeon's finger in order to gain maximal access round the heart.

This technique is not commonly used, however, as intraoperative TOE is of excellent quality.

Postoperative assessment (Intensive Care)

The intensive care unit can be quite an intimidating situation for an echocardiographer from another department. In most units space is at a premium and there is very little room to manoeuvre an echo machine beside the patient's bed. It is sensible to have a small, mobile machine of reasonably high quality dedicated to the unit. As intensive care units are open plan, the patient being scanned should be screened off to maximise privacy. The area should be made as dark as possible by switching off lights and closing any blinds or curtains at the window. If it is possible to get the patient turned even a little onto their left side, this will help, although this may not be possible if the patient is unstable and connected to a ventilator. The central sternal dressing often obscures a parasternal window and may need to be peeled back if the nursing staff are agreeable. Unfortunately, most heart surgery patients are large men, supine and ventilated with drains in situ, all of which mitigate against obtaining an optimal scan. The views obtained may not be the standard ones. It is important that the heart can be viewed from two positions at 90° to each other. Doppler studies still need to be performed parallel to the direction of blood flow.

For the first 24 hours after surgery, a patient may have no available imaging windows. This is thought to be due to a combination of oedema and air within the anterior chest wall. A TOE may be needed if obtaining echocardiogram is necessary during this time.

Echocardiograms of intensive care patients are most commonly requested for:

- diagnosis or exclusion of pericardial effusion/tamponade
- assessment of left ventricular function
- assessment of the function of a new prosthetic valve
- diagnosis or exclusion of thrombus (in cases of cardiovascular accident, or intra- or postoperative myocardial infarction(MI))
- to check intracardiac repairs (e.g. to check that a repair of a ventricular septal defect is intact).

Pericardial effusion/tamponade

After surgery, a small amount of pericardial fluid can be noted; a diameter less than 5 mm is normal (see Chapter 6). The anterior pericardium is not normally sewn together after surgery; therefore, any fluid collection is usually noted around the left ventricle. Only if the amount of fluid is large does it extend anteriorly. If an effusion is composed of blood it may clot, compressing the chambers and causing tamponade. This can be a difficult diagnosis, as haematoma has similar echogenicity to the normal tissue surrounding the heart. What can be observed is small chambers compressed by the extrinsic collection. TOE can often help in this case. Subcostal views are almost impossible to obtain due to the presence of drains and stitches.

Left ventricular function

The ventricular septum is typically dyskinetic and hypokinetic after coronary artery bypass grafting (CABG) and valve replacement. Initial function may be poor due to ischaemia during surgery. If these patients are followed up, after a matter of only days the left ventricular function can usually be seen to improve. The new grafts may thrombose after surgery causing a myocardial infarction which results in poor function. Hypotension after surgery will result in an ischaemic heart which also leads to poor contractility. Inotropic support tends to give the ventricles a jerky contractile action. The ventricles can also give a false impression of contractility. Medical staff may switch off inotropes or a balloon pump during the recording of echocardiogram in order to be able to see any changes.

After apical aneurysectomy the apex should be seen to taper, although it often remains akinetic. The suture site cannot be seen.

Prosthetic valves

The main things to check for in a newly replaced valve are paraprosthetic leaks and dehiscence, which will be demonstrated by a rocking movement of the valve. While the patient is in the intensive care unit, this preliminary scan should not be used as a baseline scan, as images are not at their best in this situation and, more importantly, most velocities will be raised due to the increase in cardiac output caused by inotropic support. For a range of normal measurements for replaced valves, see the section on prosthetic valves in Chapter 5.

Thrombus

Following CABG surgery the patient is not on anticoagulants. Therefore, if the patient suffers an intraoperative or postoperative myocardial infarction, thrombus can form. See Chapter 6 for a description of the echocardiographic appearance of left ventricular thrombus.

Repair of ventricular septal defects

A ventricular septal defect patch is typically checked after surgery to assess for any leak across the repair site. The area of the patch will be akinetic and will appear brighter than normal myocardium. The incident beam needs to be as close to 90° to the patch as possible in order to maximise imaging as well as Doppler studies. The repair site should be assessed using both continuous wave and colour flow Doppler techniques. Any leak will be from the left to right ventricle, unless the right ventricle is at a higher pressure than the left (e.g. in cases of severe pulmonary hypertension).

A catheter line in the right side of the heart can often be noted in patients up to a couple of days after operation. This is typically a Swan–Ganz catheter used to measure right-sided pressures.

To prevent cross-infection between patients in the intensive care unit, the transducer should be cleaned with an alcohol wipe or equivalent and hands washed thoroughly after each examination. The results of the scan should be related to the doctor in charge of the patient, a brief report should be added to the patient's notes and a full report recorded in the normal way.

Follow-up after cardiac surgery

Patients do not require follow-up scans after coronary artery bypass grafting unless there is renewed ischaemic disease.

Patients with replacement valves should have a baseline scan before leaving hospital or at their first outpatient appointment (see Chapter 5). If the prosthesis is mechanical, no further scans are required unless the patient's symptoms suggest that one is necessary. Patients with porcine valves should start to have regular scans at 5 years after valve insertion or sooner if symptoms indicate.[2] The septum usually remains hypokinetic in patients with a mitral or aortic valve replacement.

If a mitral valve has been repaired, the posterior leaflet is usually seen to be fixed. Although the valve has been repaired, it is likely that further degeneration will occur over a period of time, and the valve will eventually need to be replaced.

Aneurysms of the ascending aorta may form at the site of aortotomy months after the operation (see Chapter 6). If there is a small connection between the false aneurysm and the aorta, the colour flow Doppler image will show an obvious connection site. If the hole is large, it will be difficult to visualise on the colour flow image as pressures will be similar, but spontaneous contrast may be noted.

References

1. Lee EM, Shapiro LM and Wells FC. Echocardiography in mitral valve repair for mitral regurgitation: the surgeon's needs. *J of Heart Valve Dis* 1997; **6**: 228–233.

2. Chambers J, Fraser A, Lawford P, Nihoyannopoulos P, Simpson I. Echocardiographic assessment of artificial heart valves: British Society of Echocardiography position paper. *Br Heart J* 1994; **71** (suppl): 6–14.

11

CLINICAL OVERVIEW

Learning echocardiography

The aim of any echocardiographic study is to integrate all available information to provide the most comprehensive and reliable clinical diagnosis. The operator should have many different skills, all working simultaneously to achieve this aim. These skills include:

- An understanding of imaging and Doppler ultrasound physics

- An understanding of the technical operation of the machine

- Practical skills in manipulating the patient and transducer positions

- Personal skills in communicating with the patient

- An understanding of cardiac anatomy and variations

- An understanding of cardiac pathologies and their effects

- Interpretation skills in assessing the imaging and Doppler information

- Clinical skills in understanding presenting signs and symptoms

- Clinical skills in appreciating the importance and treatment of conditions

- Communication skills in passing this information on to others

AND, MOST IMPORTANTLY

- Skill in recognising the limitations of the operator and the technique.

All this may appear daunting to new echocardiographers but they should not be disheartened. Many people from different backgrounds have achieved high levels in all these skills, and there are a number of important ways to ensure they are adequately achieved. First, training must take place in a properly structured environment with appropriate supervision. Beginners can do very little on their own and will need to work continuously with an experienced colleague to start with. Later, they will move on to semi-supervised work with frequent checking. Finally, they will become independent operators, but even then they would be well advised to consult regularly with colleagues on difficult or doubtful cases.

Who should perform the examination?

Echocardiography is suited to both medically and non-medically qualified personnel. In the case of doctors there are subgroups, each with a slightly different perspective on the subject. The cardiologist will often use the echo technique as a supporting tool in the formation or the piecing together of a clinical diagnosis or management situation. This is particularly so in the case of paediatric cardiologists, for whom the echo is their 'right hand'. He or she must beware, however, of 'fitting' the echo information to their presumed diagnosis, especially when it is giving a slightly different conclusion from their other clinical findings. The radiologist may well be more objective in the diagnostic interpretation, but must be careful to take into account the context of the findings (as the examples below may show). It is important for the radiologist (or the cardiologist who is not clinically dealing with the patient) to have full information about the patient, their clinical problem and the clinical questions that are being asked. The anaesthetist will probably be more concerned with 'management information' and will be assessing the progress of a patient in the operating theatre or intensive care unit. The anaesthetist must be careful to look out for other diagnostic possibilities in addition to the particular problem that they are focused upon.

Whilst medically qualified echocardiographers are clearly at a clinical advantage, they also have weaknesses. In general it is true to say that doctors are frequently less meticulous about the practical techniques involved, often performing examinations faster and perhaps making fewer repeat measurements or recordings. They also have weaknesses in the area of reporting and documenting their work! On the other hand, technically trained staff such as cardiac technicians, radiographers or physicists may well have more precise techniques, but may not always fully appreciate the clinical significance of their findings. There are, of course, many notable exceptions to the generalisations of this paragraph.

In the presentation of the report, it is essential to make clear who has performed the examination and who has written the report. Often this will be the same person, but in many busy departments the scan is performed by a technician, who gives a provisional report, and the definitive medical report is given by a clinician who reviews the data. In some cases the report is issued by the technician alone. In this case it is essential to make it clear on the report that it is a record of technical findings, not a medical opinion.

There are many differences in working arrangements between different departments and between different countries. In the UK and the USA it is common to have technician-led scanning, but in Europe clinician led-scanning is often the usual arrangement.

Training, examination and accreditation

Training and accreditation have become vitally important with the increasing role played by echocardiography in the management of patients. In previous years the echocardiography department in each hospital adopted its own style of work and training, and hence the standards and quality of work varied tremendously from place to place. In most countries there have been strenuous efforts to standardise the training and accreditation requirements for echocardiographers, so that a uniform quality of work can be expected.

Each country has its own arrangements. In the UK the lead has been taken by the British Society of Echocardiography (BSE) a multidisciplinary organisation with many senior figures in echocardiography participating in it. Its aims are many, but training and accreditation are high on its list of priorities. A training syllabus can be obtained from the society, and regular accreditation examinations are held. At present this examination is a voluntary one and is held for the benefit of Society members, but increasingly employers are seeking some form of documentation of echocardiographic skills and the 'BSE exam' is proving to be very useful in this respect. The training of medical specialists is also becoming more structured and many specialist registrars in the UK are taking the 'BSE exam' to demonstrate their competence in this field.

More information, including details of training requirements and an 'exam pack' can be obtained from the Society at:

British Society of Echocardiography
9 Fitzroy Square
London W1P 5AH

Clinical Contexts

Listed below are a few examples showing how important it is to correlate clinical signs, symptoms and other information with the different types of information that may be derived from within the echocardiographic examination. These examples are not meant to be comprehensive, but rather are intended to highlight the way echocardiography works as a clinical tool, inter-relating with good overall clinical assessment and management.

Aortic stenosis and left ventricular function

The operator will have learned the techniques of estimating the severity of aortic stenosis by measuring the peak velocity of flow through the valve, taking care in particular to get proper alignment of the ultrasound beam with the peak velocity jet. Even if this has been achieved by meticulous technique the operator must be aware of pitfalls and traps. If the left ventricle is severely impaired and there is a reduced cardiac output or stroke volume, then the velocity of flow through the valve may well be reduced, even though the valve is still severely narrowed. The operator must therefore recognise this situation and assess the valve by imaging techniques, possibly even by transoesophageal echo, to see if the orifice really is very narrow. In some cases the calculation using the continuity equation may be needed to assess the valve orifice size. If all else fails, the inconsistency between findings should be reported clearly, so that other investigations, for example cardiac catheterisation, may be considered.

Volume overload and left ventricular function

In a number of conditions there will be left ventricular volume overload associated with an important haemodynamic lesion. In the case of either mitral or aortic regurgitation, the left ventricle will have to eject more blood with each contraction in order to make up for the leak . In assessing severity, the operator must be aware that severe valve regurgitation is almost always associated with left ventricular volume overload. In other words, do not lightly diagnose severe regurgitation on colour flow Doppler examination alone, be sure you can also see the dilated and hyperdynamic action of the ventricle. Conversely, if you see a volume overloaded ventricle with a large stroke volume, be sure to look for the cause of the volume overload. You should always be suspicious about diagnosing a severe valve regurgitation if there is no sign of volume overload.

Heart murmur of unknown origin

Who has referred the patient? What is the type of murmur? What is the clinical background?

If a pregnant woman is referred because of a soft murmur of recent onset, then it will not be surprising to find a normal heart as the increased cardiac output of pregnancy can often produce 'innocent' flow murmurs (although this is no excuse for an incomplete examination). If, however, an experienced cardiologist has referred a young patient with a loud and harsh systolic murmur, it would be exceptional if the echocardiographic study did not reveal a clear cause, such as a ventricular septal defect or a valve lesion, and the echocardiographer should be careful to determine its cause. In other words, the examination should be carried out with a good understanding of the clinical context.

Transient ischaemic attack

In the case of a patient with transient neurological symptoms (a temporary, or 'mini', stroke lasting less than 24 hours) the diagnostic possibilities are very different in the different age groups. In an elderly patient there can be many causes of stroke and they are often not be related to the heart as a source of possible embolus. In this group the clinical work-up may involve echocardiography, but will be directed by the physician who is managing the patient. Many other possibilities will have to be considered. In young patients with sudden onset of neurological symptoms, the echocardiogram will be an urgent early examination, and if no abnormality is found the investigation may have to proceed on to transoesophageal studies. Complex cases of this sort will often be managed by good consultation between the clinician and the echocardiography department.

Suspected infective endocarditis

It is very common for a patient to be referred for diagnosis of infective endocarditis, but it should be remembered that this diagnosis, while aided considerably by echocardiography, is essentially a clinical one made on the basis of clinical signs and microbiological tests. If a patient has the clinical signs of infective endocarditis and is unwell, then failure to find an obvious vegetation or valve lesion does not mean that there is no endocarditis, it just reduces the possibility of the diagnosis. An echogenic lesion on the leaflet of a mitral valve of a patient who is fit, well and active should be assessed with caution. It might be a vegetation, but it may well be another abnormality, possibly of long standing.

Follow-Up Surgical Assessment

In this circumstance, skilled echocardiography must be combined with particularly good clinical communication. It is important to know precisely what operation has been done. For example, has a valve prosthesis been implanted and, if so, what type is it? Without this knowledge it is harder to assess its function. In many centres it is routine practice to study all patients who have had valve surgery a few weeks after surgery. This allows a 'baseline' to be established so that any future change in valve function will be easier to diagnose. It is also very important to know if any previous echocardiographic studies have been done, either before or after surgery, so that changes in valve function and ventricular function can be documented. In a patient who has undergone coronary artery bypass grafting and has a poorly functioning left ventricle it is very important to know the preoperative condition of the ventricle so that it can be seen whether the deterioration is related to the surgery or occurred beforehand. In serial follow-up examinations it is particularly important to use a consistent technique so that scans can be compared with previous studies.

Communication and Reporting

At all times there should be appropriate reporting and communication with referring clinicians. If you have examined a patient for a GP or family doctor who is suspicious that his patient may have an important heart problem, do not send him a complex technical report full of measurements and derived indices. By all means include this information if you wish, but make sure you have explained in simple and straightforward terms what you have found. In addition, bear in mind that you may be more familiar than the GP with the usual management of any problem you have diagnosed. Give him appropriate advice, particularly about when to seek specialist help (but do not offer advice beyond your own level of knowledge). On the other hand, a cardiologist referring a patient with a complex problem will no doubt want accurate quantitative answers about the condition he or she is managing.

Speed of response is also important. Of course it is helpful to return a report as soon as possible but usually 2 or 3 days will pass while the report is typed and sent out. If, however, you have discovered a new finding that is clinically important and urgent, then it is your responsibility to pass on the information immediately. Sometimes a telephone call is appropriate, but in some cases you may ask an appropriate clinician to come and see the patient immediately. If you are the first person to diagnose an atrial myxoma, then you have the responsibility to inform a cardiologist immediately.

Conclusion

Echocardiography is one of the most challenging but rewarding investigations in medicine. It involves so many skills, but when you have gained enough experience they will all begin to 'click' together. Those people who like a challenge, who always strive for something a little better, who are both practical and technical and who enjoy working with people will make the best echocardiographers.

Appendix
I

Report writing

Probably the most important concept to keep in mind when writing a report is to answer the clinical reason for referral. Just as a full examination should be performed on every patient, so a full report should be written. This should include both normal and abnormal findings. It is important to get the balance right: reports that are unnecessarily long are difficult to read and gleaning of the significant points can be tedious. Conversely, reports that are too brief will give the impression that a complete study has not been performed.

The report should be written directly following the examination when the information is fresh. Even leaving all reporting to the end of a session can causes confusion and information and interpretation of results formed at the time of scan can be forgotten.

It is useful to have a standard reporting form for all reporters. This will keep a degree of consistency and standard of report and will ensure that information is not left out of the report. Figure I.1 shows typical report worksheet.

General aspects

1 Correct patient identification is essential.
2 The date of examination is essential.
3 If the operator is different to the reporter this should be highlighted. If queries arise at a later date it will be necessary to know who performed the scan.
4 Good documentation is necessary in a busy department. Being able to quickly identify a video tape will save a lot of time, rather than looking back through the day book.
5 Technical quality should be mentioned at the beginning of a report (and maybe again in the summary if particularly bad) so that the report may be read in context.
6 Referral history has two functions. The first is to prompt the operator/reporter to ensure the clinical question is answered. The second purpose is that the report will be read in years to come when the original reason for referral may have been forgotten.

Clinical aspects

7 The left ventricle should be described in terms of size, shape (e.g. globular) and contractility. Be aware of volume overload, (ventricles which are dilated but show vigorous contractility). Contractility can be further split into the different regions (see chapter 4). An estimate of overall function is a useful guide if there are varied regional wall abnormalities but this is rather subjective and depends a lot on experience. Some departments choose not to quote an ejection fraction in every patient due to inaccuracies in its calculation, particularly in patients with regional wall motion variations.

The degree of any hypertrophy should also be recorded. Any other myocardial abnormalities should also be noted – e.g. thinning, altered echo pattern. Intracavity gradients or any other unusual feature in the ventricle should be recorded in this section.

8 The mitral valve should be described firstly from the two-dimensional images. This includes thickness and movement of the leaflets. Any prolapse or buckling of the leaflets on closure should be noted. If annular thickening is present, this should also be included.

Doppler findings should then be described. If pressure half time and forward velocity are well within normal limits, some operators may choose not to quote the exact figures. Simply 'normal mitral valve Doppler examination' would cover this situation. Any mitral stenosis should be graded and the estimated valve area stated. Mitral regurgitation should be noted in terms of colour flow appearances (i.e. size, distribution and intensity of jet, and size of left atrium).

If the left atrium is dilated measurements should be quoted. Atrial fibrillation is often the result of a dilated left atrium, so the size of the atrium is necessary in such patients.

9 The aortic valve should be described in a similar fashion to the mitral valve. The number of leaflets should be noted where possible. Describe the degree of thickness and movement of the leaflets. The peak and mean pressure drops across the aortic valve need only to be quoted if they are outside the normal range, with the estimated degree of stenosis alongside. Valve area may be calculated and included in cases of stenosis. Quantify aortic regurgitation. This must be described by the different methods used to quantify it, e.g. 'Severe aortic regurgitation on colour flow confirmed by degree of reversed flow in descending aorta'.

The presence of a left ventricular outflow tract gradient should be included here.

The aortic root needs a brief mention in terms of appearance and size. The ascending aorta only needs to be commented on if the reason for referral includes the aorta or if an abnormality is found.

10 The right ventricle is described in terms of size and contractility and the presence of any hypertrophy.

HOSPITAL NAME
Echocardiogram Report

Patient Name		Date ②	Operator ③
①			
Hospital No.　　　　DOB		Tape No. ④	
Referred by	History		
Technical quality			
⑤	⑥		

LEFT VENTRICLE (Normal ranges: EDD 37mm to 51mm, ESD 23mm to 36mm, wall thickness 7mm–11mm, EF 55–80%)

EF%	EDD	mm ESD	mm septum	mm inf wall	mm
		⑦			

MITRAL VALVE/LEFT ATRIUM　⑧

AORTIC VALVE/ASCENDING AORTA　⑨

RIGHT SIDED STRUCTURES　⑩

PERICARDIUM & EXTRACARDIAC　⑪

SUMMARY　⑫

Reported by:　PRINT _____　　　Checked by:　PRINT _____

　　　　　　　Signed _____　　　　　　　　　　　Signed _____

MITRAL VALVE/LEFT ATRIUM (Normal P/2t<70ms=area 3+cm², LA 52mm × 44mm)
AORTIC VALVE/ASCENDING AORTA (Normal AV PPD<25mm Hg, aortic root diameter<39mm, asc aorta<34mm)
RIGHT SIDED STRUCTURES (Normal RV diameter<35mm, TR PPD<25mm Hg, PA acc. time>100ms)

Figure I.1 – Typical report worksheet. Refer to text for details.

Tricuspid regurgitation should always be sought and the jet velocity measured wherever possible. The estimated pressure drop of tricuspid regurgitation only needs to be quoted if it is greater than 25 mmHg, along with the degree of pulmonary hypertension indicated. If the right atrium is dilated quote its measurements.

The presence of a VSD/ASD can be included in this section, and should state position and size. If the pulmonary valve and/or pulmonary artery have been assessed, include the findings here.

11 The pericardium and extracardiac section only needs to be filled in if abnormalities are found, (e.g. pericardial effusions/masses, pleural effusions, coarctation, IVC/abdominal aorta pathology).

Summary

12 The summary should be kept as brief as possible but it is a crucial part of the report and should bring together the essence of the examination. The writing of a good summary is an important skill to acquire. Some guidelines are given below:

- Any unusual pathology should be noted first with its size and location and any haemodynamic effect it may be causing. Unsuspected pathology needs to highlighted.

- Trivial abnormalities (e.g. valve regurgitation) need not be repeated in the summary. Normal anatomy need not be commented on unless directly queried in the referral letter or if it is an important negative finding.

- Comparisons with previous studies should be included in the report (N.B. the video from the previous scan should be viewed at the time of the current examination because inter-operator interpretation can vary widely).

- If anatomy cannot be seen due to poor imaging it is better to state that it could not be visualised than leave it out of the report as any anatomy omitted might be assumed to be normal by the reader of the report.

- The reporter should be aware of the clinical significance of threatening or prognostically serious conditions and should be able to advise the referring clinician immediately if there is a worrying problem.

- If the reporter is medical, a clinical opinion can be given which may include advice about further diagnosis or treatment. If the report is issued by a non-medical person, that is a technical report, care must be taken when wording the conclusion so as not to give inappropriate clinical advice.

- The summary should be written in a way that is appropriate for the reader of the report. A highly technical summary with much quantitative data may be useful for an expert cardiologist but would be very confusing for a general practitioner.

- The reporter's name, position and title should be clearly stated.

If in doubt always seek a more senior opinion.

Biological effects of ultrasound

Mechanical interactions

As a wave of ultrasound passes through tissue it causes the tissue particles to vibrate. Microstreaming can result, fragmenting macromolecules.

Thermal interactions

As a wave of ultrasound passes through tissue it loses energy in the form of heat. The rate of temperature rise of the insonated tissue is related to the intensity of the ultrasound beam, the attenuation coefficient of the tissue (see chapter 3), the cross-sectional area of the beam, the exposure time and the method of heat dispersion (blood flow and thermal conductivity of the tissue). This is particularly important in TOE examinations.

Cavitation interactions

As ultrasound passes through tissue the sinusoidal pressure wave causes localised regions of increased and decreased pressure. These pressure differences cause bubbles of gas to form within the tissues, termed cavitation. Cavitation causes damage to biological molecules.

Safety

Currently, no biological effects have been observed in humans at diagnostic ultrasound intensity levels. However, as ultrasound is a relative new modality, there is not enough data to categorically state the absolute safety of diagnostic ultrasound.

A clinical safety statement is issued every year by the European Federation of Societies for Ultrasound in Medicine and Biology (EFSUMB). The 1998 statement cautions against the use of pulsed and colour flow Doppler during fetal examinations at the time of fetal organogenesis, and keeping power output in Doppler studies to a minimum during later pregnancy.

Of more relevance to the cardiac sonographer is that recent studies have shown localised extravasation from alveolar capillaries at diagnostic ultrasound levels. EFSUMB therefore recommends high output settings (pulse amplitudes above 1 MPa) 'should be avoided if possible during examinations which might expose lung surfaces.' Output settings of individual machines should be available from the manufacturer.

Physics

Transducers

There are two different kinds of transducer used for the majority of cardiac ultrasound. These are electrical and mechanical. These terms describe the way the ultrasound beam is steered through an arc to produce a plane of ultrasound.

ELECTRICAL SECTOR TRANSDUCERS

The electrical transducers used for cardiac ultrasound are called phased array transducers. The transducer is made up of a small number of crystal elements. Each crystal has separate electrical connections through which a voltage can be applied. Steering of the ultrasound beam to produce a sector is accomplished by applying an excitation voltage to each crystal in different sequences. This is achieved by delays which are controlled by the system's microprocessor. The delays are changed rapidly, and by small amounts so that each scan line is produced at a slightly different angle until the entire sector has been completed (Figure I.2). Focusing of the ultrasound beam is also achieved by alteration of the delay times.

There are no mechanically moving parts in a phased array transducer and this allows the property of an 'agile beam'. This means that two successive ultrasound pulses can, if required, be sent out in very different directions. This includes pulses for different modalities (e.g. imaging, M-mode or Doppler). This means that the system can share the time available between modalities to interlace different functions. For example a 'live' 2-D image can be viewed at the same time as the M-mode or Doppler trace derived from that image. If optimum quality is required, then sharing functions should be avoided but in clinical practice this facility is often very useful.

MECHANICAL SECTOR TRANSDUCERS

There are a variety of different forms of mechanical sector scanners but all involve physical movement to sweep the ultrasound beam through an arc.

Rocking transducer – One crystal is mounted on an oscillating mechanism that sweeps the beam (Figure I.3a).

Rotating transducer – Three to four transducer crystals are mounted on a rotating wheel and so are able to operate at a fast frame rate (Figure I.3b).

Rocking mirror – One stationary transducer is aimed towards a rocking mirror which reflects the beam into the patient (Figure I.3c).

In each of the systems the transducer crystals are surrounded by an alcohol/water mixture, or oil, and are housed in an echolucent casing. The face of the transducer is very rounded and fits nicely between ribs, although much jelly is needed to maintain contact of the entire face. Due to the mechanics contained in the probe it tends to be heavy and bulky, and although they are well insulated, a small amount of vibration is transferred to the operator's hand.

ELECTRICAL VS MECHANICAL
Electrical:

- secondary lobes (side and grating lobes) produce artefacts
- focusing is not so good in small faced transducers
- light weight
- tend to be more expensive
- simultaneous functions possible

Mechanical:

- larger, bulkier, heavier
- well focused
- smaller contact area on skin due to curved face (hence reverberration artefacts at edges)
- moving parts – vibration and wear and tear

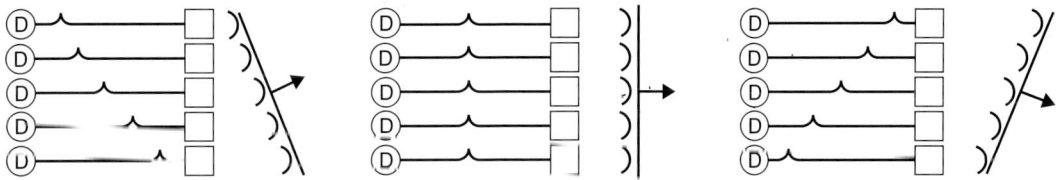

***Figure I.2** –* Beam steering in an electrical transducer, achieved with delays, Ⓓ.

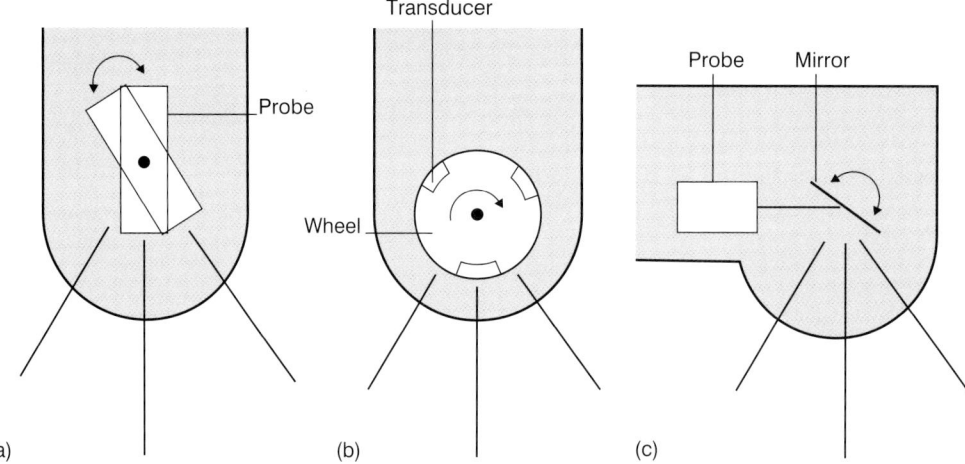

Figure I.3 – (a) Rocking transducer. (b) Rotating transducer (c) Rocking mirror

- single functions only at any time

Imaging artefacts – with particular reference to cardiac ultrasound.

An imaging artefact refers to anything that is, or is not, visible on an image that does not correlate directly with the actual tissue being insonated. This includes:

1. Objects perceived on the scan that are not actually present.
2. Objects that should be visible but are not
3. Misregistration of objects (objects that are present but the location is plotted incorrectly).

The most common artefacts are described below.

REVERBERATION (Figure I.4)

This occurs at highly reflective interfaces perpendicular to the incident beam. Ultrasound is reflected between two surfaces (e.g. two reflective objects or a reflective object and the face of the transducer) causing multiple echoes to be displayed at regular intervals relating to the distance between the two reflectors.

Reverberation is very often seen in the apical four chamber view in the apex of the left ventricle. It is very important not to confuse these artefactual echoes with thrombus.

This artefact is also partly responsible for obscuring the left atrium when a mechanical mitral valve replacement is in situ. It can be a useful artefact to identify the needle tip in a pericardial effusion when draining.

COMET TAIL (Figure I.5)

Similar to reverberation artefacts are comet tail artefacts. These occur when there are multiple reflections *within* a small structure. They tend not to be constant or impede the image and are easily identifiable.

SHADOWING

Shadowing occurs behind an object which is highly reflective or attenuating. The object reduces the intensity of the ultrasound beam both to and from the structures behind it.

Shadowing can be seen behind valve sewing rings (Figure I.6) and areas of calcification. The most noticeable shadowing occurs with mechanical prosthetic

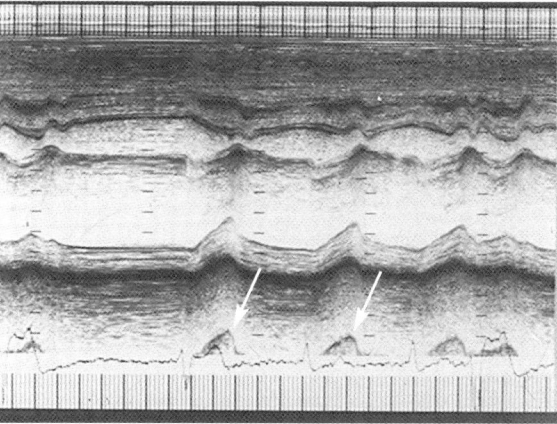

Figure I.4 – Image of reverberation posterior to the left ventricular wall on an M-mode trace (arrowed).

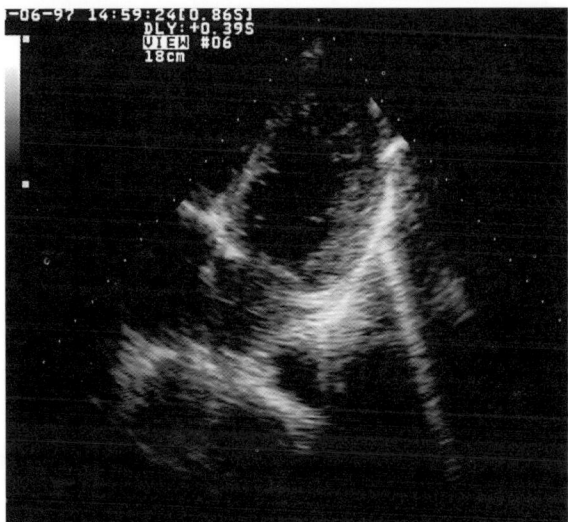

Figure I.5 – 'Comet tail' artefact in apical four chamber view. Thin, bright lines appear intermittently during real-time scanning.

valves, totally obscuring structures that are behind them. Shadowing not only obscures structures, but can lead to rather spurious images.

ENHANCEMENT

If ultrasound passes through a depth of fluid which has little attenuation then the surfaces beyond this will be shown brighter as the system has assumed a uniform tissue attenuation. This is particularly noticeable with fluid filled cysts but the effect is always present beyond blood filled cardiac chambers and is usually compensated for by non linear settings of the time/gain compensation controls.

MIRROR IMAGE

Mirror image artefacts occur when an object lies directly in front of a highly reflective surface. If the scale is set small enough, this can often be seen in slim patients on the parasternal long axis view. The heart sits directly on the diaphragm which is extremely reflective. Due to multiple reflection, a second, mirror image of the heart is produced below the diaphragm.

LATERAL AND AXIAL RESOLUTION CAUSING ARTEFACTS

Objects smaller than the axial or lateral resolution of the system (e.g. less than 2 mm) may not appear on the image. Alternatively, they may be registered but will be displayed at the systems smallest resolution, (e.g. In a

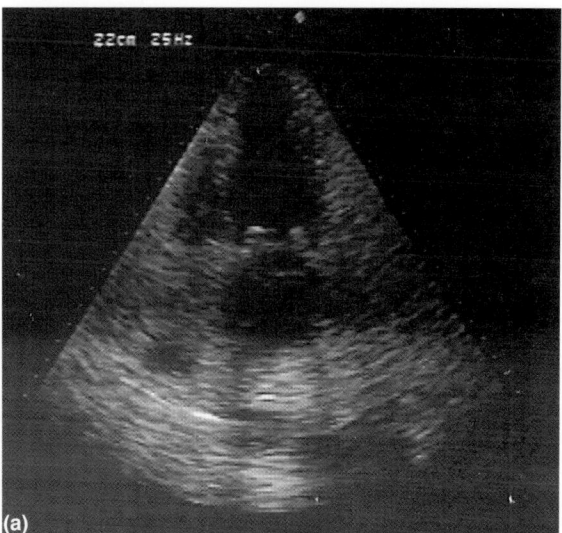

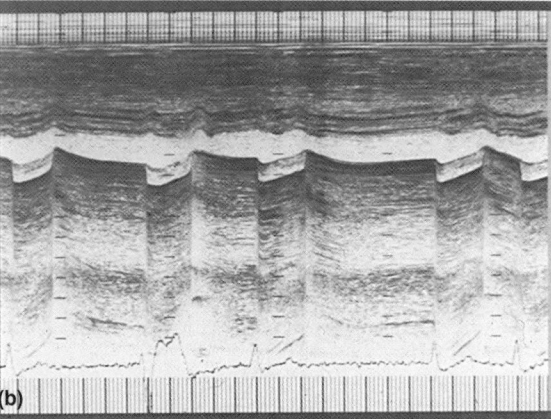

Figure I.6 – (a) Image of MV sewing ring with shadowing. The radial lines of acoustic shadowing passing through the posterior left atrial wall caused confusion about the possibility of an abnormal mass. (b) Combined acoustic shadowing and reverberation on an M-mode trace caused by strong reflections from the tilting disc of a mechanical mitral prosthesis.

system with a resolution of 2 mm, a 1 mm object will be displayed as being 2 mm).

Two objects that are spaced closer together than the resolution of the system will be displayed as one object.

Some ways in which the lateral and axial resolution can affect the cardiac images are:

1. Loss of echoes from the interatrial septum in the apical four chamber view.
2. Tiny vegetations are not displayed.

3. Tiny 'holes' in the heart (e.g. small VSDs, perforations in valve leaflets) will not be identified on imaging.

SLICE WIDTH AND PARTIAL VOLUME EFFECT

It is easy to (wrongly) assume that the width of an ultrasound beam is paper-thin. In reality, all beams have width, predetermined at manufacturing stage of the transducer by crystal size and focusing.

The effects of this are most typically seen when scanning vessels rather than the large cardiac chambers. If the beam slice passes through both solid tissue and echo free tissue (e.g. vessel) at the same level, echoes from the solid tissue around the vessel will be plotted within the vessel on the image, filling it in, and could possibly represent a mass within the vessel (Figure I.7). Scanning a vessel in this situation in two planes, as should always be performed regardless, can help to identify this artefact.

SIDE LOBES AND GRATING LOBES

Electrical transducers can give rise to artefacts from side and grating lobes. Due to the way the ultrasound beam is focused and steered in an electrical transducer, small beams (or 'lobes') outside the main beam can form. Although the intensity of these lobes is low and hence returning echoes on the whole are ignored, if one of these lobes passes through a highly reflective structure the returning echoes will be plotted on the image as if they had returned from the main beam. Scanning a structure from multiple different projec-

tions can help to eliminate misinterpretation of these artefacts.

Spectral Doppler artefacts

CARDIAC AND RESPIRATION MOVEMENT

Cardiac and respiration movements can swamp a spectral Doppler trace as they produce high intensity movement. The majority of cardiac movement is low velocity and so can be removed by filtering out the low velocities from the trace. Respiration movement is more difficult to eliminate. Altering the transducer position or asking the patient to hold their breath may help.

MIRRORING

Mirroring or 'cross talk' of a spectral trace occurs in cases of high intensity flow (Figure I.8). Increasing the Doppler filter and/or lowering the Doppler power and gain can help. Mitral regurgitation can be falsely reported and care needs to be taken when interpreting a spectral trace.

TURBULENT FLOW

Although turbulent flow is not really an artefact, it can cause confusion in the interpretation of the spectral trace. Very turbulent flow (such as severe mitral

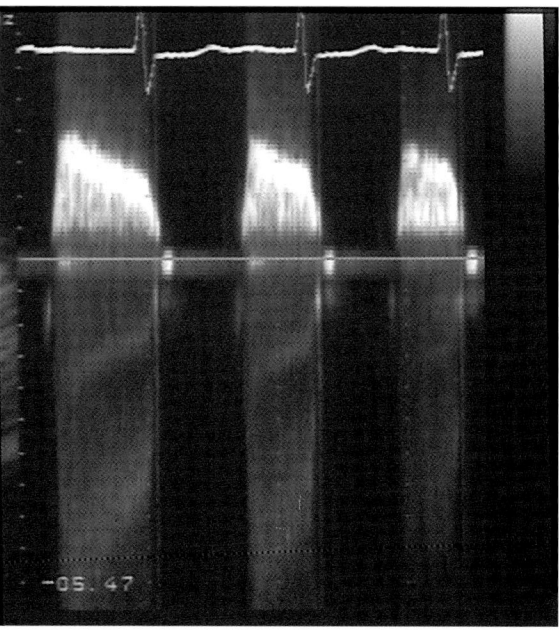

Figure I.8 – Crosstalk. Mitral valve pulsed Doppler trace. The signal gain is set too high, causing a mirror image (less intense) of the mitral flow signal below the zero baseline.

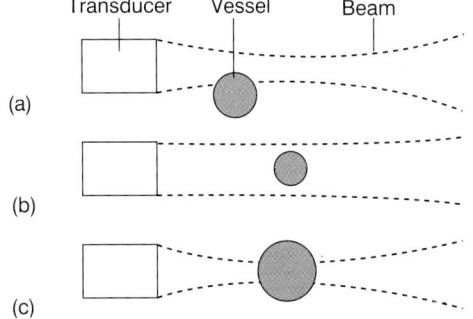

Figure I.7 – Where vessel and soft tissue are included in the beam (a) or when using a wide beam (b), the vessel cannot be resolved from the surrounding soft tissue and will appear solid. In example (c), the vessel will appear echo-free.

regurgitation or flow through a VSD) will usually cause a harsh audible sound. The spectral trace will display flow both above and below the zero line, due to the multiple directions in which blood is spraying through the valve or defect. The envelope of the trace is often indistinct and measurement of the peak velocity can be overestimated, especially in cases of aortic stenosis (Figure I.9).

The spectral trace can be improved by increasing the Doppler filter, lowering the compression and the Doppler gain and also reducing the output power. Try to determine the real peak from the artefact before measuring the maximum velocity.

ALIASING (SEE CHAPTER 3)

Aliasing occurs when using pulsed wave Doppler if the velocity of blood that is being interrogated is higher than the velocity limit of the system. It causes incorrect plotting of the resultant velocity on the spectral trace (refer to Figure 3.14 in Chapter 3). There are several ways to overcome this problem.

1. Move the zero line (base line) to either the top or bottom of the display (depending on direction of flow). This will give double the maximum velocity that can be displayed.
2. Increase the velocity range, which increases the pulse repetition frequency (PRF). Most echo machines have an option to raise the PRF, typically called high PRF (HPRF). This increases the sampling rate by introducing more sample volumes. Some range ambiguity is then introduced as flow from every sample volume is displayed on the same trace.

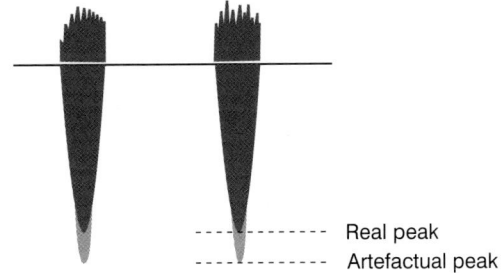

- - - - - - - Real peak
- - - - - - - Artefactual peak

Figure I.9 – Turbulent flow (e.g. through a VSD or aortic stenosis) recorded on continuous wave Doppler studies typically displays velocities in all directions. The envelope is usually not smooth. Measure the peak velocity where a definite top to the envelope is seen, not to the higher, artefactual peak.

3. If the blood flow that is being interrogated is very high velocity, continuous wave, rather than pulsed wave Doppler, should be used.
4. A lower frequency transducer can display higher velocities before aliasing occurs (see Doppler equation in Chapter 3).

Colour Doppler artefacts

Because colour Doppler images are superimposed on grey scale images, some artefacts affecting the grey scale image can also affect the colour display. These include mirror image, reverberation and misregistration from side and grating lobes. A mirror image artefact can be typically detected when trans oesophageal echocardiography is used to visualise the descending aorta. The wall of the aorta is highly reflective and flow is displayed both within and outside the aorta. It is important in such cases not to falsely diagnose a dissection. Acoustic shadowing will also prevent the display of colour flow behind highly reflective structures (for example, mitral regurgitation behind a mechanical mitral valve replacement).

GREY SCALE GAIN TOO HIGH

If grey scale gain is set too high when colour Doppler studies are performed, the echo free pools of blood (for example, within a cardiac chamber) which should appear as black areas, are displayed as grey. Two problems then arise:

1. The pixels on the monitor which should be filled with colour are instead filled with grey scale information.
2. The contrast between the colours and the background echoes is reduced and it is more difficult to visualise subtle flow, or to underestimate the volume of flow.

COLOUR GAIN TOO HIGH

If the colour gain is set too high, colour noise is displayed. This means that areas with no or low velocity flow as well as myocardium are filled with colour pixels. It is then more difficult for the operator to visualise actual flow. In practice, each time colour flow Doppler is applied to an image, the colour gain should be turned up until colour noise is displayed, then slowly lowered to a point when the noise just disappears. This will then ensure that the colour gain is set at its optimum level.

COLOUR GAIN TOO LOW

If the colour gain is set too low, low velocity and small volume flow will not be displayed and hence flow is underestimated, or missed altogether.

ALIASING (SEE CHAPTER 3)

Colour aliasing occurs if the velocity of blood that is being interrogated is higher than the velocity range of the colour display. It causes a 'wrap-around' of colour, displaying both blue and red within the same jet, even though all blood is moving in the same direction. Although in most circumstances artefacts hinder interpretation, aliasing can be beneficial in identifying fast flow within the heart when using colour flow imaging. With practice, the operator's eye is automatically drawn to these areas of aliasing (sometimes described as mosaic) and further interrogation of this flow with spectral Doppler studies can be performed.

FLOW PERPENDICULAR TO ULTRASOUND BEAM

The basic principles of flow identification by Doppler studies depends on the angle between the incident beam and the direction of blood flow (cos θ). If flow is perpendicular to the incident beam (cos $90° = 0$), then no flow is recognised by the ultrasound system. A good example of this is when colour flow is applied to the arch of the aorta on the suprasternal view. Flow can be seen in the ascending and descending aorta, and, although we know that blood is flowing around the arch at approximately the same velocity as in the ascending and descending aorta, no flow is displayed (see Figure 3.19 in Chapter 3).

INCORRECT FILTER SETTINGS

Some ultrasound systems give the operator the facility to alter the colour velocity filters. Some have presets for abdominal flow (low velocity) and cardiac flow (high velocity). If the filter is set to remove low velocity flow, flow through the IVC and hepatic veins will not be displayed. If abdominal presets are used when scanning the heart only low velocity flow is displayed and high velocity flow is ignored, and thus very little flow within the heart will be detected. If you are able to alter these filters on your machine, check the settings before you start your session.

DEPTH AMBIGUITY

Colour Doppler signals returning from a great depth will be plotted incorrectly on the grey scale image due to the time taken for these signals to return. For this reason, most systems limit the depth at which the colour flow Doppler box can be positioned (as well as to maintain an acceptable frame rate).

LOW FRAME RATE

The frame rate of most systems drops when colour flow Doppler is applied due to the time needed to collect the information (see Chapter 3). If the frame rate drops to less than about 15 frame/second (depending on the heart rate), continuous flow cannot be monitored. For example, rather than having five or six frames to follow a jet of mitral regurgitation to the back of the left atrium, only one frame of colour may be visualised with flow just at the back of the left atrium. In another heart cycle, it may only display one frame of colour at the orifice of the mitral valve, making it extremely difficult to estimate the amount of regurgitation. Decreasing the depth at which the colour flow box is applied, reducing the size of the colour box and reducing the size of the grey scale image can all be used to increase the frame rate.

COLOUR FLASH

This is a burst of colour that lasts for one frame only, rather than for a complete systole or diastole. It is usually a single tone blue or red with no aliasing. It is thought to be due to cardiac movement or respiration. It is very commonly seen in patients with a mechanical mitral valve replacement, when flashes of colour can be seen within the left atrium. Care needs to be taken not to confuse these flashes of colour with mitral regurgitation. True mitral regurgitation should be visualised throughout systole (not just for one frame) and is often accompanied by flow convergence in the left ventricle (see Figure 5.31 in Chapter 5).

COLOUR BLEED

Colour bleed is the extension of colour flow into adjacent tissue. A typical example of this is flow through a tiny VSD. The VSD cannot be visualised on imaging (due to lack of resolution) but the colour jet may appear relatively quite wide.

ENVIRONMENTAL ARTEFACTS

Colour flow images are more susceptible to electrical interference than grey scale images. Problems are usually encountered in the operating theatre when the diathermy is used.

Measurement calculations

Most present commercially available cardiac ultrasound machines have cardiac measurement packages programmed into them. From just a few basic measurements made by the operator, standard calculations are made regardless of the pathology or blood flow dynamics that are involved. If you have an understanding of how the calculations are performed you will have an idea of inaccuracies that are introduced and whether to religiously quote all numbers the machine's software gives you or to make your own interpretation of the results.

Ejection fraction calculations

$$EF(\%) = \frac{EDV - ESV}{EDV} \times 100$$

EDV = end diastolic volume
ESV = end systolic volume.

TEICHHOLTZ METHOD

The Teichholtz method is probably the most widely used (and easiest to perform, although not necessarily the most accurate) method for calculating a left ventricular volume. The volume is calculated from a one dimensional diameter as follows (Figure I.10):

$$\text{Volume of LV} = 4/3\pi \times L/2 \times D_1/2 \times D_2/2$$

The Teichholtz method assumes that:

$$L = 2 \times D_1, \text{ and } D_2 = D_1$$

$$\therefore \text{Volume} = D_1^3, \text{ i.e. that the LV is a cube!}$$

This method does not take into account unusually shaped ventricles, for example globular shaped. It also assumes that the ventricle is of uniform contractility and so does not take regional wall abnormalities into account. For example, if the base of the left ventricle is contracting well but the apex is dilated and akinetic, it will vastly overestimate the ejection fraction. Therefore in cases of regional wall abnormalities, an ejection fraction should not be quoted directly from the Teichholtz method.

AREA LENGTH

This volume measurement calculates the left ventricular volume from two-dimensional measurements (Figure I.11). It takes into consideration unusually shaped ventricles and some regional wall abnormalities. The biggest drawback of this calculation is that excellent quality images have to be gained for accurate tracing to be performed.

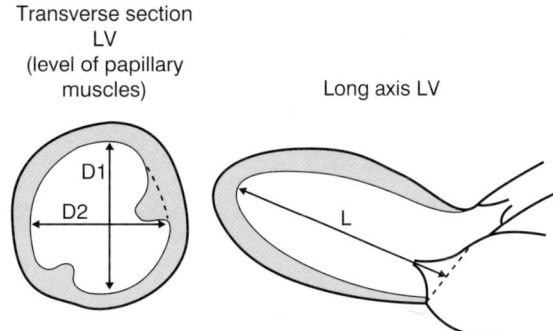

Transverse section LV (level of papillary muscles)

Long axis LV

Figure I.10 – Theoretical measurements needed to calculate LV volume from the Teichholtz method. D1 = AP diameter, D2 = transverse diameter, L = length of LV.

$$\text{Volume} = \frac{0.85 \times (\text{area})^2}{\text{length}}$$

MODIFIED SIMPSON'S RULE

To measure volume using Simpson's rule, multiple diameters, equally spaced, along the left ventricle must be measured which are converted to an area measurement and are then added together to obtain a volume. The modified Simpson's rule takes three to four diameters along the length of the left ventricle on both the long and short axis views. This obviously is quite time consuming and excellent quality images of the entire length of the ventricle are required.

Fractional shortening

Fractional shortening (FS) reflects left ventricular function. It is not a volume measurement and is derived directly from the EDD and ESD measurements. It is not dependent on heart rate.

$$FS\ (\%) = \frac{EDD-ESD}{EDD} \times 100$$

This is not a widely used measurement as it has been shown to only be helpful in normally shaped ventricles ventricles with uniform function.

Stroke volume

Stroke volume (SV) is the amount of blood ejected from the left ventricle during each systole. The usual way to calculate this volume is as follows:

Apical 4 chamber view

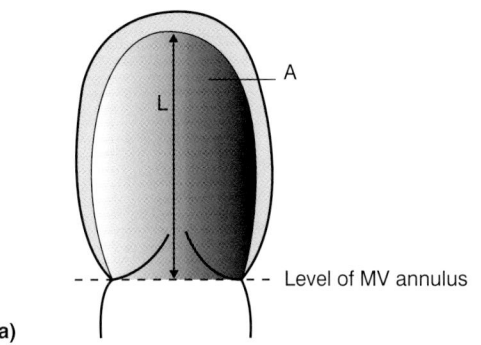

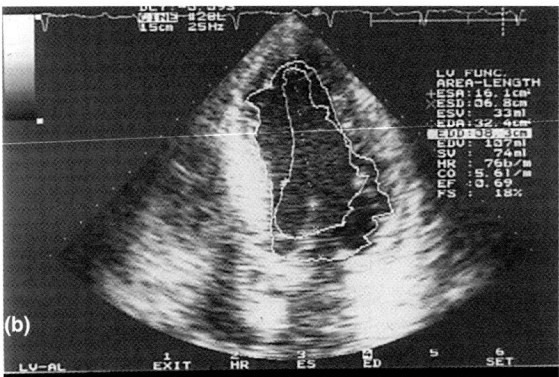

Figure I.11 – Measurements required for area length calculation of LV volume. (a) L = length of LV, A = area of maximum cavity in apical four chamber view. (b) Two-dimensional image showing tracing of left ventricular endocardium in systole and diastole to calculate volume by area length method.

$$SV \text{ (ml)} = EDV - ESV;$$

the volumes being calculated from one of the above methods.

In this calculation, any errors present in the calculation of ventricular volume will be enhanced as the difference between one erroneous value and another will be even more erroneous.

Aortic ejection volume

This method is slightly more complex and measures the blood flow in the left ventricular outflow tract (LVOT). This equates to stroke volume in the absence of valvular severe regurgitation or VSD. If there is mitral regurgitation, for example, the stroke volume of the ventricle may be large, but the ejection volume may be small, the difference being accounted for by blood being ejected into the left atrium.

$$SV \text{ (ml)} = A \text{ (cm}^2) \times V_{mean} \text{ (cm/s)} \times ET \text{ (s)},$$

where A is the area of the LVOT, V_{mean} is the mean velocity in the LVOT measured from the spectral trace of pulsed wave Doppler in the LVOT, and ET is the ejection time (time measured on the same spectral trace as above from start of flow to end of flow).

It should be remembered that stoke volume will be increased in cases of significant mitral and aortic regurgitation.

Cardiac output

Cardiac output (CO) reflects cardiac function. It is the volume of blood pumped by the heart in one minute. A normal adult needs a cardiac output of about 5 litres/minute, at rest, to meet the demands of the body.

$$CO \text{ (l/min)} = \frac{SV \text{ (ml)} \times \text{heart rate (bpm)}}{1000}$$

Be careful not to overestimate cardiac output in the presence of mitral and aortic regurgitation, when stroke volume does not equal ejected volume.

Left ventricular mass

The principle of this calculation involves derivation of left ventricular volume internally (endocardium to endocardium) and externally (right side of interventricular septum to epicardium of posterior left ventricular wall). Once this has been done using standard techniques, subtraction of the former from the latter will give muscle volume.

Then, LV Mass = myocardial volume × 1.03

It is essential to appreciate potential for error using this technique and it must not be used unless the examination is of high quality.

Proximal Isovelocity Surface Area (PISA)

This technique has been used to calculate flow, particularly mitral regurgitation, by observing the colour flow pattern of the converging and accelerating blood that moves towards the regurgitant orifice. In simplified terms, the blood accelerates as a hemisphere with delineation of the velocity by the hemispheric layers of colour aliasing. Knowledge of the size of the hemisphere and the aliasing velocity allows calculation of volume flow.

This technique requires meticulous attention to detail and should only be performed when the operator has fully studied the method and its pitfalls in detail.

Developing and future applications of echocardiography

Ultrasound is a very rapidly expanding and advancing field. Because of the non invasive and non harmful nature of ultrasound it is likely to continue to draw interest from many researchers, with the possibility of making some of the older, more invasive procedures obsolete. Hand in hand with this is the need for operators to continue to be updated from courses and literature, and for echocardiography departments to update its equipment on a regular basis.

Harmonic imaging

Many manufacturers have recently introduced harmonic imaging into echocardiography machines. This takes account of the principle that a reflected sound wave will contain second degree harmonics which are waveforms that have twice the frequency (or half the wavelength) of the original waveform.

This allows the system to emit ultrasound energy at a lower than usual frequency but receive the returned energy at the higher harmonic frequency. The advantage of this is that the benefits of deeper penetration with lower frequency ultrasound are retained, without the loss of image quality normally associated with these lower frequencies. Typically, emitted frequencies of 1.6 – 2.0 MHz are used, with returned frequencies of 3.0 – 4.0 MHz being used for image formation.

This technology allows much improved imaging in 'difficult' patients but care must be taken to avoid overuse of this technology as there can be an unusual texture to the images produced. This technology is currently in its early stages of clinical application.

Contrast echocardiography

The use of contrast in echocardiography is still an emerging field. In its most basic form it has been used for some time to demonstrate shunts by injecting agitated saline intravenously.

Contrast agents are manufactured commercially and include free gas bubbles, encapsulated gas bubbles, suspensions and emulsions. New agents are now manufactured to cross the cardiopulmonary barrier so that contrast injected intravenously will cross to the systemic circulation.

The presence of tiny air bubbles increases backscatter and hence tissues containing contrast agents will be highlighted.

There are three main areas in which contrast can be used within the heart.

CAVITY FILLING

This is especially useful to visualise the blood pool in the left ventricle since the borders between the blood and myocardium are highlighted.

MYOCARDIAL PERFUSION

Contrast is introduced by intracoronary injection. It delineates the myocardium supplied by each of the coronary arteries. It can be combined with stress echocardiography to monitor changes with increased work load.

FLOW ENHANCEMENT

If Doppler signals are poor, contrast can be injected to increase the number of reflectors and hence increase the intensity of the resultant spectral trace. This is the case for both colour flow and spectral Doppler studies.

Harmonic contrast imaging

Harmonic imaging further enhances contrast Doppler and imaging studies by ignoring tissue echoes. The contrast microbubbles are all an exact size, manufactured to resonate at both the frequency of the transducer and twice that frequency. Specialist equipment is required to tune in to listen to twice the incident frequency only. Since tissue echoes return at the incident frequency they are not recognised.

Three dimensional echocardiography

Currently the most work in three dimensional (3D) ultrasound is performed in conjunction with transoesophageal and intravascular (see later) ultrasound. Information required for 3D reconstruction from transoesophageal scans is obtained by fixing the transoesophageal transducer in one place and then rotating the beam through 180°. Commercially available 3D reconstruction machines with highly sophisticated computer software are available to attach to most current cardiac ultrasound machines (Figure I.12). Excellent images in all panes are required to create a good 3D reconstruction, explaining why transthoracic echocardiography is not really suited to 3D scanning. The images gained also have to be ECG gated. Reconstruction times are getting shorter and it will only be a matter of time before real time 3D scanning can be performed.

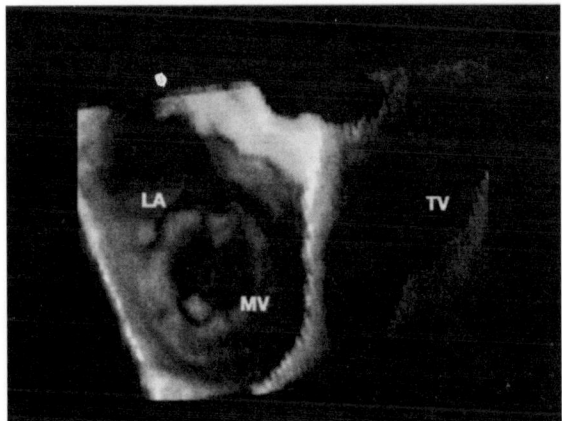

Figure I.12 – Three-dimensional image of a prosthetic mitral valve using reconstruction with a special Echo-CT transoesophageal pullback probe (courtesy of Tomtec).

Intravascular ultrasound (IVUS)

Although IVUS is not, strictly speaking, a branch of echocardiography, it is associated in the sense that many IVUS examinations are performed on coronary arteries (Figure I.13). A tiny transducer of very high frequency (20 – 30 MHz) is incorporated into a catheter. Most transducers are mechanical and rotate to give a 360° field of view. The resultant image gives high quality detail of the wall and lumen of the vessel. Plaques that

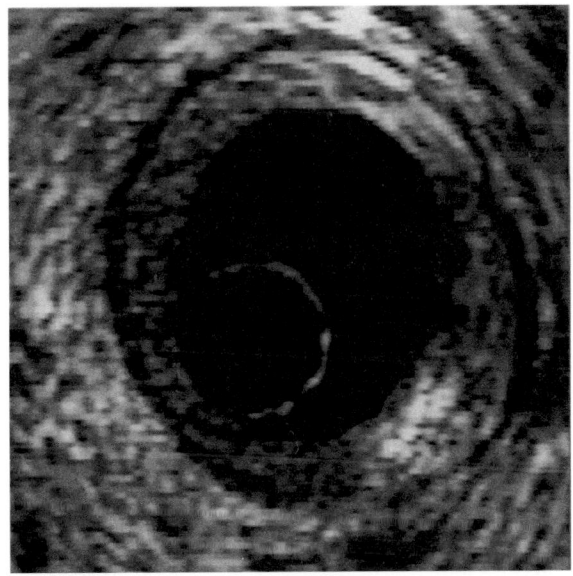

Figure I.13 – IVUS image showing the arterial wall (courtesy of CVIS).

may be missed on conventional angiography can be clearly identified. This is an invasive catheter laboratory technique which utilises expensive single-use intravascular transducers.

Wall motion detection

Most echocardiographers agree that quantifying left ventricular wall motion is one of the most difficult aspects of echocardiography. For this reason, many different forms of wall motion detection packages have been devised. A few of the commercially available ones are listed below.

ON LINE BOUNDARY DETECTION

By detecting the difference between echoes produced by myocardium and blood, a line can be traced, by the machine's software, around the border of the myocardium in real time (Figure I.14). This, then, allows the machine's software to automatically calculate an ejection fraction.

DOPPLER TISSUE IMAGING (DTI)

The Doppler principle can be applied to all moving structures. If the high velocity, but low intensity Doppler signals from blood movement are filtered out by the ultrasound machine, the high intensity but low velocity movement of the myocardium remains. In this way, both wall direction and velocity are colour coded in much the same way as blood flow. It is angle dependent and relies on good images to obtain a good colour image (Figure I.15).

POWER MOTION

This is an amplitude based Doppler examination rather than velocity and direction based to create a colour image. Brightness of the one colour hue increases with an increase in amplitude, that is, an increase in movement. It is more sensitive to low velocity movement and is less angle dependent than tissue colour Doppler applications (Figure I.16).

COLOUR KINESIS

Colour Kinesis is a way of monitoring the amount of movement made by the endocardial border. By differentiating between myocardium and blood, the machine's software (in real time) colour codes the amount of movement of the endocardial surface, displaying the movement as a series of coloured contours. For example, normal contractility is displayed as several differently coloured thick bands, whilst reduced con-

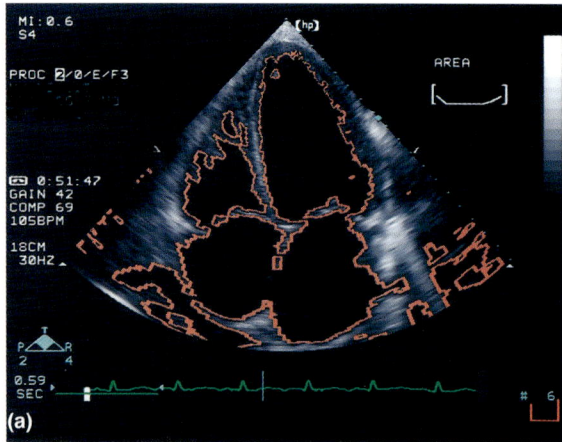

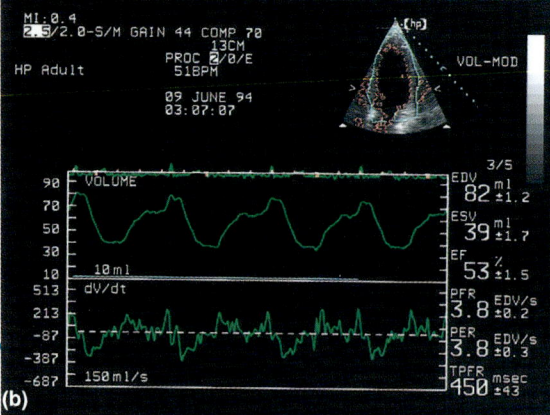

Figure I.14 – (a) Automated real-time boundary detection allowing accurate measurement of volumes and regional wall motion. (b) On-line real-time volume calculation using automated edge detection (courtesy of Hewlett-Packard).

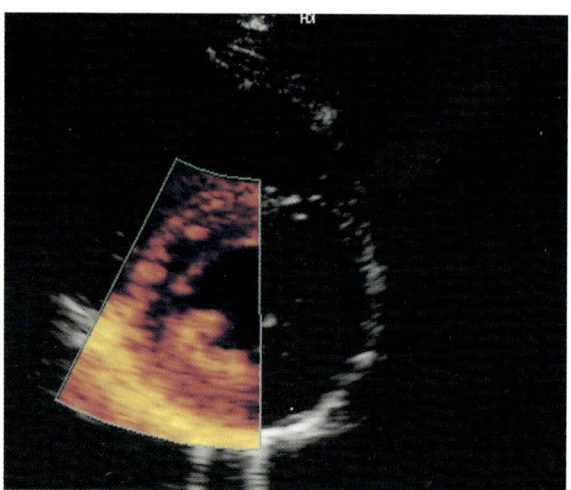

Figure I.16 – Power motion imaging in a short axis view of the left ventricle (courtesy of ATL).

tractility is displayed as thin bands of fewer colours (Figure I.17).

Cardiac output measurements

Cardiac output is one of the most commonly asked questions by clinicians which is given indirectly by the echocardiogram when we assess the left ventricular function. New methods for calculating cardiac output are always being researched. One recently described method is to measure the cardiac output from detailed assessment of colour flow in the left ventricular outflow tract. Unaliased colour is necessary for the software to

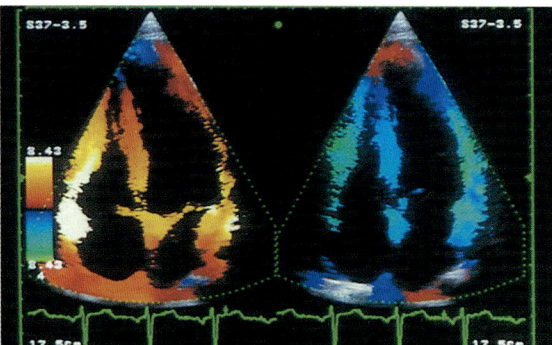

Figure I.15 – Doppler tissue imaging of a normal heart in the four chamber view. Colours show contraction towards the centre of gravity. Diastole on the left, systole on the right (courtesy of Toshiba).

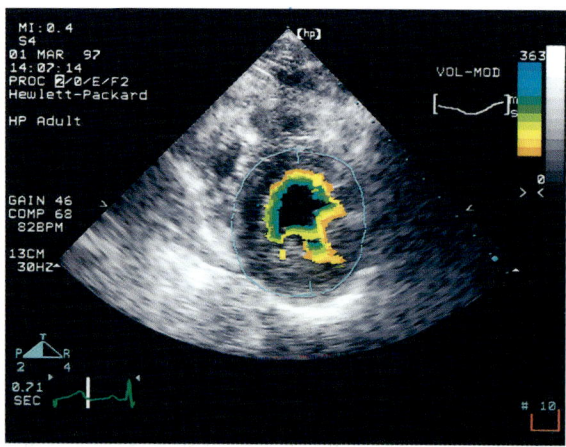

Figure I.17 – Short axis left ventricular image with colour kinesis showing circumferential contractility. The outline includes the two papillary muscles (courtesy of Hewlett-Packard).

obtain an accurate velocity measurement. The area of the outflow tract can also be calculated by the software as the area filled with colour pixels. These two measurements are then used to calculate cardiac output (Figure I.18).

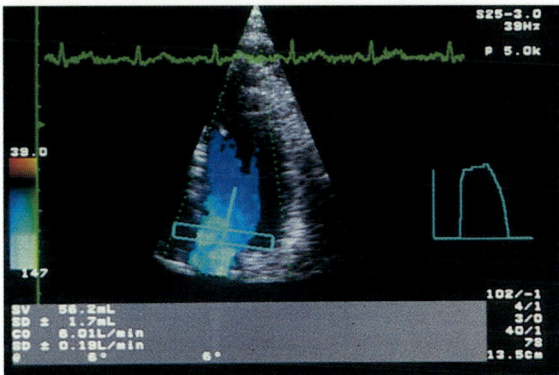

Figure I.18 – Automated cardiac output using colour flow Doppler technique (courtesy of Toshiba).

Appendix
II

Commonly used clinical and echocardiographic abbreviations

AA	aortic aneurysm		EF	ejection fraction
AF	atrial fibrillation		ESD	end-systolic diameter
AI	aortic insufficiency		ESM	ejection systolic murmur
AO	aorta		ET	ejection time
AR	aortic regurgitation		FS	fractional shortening
AS	aortic stenosis		HF	heart failure
ASD	atrial septal defect		H(O)CM	hypertrophic (obstructive) cardiomyopathy
AV	aortic valve			
AVD	aortic valve disease		h/o	history of
AVR	aortic valve replacement		HPRF	high pulse repetition frequency
AVSD	atrioventricular septal defect		HR	heart rate
BP	blood pressure		HS	heart sounds
BPM	beats per minute		HT	hypertension
CABG	coronary artery bypass grafting		ICU	intensive care unit
CAD	coronary artery disease		IDDM	insulin-dependent diabetes mellitus
CCF	congestive cardiac failure		IE	infective endocarditis
CFM	colour flow mapping		IHD	ischaemic heart disease
CHD	congenital heart disease		ITU	intensive therapy unit
CHF	chronic heart failure		IVC	inferior vena cava
CO	cardiac output		IVS	interventricular septum
c/o	complains of		JVP	jugular venous pressure
COAD/COPD	chronic obstructive airways/pulmonary disease		LA	left atrium
			LV	left ventricle
CRF	chronic renal failure		LVF	left ventricular failure
CVA	cerebrovascular accident		LVH	left ventricular hypertrophy
CVP	central venous pressure		MI	myocardial infarction *or* mitral insufficiency
CW	continuous wave Doppler examination			
CXR	chest X-ray		MR	mitral regurgitation
DCM	dilated cardiomyopathy		MS	mitral stenosis
DM	diabetes mellitus		MV	mitral valve
DVT	deep venous thrombosis		MVD	mitral valve disease
EA	emergency admission		MVP	mitral valve prolapse
ECG	electrocardiograph		MVR	mitral valve replacement
EDD	end diastolic diameter		NDDM	non-insulin dependent diabetes mellitus

(M)PA	(main) pulmonary artery	SOB	shortness of breath
Palps	palpitations	SOBOE	shortness of breath on exertion
PDA	patent ductus arteriosus	SV	stroke volume
PE	pulmonary embolus	SVC	superior vena cava
PFO	patent foramen ovale	SVT	supraventricular tachycardia
PMH	past medical history	TAPVD	total anomalous pulmonary venous connection
PND	paroxysmal nocturnal dyspnoea		
PR	pulmonary regurgitation	TEE	transesophageal echocardiogram (American spelling)
PRF	pulse repetition frequency		
PS	pulmonary stenosis	TGA	transposition of the great arteries
PV	pulmonary valve	TIA	transient ischaemic attack
PVB	premature ventricular beats	TOE	transoesophageal echocardiogram (British spelling)
PW	pulsed wave Doppler examination		
QP/QS	systemic-to-pulmonary flow ratio (intracardiac shunt)	TR	tricuspid regurgitation
		TS	tricuspid stenosis
RA	right atrium	TTE	transthoracic echocardiogram
RhF	rheumatic fever	TV	tricuspid valve
RV	right ventricle	USA	unstable angina
SBE	subacute bacterial endocarditis (*now called* infective endocarditis)	VF	ventricular fibrillation
		VSD	ventricular septal defect
SOA	swelling of ankles	VT	ventricular tachycardia

Appendix

III

Glossary

absorption changing of ultrasound energy into other forms of energy, mainly heat.

akinetic complete absence of ventricular wall contractility.

aliasing misinterpretation of high Doppler frequencies, inherent to pulsed wave and colour flow Doppler signals.

aortotomy site of surgical opening of the aorta.

atrial fibrillation rapid, irregular contractions of the atria working independently of the ventricles.

attenuation reduction in intensity of the ultrasound beam due to absorption and reflection.

autograft an individual's heart valve used as a valve replacement at a different site in their own heart (most commonly pulmonary valve used as an aortic valve replacement).

axial resolution ability of a system to resolve two closely spaced reflectors along the axis of the beam.

B-mode brightness mode – typically two-dimensional scanning.

baseline zero velocity line for spectral Doppler trace.

beam width diameter of the ultrasound beam at any point along its length – changes along length with focusing and divergence.

Bernoulli equation describes acceleration of flow through a restriction.

bradycardia slow heat rate (less than 60 beats per minute (bpm).

dehiscence an area around a valve replacement where the sutures have pulled away from the tissue causing rocking movement of the valve and associated regurgitation.

diastole relaxation period of the heart cycle when the ventricles fill.

dynamic range range of signal amplitudes (levels of grey) that can be displayed on an ultrasound system.

dyskinetic disordered contractility.

Ebstein's anomaly malformation of the tricuspid valve – posterior and septal leaflets attached to wall of right ventricle, anterior leaflet attached to tricuspid annulus.

eccentric not central; blood flow directed to one side.

embolism clot that has formed at one site in the body and travelled to another causing obstruction.

endocardium inner surface of the heart muscle wall.

envelope outside edge of a spectral Doppler trace.

epicardium outer surface of the heart muscle wall.

Fallot's tetralogy congenital heart disease that has 1. VSD, 2. crossing of the aorta over both right and left ventricles, 3. pulmonary stenosis and 4. right ventricular hypertrophy.

filter process to remove low frequencies from a Doppler signal.

flow convergence a 'rainbow' of colour proximal to a site of obstruction or regurgitation displayed on colour flow Doppler images as the flow accelerates.

focus the area of an ultrasound beam where the beam width is at its narrowest and beam intensity is maximised.

Fourier analysis mathematical method by which reflected echoes are separated into individual frequencies for Doppler display and interpretation.

frame image produced by one complete sweep of an ultrasound beam.

frame rate number of frames produced every second.

gain control to amplify returning signal without increasing patient dose.

homograft donor human tissue valve replacement.

hyperkinetic/hyperdynamic increased contractility of ventricles.

hypokinetic reduced contractility of ventricles.

infarct tissue death due to interrupted blood supply.

interface where two tissues of different acoustic properties meet and hence echoes formed.

laminar flow organised blood flow (all flow is at a similar velocity at any point in time).

lateral resolution ability of an ultrasound system to resolve two closely spaced reflectors at the same distance from the transducer face.

misregistration inaccurate display of an echo within an image due to artefact such as refraction or side lobes.

M-mode motion mode. Display of an interface's position and velocity over time.

Nyquist limit maximum measurable frequency shift that can be displayed on pulsed wave and colour flow Doppler traces before aliasing occurs.

pansystolic throughout systole.

paradoxical myocardial movement opposite to the correct direction.

paroxysmal every now and then.

pericardiocentesis drainage of fluid from the pericardial space.

piezo electric effect the ability of a material to convert a pressure wave (e.g. sound wave) into an electrical signal and vice versa.

primum atrial septal defect incomplete form of atrio-ventricular septal defect where there is no septum at the base of the defect between the mitral and tricuspid valves.

range gate a small area at a distance from the transducer at which Doppler signals are collected for a required pulsed wave Doppler trace.

refraction bending of a sound wave as it passes across boundaries of tissues with differing sound velocities. Causes artefacts by misregistration.

reject electronic pre or post processing that ignores signals outside a selected level resulting in an image or spectral trace of maximum diagnostic quality.

reverberation artefact caused by multiple reflection of the ultrasound beam between the transducer face and a highly reflective structure, or two highly reflective structures.

scan converter a computerised device that stores returning echo signals in digital format to create the resultant grey scale, two-dimensional image.

scattering the reflection of a sound wave in multiple directions and intensities from a small interface.

secondum atrial septal defect common type of defect in the atrial septum

shadowing loss of echo signal behind a highly reflective or highly attenuating structure.

shunt a connection that diverts blood flow from one pathway to another – may occur naturally or by surgical intervention.

side lobes (grating lobes) secondary ultrasound beams outside the main beam inherent in electrical transducers. Causes artefacts by misregistration.

spectral analysis technique for displaying the different frequency components of a Doppler signal.

spectral broadening presence of multiple simultaneous frequency components in a Doppler signal.

spectral Doppler the display of the frequency components of a Doppler signal in real time graphical form for pulsed and continuous wave Doppler signals.

sternotomy surgical opening of the chest, usually vertically down the centre of the sternum.

syncope fainting.

systole period of contraction of the ventricles.

tachycardia rapid heart rate (faster than 100 bpm).

tamponade compression of the heart by a pericardial collection of fluid.

thoracotomy operation to open the chest, usually between the ribs.

thrombus blood clot.

time gain compensation (TGC) operator variable control of amplification of returning echo signal strength at multiple distances from the transducer face, to compensate for attenuation.

turbulence disturbed blood flow.

xenograft animal tissue valve replacement.

INDEX